Color Atlas of

SMALL ANIMAL DERMATOLOGY

—A GUIDE TO DIAGNOSIS—

Second Edition

Color Atlas of

SMALL ANIMAL DERMATOLOGY

—A GUIDE TO DIAGNOSIS—

Second Edition

George T Wilkinson
Scalby
Scarborough
North Yorkshire

Richard G Harvey
The Veterinary Centre
Cheylesmore
Coventry

Mosby-Wolfe

London Baltimore Barcelona Bogotá Boston Buenos Aires Caracas Carlsbad, CA Chicago Madrid Mexico City
Milan Naples, FL New York Philadelphia St. Louis Seoul Singapore Sydney Taipei Tokyo Toronto Wiesbaden

Copyright © 1994 Times Mirror International Publishers Limited
Published in 1994 by Mosby–Wolfe an imprint of Times Mirror International Publishers Limited
Printed by Grafos S.A. Arte sobre papel, Barcelona, Spain.
ISBN 0 7234 1898 5
Reprinted 1995

For full details of all Times Mirror International Publishers Limited titles please write to Times Mirror Interrnational Publishers Limited, Lynton House, 7–12 Tavistock Square, London WC1H 9LB, England.

A CIP catalogue record for this book is available from the British Library.

Library of Congress Cataloging-in-Publication Data has been applied for.

Contents

Acknowledgements

The authors wish to thank the following colleagues for their generous loan of illustrations.

L. Bellstrom, nos. 646-650.

R. Bond, nos. 69, 112 and 270.

E. B. Breitschwerdt, no. 282.

O. M. Briggs, no. 749.

C. J. Chesney, no. 186.

Ferrer, L. Rabanal, R., Fondevila, D., Ramos, J. A., and Domingo, M. (1988). Skin lesions in canine leishmaniasis. *Journal of Small Animal Practice*, **29**: 381–388. No. 83.

M. R. Geary, nos. 98 and 99.

C. E. Griffen, nos. 580, 588 and 685.

R. E. W. Halliwell, nos. 744 and 745.

M. E. Herttage, no. 783.

J. M. Keep, nos. 298 and 780.

W. R. Kelly, no. 125.

G. A. Kunkle, nos. 765–768.

M. P. C. Lawton, nos. 518, 522 and 602.

C. P. Mackenzie, nos. 107–109.

D. C. Mactaggart, no. 192.

N. A. McEwan, nos. 530–532.

I. S. Mason, nos. 712 and 713.

K. V. Mason, no. 711.

K. A. Morello, no. 236.

G. H. Muller, nos. 106, 324 and 806.

Post, K., Dignean, M. A., and Clark, E. G. (1988). Hair follicle dysplasia of Siberian huskies. *Journal of the American Animal Hospital Association*, **24**: 659–662. No. 720.

D. J. Prieur and L. L. Collier, nos. 753 and 754.

D. H. Scarff, no. 526.

D. W. Scott, nos. 419, 425 and 436–440.

Scott, D. W. (1980). Feline Dermatology 1900–1978: A monograph. *Journal of the American Animal Hospital Association*, **16**: 331–459. Nos. 182 and 183.

R. Sutton, nos. 631 and 632.

K. L. Thoday, nos. 714 and 715.

A. H. M. Van Den Broek, no. 529.

Wilkinson, G. T. and Bate, M. J. (1984). A possible further clinical manifestation of the feline eosinophilic granuloma complex. *Journal of the American Animal Hospital Association*, **20**: 325–331. Nos. 201–205.

Wilkinson, G.T. and Leong, G. (1988). Prototkecosis in a dog. *Australian Veterinary Practitioner*, **18**: 47–49. Nos. 318–321.

Wilkinson, G.T. and Kristensen, T. S. (1989). A hair abnormality in Abyssinian cats. *Journal of Small Animal Practice*, **30**: 27–28. Nos. 730 and 731.

J. A. Yager, nos. 434, 435, 462, 479, 523, 524, 527, 659 and 675.

Introduction

Since the publication of the first edition of *A Colour Atlas of Small Animal Dermatology* in 1985 there has been a great upsurge of interest in veterinary dermatology. This has been reflected in the formation of Colleges and Associations for the study of the subject in many countries and also in the publication of a succession of colour atlases and textbooks devoted to the speciality. Concurrent research has led to a greater understanding of small animal skin disease and to reclassification of several conditions. For these reasons it was felt that a second edition was required, but that this should be designed more as an aid to that most difficult of tasks, the formulation of a diagnosis, rather than just another atlas of dermatology.

The most difficult step to accomplish in the management of a dermatological case is the reconciliation of a theoretical appreciation of the possible aetiologies and the formulation of a practical differential diagnosis. It has been said that the dermatologist is in a very privileged position in that the entire organ of the skin is available for direct examination by all the senses. Yet, paradoxically, it is this very availability which can prove so daunting. When faced with a dog which is scratching, shedding scale and is covered in spots it can be difficult to know where to start. The aim of this book is to provide a bridge. A bridge between the reality of the consulting room and the making of a diagnosis, between the theory and practice of dermatology and between the desire to learn and the deterrent size of today's standard textbooks.

The text covers the basics of history taking, clinical dermatological examination and the subsequent use of laboratory and other investigative techniques. A comprehensive collection of colour illustrations constitutes the 'colour atlas' portion of the book, detailing clinical presentations and, where suitable, the diagnostic tests that may be employed. The book is mainly concerned with skin disease in the dog and cat, but small mammals are also covered. It is hoped that the book will prove of value to veterinary students and clinicians.

Chapter 1

The history and physical examination

Much is made of the luxury that the clinician enjoys when examining a dermatological case. The whole organ is open to visual examination and palpation and thus a definitive diagnosis will surely follow. The reality is that reliance upon clinical examination alone will not be satisfactory; the limited range of the cutaneous response to insult and the frequent occurrence of non-diagnostic secondary lesions combine to confuse the clinician. The clinical examination is only one of three facets upon which a diagnosis is made. A comprehensive history and the analysis of the results obtained from various laboratory tests are equally important to making a definitive diagnosis.

Some clinicians like to make a brief examination of the animal before taking a history while others prefer the opposite approach. Whichever is adopted the initial workup is concluded with the taking of appropriate samples to define a diagnosis or to produce a limited list of differential diagnoses to which further tests may be applied.

This chapter covers an approach to the taking of a history and guidelines for a clinical examination. The following two chapters deal with primary and secondary lesions, and with laboratory investigations.

The collation of the animal's history begins with the breed, age and sex (signalment), considers the environment of the animal and then concentrates on the details of the disease in question with any progression of the dermatosis and the response, if any, to treatment being noted. The presence of contagion or zoonoses should be assessed.

Many clinicians use printed forms with checkboxes to ensure that information is recorded in a routine and efficient manner. An example of one is illustrated (pp. 10 and 11). Clients may be provided with similar forms and encouraged to fill in the answers to many of these questions while they are waiting for their appointment.

History

Signalment (Breed)

A number of dermatoses have an identified heritable basis and certain diseases are noted to occur more frequently in some breeds than in others, which suggests an heritable component. Furthermore, some breeds, such as the German shepherd dog and Chinese Shar pei, for example, appear to suffer disproportionally from skin diseases compared with other pure-bred and cross-bred animals. Breed predisposition for a given disease will vary both with the environment and the local gene-pool and thus a list matching breeds with diseases such as atopy may be inappropriate. Nonetheless, correlations such as those in **Table 1** are reasonably firm.

Table 1 *Examples of some dermatoses with predisposed breed of dog*

Hypothyroidism	**Generalised demodicosis**	**Atopy**
Boxer	Cairn terrier	Boxer
Cocker spaniel	West Highland White terrier	English Bull terrier
Doberman pinscher		English setter
Labrador retriever		German shepherd dog
miniature Dachshund		Labrador retriever
Shar pei		West Highland White terrier
Canine acne	**Defects in keratinisation**	**Sebaceous adenitis**
Boxer	Basset hound	Hungarian Vizsla
bulldog	Cocker spaniel	Standard Poodle
Doberman pinscher	Irish setter	
Great Dane	Springer spaniel	
Labrador retriever	West Highland White terrier	

DATE

OWNER:
ADDRESS:

TEL: home
work

ANIMAL:
BREED: AGE: SEX: Wt:

SOURCE:

CONTACTS:

MANAGEMENT DETAILS:
DIET:

HOUSING AND EXERCISE:

ROUTINE SKIN CARE:

VACCINATION: up to date:___   WORMING: up to date: ___

MEDICAL DETAILS:
APPETITE, THIRST:

GASTRO-INTESTINAL:

RESPIRATORY, CARDIOVASCULAR:

ORTHOPAEDIC, EXERCISE TOLERANCE:

URINOGENITAL:

NOTES:

CURRENT MEDICATIONS:

NOTES:

DERMATOLOGIC DETAILS:

PRURITUS: absent: ___   moderate: ___   severe: ___   unremitting: ___
LESIONS: primary:

              secondary:

DISTRIBUTION:

SKIN SCRAPES:

CYTOLOGY:

TAPE STRIPS:

TRICHOGRAM:

DIFFERENTIAL DIAGNOSIS AND DIAGNOSTIC PLAN:

Age

A number of diseases such as atopy, demodicosis and dermatophytosis occur more frequently in the younger animal whereas endocrinopathies and neoplasia are typically seen in middle-aged and elderly animals. Other diseases, such as ectoparasitism (apart from demodicosis) and dietary hypersensitivity are seen in no particular age group.

> • It is important that a distinction be made between the age at which an animal is presented and the age at which the disease was first apparent. Most pruritic disorders are gradual in onset although a few, such as acute pyotraumatic dermatitis or drug eruption, may be very rapid in progression. Knowledge of the age of onset of the clinical signs and the rate of progression of the signs may therefore be of rather more help than the age at presentation.

Sex

Patently, disorders such as Sertoli-cell tumour or hypo-oestrogenism can only occur in their respective sexes. The clinician should be aware that the sex of an animal may be associated with certain lifestyles which in turn may predispose to disease. Thus entire male cats are predisposed not only to cat bite abscess but also to infection with feline immunosuppressive virus infection, both a consequence of bite wounds.

Environment, diet, health status and lifestyle

Environment

It is important to have a knowledge of the environment of the animal. The presence of other animals is of great interest because if they are unaffected by the disease it suggests that the dermatosis may not be contagious. Conversely, the presence of another animal, such as a cat, prompts suspicion of an ectoparasitic disease, in particular flea infestation. Lesions on the human contacts may be particularly useful in arriving at a diagnosis (see Chapter 19).

Diet

The diet of the patient has great relevance. Although absolute dietary deficiencies are very rare some of the dietary-responsive dermatoses, such as zinc-responsive dermatosis, are rather more common. Dogs fed complete diets may be presented with mild defects in keratinisation which respond to supplementation with sunflower oil, for example. Dietary hypersensitivity should also be borne in mind. Although one cannot diagnose this disorder simply from a knowledge of the diet, one needs to know the components in order to suggest an appropriate exclusion diet.

Health status

General enquiries into the health of the animal may help to define whether there is internal disease present. Thus appetite and water intake, exercise tolerance, changes in body weight or conformation and assessment of mental attitude are all potentially relevant. For example, a hypothyroid dog may have reduced exercise tolerance and weight gain associated with anoestrus and a degree of mental dullness. The regularity of a bitch's oestrus should be assessed and knowledge of the level of fertility of stud dogs may be useful. Evidence of change in sexual or dog-to-dog social conduct may suggest gonadal aberration. Dogs with severe pruritus such as that due to scabies often lose weight. Changes in body conformation may accompany hyperadrenocorticism.

Lifestyle

The lifestyle of the animal will also give clues to diagnosis. Thus a solitary cat which never leaves the house will not be at risk from contagious ectoparasites. A short-haired dog, particularly a Doberman pinscher, maintained in a dry environment, may rapidly develop a mild scale. A short-haired pointer which works at weekends may present on Tuesdays with florid pustules on the flanks and the anterior aspects of the limbs due to the traumatic inoculation of bacteria by vegetation, hunting dog pyoderma.

A knowledge of the immediate environment may also be important if allergic- or irritant-contact dermatitis is suspected. Irritant-contact dermatitis may be suspected from the distribution of the lesions (confined to the feet or ventrum) and the demonstration of access (building work, for example). If allergic-contact dermatitis is suspected then exclusion trials will rely on a knowledge of the immediate environment.

The country of origin should be established since diseases common in one country may be rare in another. Thus Leishmaniasis is common in the Mediterranean basin but rare in Northern Europe. The disease may, however, occur if the dog originates from a country where it is endemic.

History of the disease

The particular history of the disease is very important. The clinician will wish to know where the initial lesions were? Was there pruritus at this point? Is there pruritus now? How has the disease progressed in extent and severity? A knowledge of the nature of any primary lesions is often of great value. Many owners will describe the natural history of a pustule with great accuracy without knowing what they are describing. Knowledge of any cyclic or seasonal pattern to the pruritus is useful. Thus many atopic dogs are only seasonally pruritic at first, before becoming perennially affected.

The predilection sites of atopy are the face, ears, ventrum and feet. Pruritus is typically moderate and is infrequently apparent in the consulting room. In contrast, sarcoptic mange is highly pruritic from the outset and the pruritus is usually very apparent during the examination. The disease typically follows a progression with initial lesions appearing at launch points; the elbows, hocks and pinnae. However, in contrast to atopy, there is rapid extension to the adjacent areas of the body and zoonotic lesions are common.

Response to previous treatments

There is little to be gained from a knowledge that the pruritic pustular condition of a two-year-old German shepherd dog responds temporarily to a combination of antibacterial, glucocorticoid and antiparasitic treatment. There is much to be gained from the knowledge that either antibacterial agents or glucocorticoids suppressed the clinical signs but that ectoparasitic treatment was of no value. Such details suggest that a pruritic bacterial disease is at least partly responsible for the clinical signs. This suggests a recurrent superficial folliculitis and should prompt a search for the underlying cause, typically atopy.

Previous therapeutics may also have an effect on certain diagnostic tests and thus a knowledge of recent medication is desirable. For example, intradermal skin testing is of no value if the patient has received a depot glucocorticoid injection the week previously. Bacterial culture and sensitivity testing may be greatly affected by recent antibacterial therapy.

Physical examination

All animals should be subjected to a complete physical examination before the detailed examination of the skin takes place. This precaution will help to ensure that systemic disease is detected and will eliminate any tendency to jump to the wrong conclusion.

General examination

This should include examination of the oral cavity and ears, palpation of the superficial lymph nodes, auscultation of the heart, palpation of the abdomen and measurement of rectal temperature. The animal should be weighed. Early clues to hypothyroidism may be lack of the expected tachycardia that often occurs during a physical examination and a rectal temperature less than 101°F (38.3°C). Similarly, polylymphadenopathy and pyrexia are both features of demodicosis and deep pyoderma while polylymphadenopathy, weight loss and pruritus are common findings in scabies.

Dermatological examination

The hair and condition of the coat are assessed by observation, touch and smell. Changes in colour often occur with age but changes in colour and texture may suggest endocrine disease. Loss of hair only becomes apparent when some 30% of the coat is lost and an effort should be made to assess whether there is loss of primary or secondary coat. The skin should be examined in detail, taking account of the presence and nature of any scale or crust, the surface of the skin and the nature of any lesions.

The ability to differentiate a primary lesion (which may be a feature of the underlying disease) from a secondary lesion is important and is covered in detail in the following chapter. Primary lesions arise *de novo* in the skin and comprise macules, papules, pustules, vesicles or wheals. Secondary lesions arise as a consequence of disease or associated self trauma and include scale, ulceration, crust, excoriations, hyperpigmentation and lichenification. The distribution of the lesions should be noted.

Careful observation may allow identification of the disease in progress. Thus in the case of flea-bite hypersensitivity there may be pruritus, papules, crusted papules and scale, typically on the dorsal lumbosacral region although the perineum and groin also may be affected. In cases of superficial pyoderma there may be similar signs and distribution of lesions.

However, in the case of superficial pyoderma there may be pustules and epidermal collarettes, neither a feature of flea-allergy dermatitis. It should be remembered that pustules are not only a feature of bacterial disease as they may be seen in cases of demodicosis, dermatophytosis, and autoimmune disease.

Further reading

August, J. R. (1986). Taking a dermatologic history. *Compendium on Continuing Education*, **8**: 510–518.

Griffin, C. E. (1989). Diagnostic approach to dermatologic disease. In: Nesbitt, G. H. (Ed.) *Contemporary Issues in Small Animal Practice, 8, Dermatology*, pp. 1–19.

Chapter 2:

Primary and secondary lesions: recognition and significance

The skin of the dog and, more particularly, that of the cat has only a limited range of responses to insult and these manifest as lesions and clinical signs. Most owners will detect gross changes such as the onset of pruritus, a change of odour, the loss of hair, the presence of scale or crust or a change in pigmentation and these are the main presenting signs of dermatological disease.

However these are non-specific secondary changes which reflect not only a number of underlying aetiologies but also the effect of the cutaneous response to chronic inflammation and other influences such as self-excoriation. In themselves these changes provide few clues to the disorder which may be present. A number of diseases such as sarcoptic mange, atopy or a defect in keratinisation may present with only these secondary or evolutionary changes and in these circumstances the information obtained from signalment, history and physical examination is important to arriving at a diagnosis. Other diseases however may be characterised by the presence of more significant primary lesions **(Table 2)**.

A primary lesion arises *de novo* in the skin and usually reflects the underlying aetiology, so that while it may not be pathognomonic it can be attributed to a limited number of diseases. Primary lesions are not always present at the time of examination because they may be very transient; vesicles, for example, may only persist for an hour or two. In other cases the primary lesions may be difficult to identify among the secondary changes that will invariably be present.

It is essential to understand that although primary lesions are useful from a diagnostic point of view they should not be looked at in isolation. Many lesions undergo a sequential evolution resulting in a variety of identifiable changes to the skin and it is the presence of all these lesions, coexisting and often in close proximity, that allows the clinician to deduce the underlying pathology. Thus the recognition of a pustular phase, its precursor the papule and a non-scarring healing phase will allow the conclusion that the lesions are superficial and epidermal in origin.

It is the ability to recognise a lesion and its distribution, to appreciate its development and its evolution that is crucial to making the first step in dermatological diagnosis, formulating a differential diagnosis.

Table 2

Primary (diagnostic) lesions	Secondary (evolutionary) lesions
macule	comedone
papule	epidermal collarette
pustule	scale
wheal	crust
vesicle	excoriation
plaque	erosion
nodule	ulcer
tumour	lichenification
cyst	hyperpigmentation
	hypopigmentation
	scar

1   **Macules**. Circumscribed, small changes in skin colour.

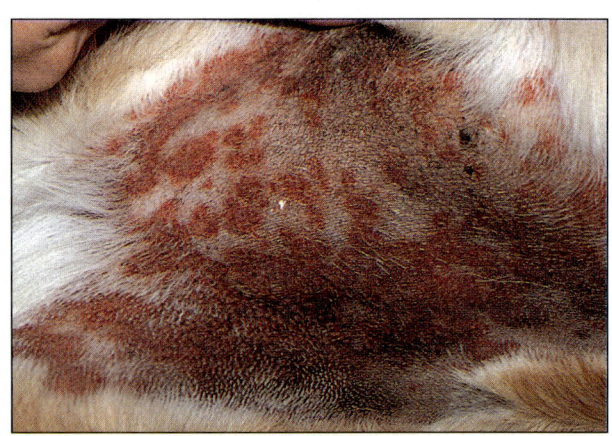

2   **Patches**. Larger than macules, often with ill-defined perimeters. In this case the patches are due to cutaneous haemorrhage, a consequence of drug eruption following administration of metoclopramide.

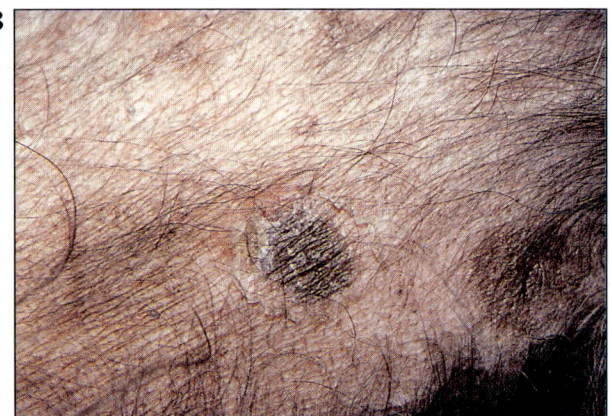

3   **Patches**. Post-inflammatory hyperpigmentation is common during the healing phases of superficial pyoderma.

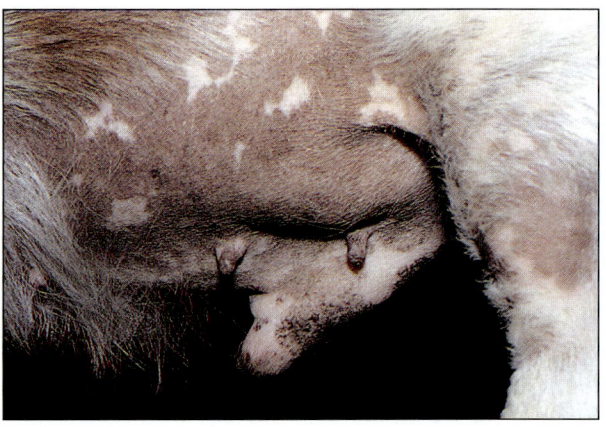

4   **Patches**. Endocrine dermatoses are often associated with increases in pigmentation. This is usually confluent, particularly in the areas of alopecia. In this example there are blotchy patches of hyperpigmentation in association with a Sertoli-cell tumour.

Macules and patches

Macules and patches are characterised by discoloration of the skin. There is no elevation or thickening of the skin. Macules (**1**) are focal, well-circumscribed and less than 1 cm in diameter whereas patches (**2**) are often less well circumscribed and are larger than 1cm diameter.

The changes in colour may be due to a variety of causes such as inflammatory erythema, haemorrhage or pigmentary aberrations. Erythema is the commonest cause and may be seen in localised inflammatory reactions destined to become papules or pustules and other conditions such as localised demodicosis. Haemorrhage into the skin is less common and suggests clotting defects, poisoning (Warfarin) or defects in vascular integrity, as may occur in Rocky Mountain spotted fever or drug eruption, for example (**2**). The distinction between hyperaemia and haemorrhage is important and may be made by diascopy (see Chapter 3, Diagnostic tests and clinical pathology).

Changes in pigmentation may be congenital or acquired and may involve both the loss, or the acquisition, of pigment. Hyperpigmentation is more common, and may be post-inflammatory, as in the healing lesions of superficial pyoderma (**3**) or a feature of a non-inflammatory disease such as

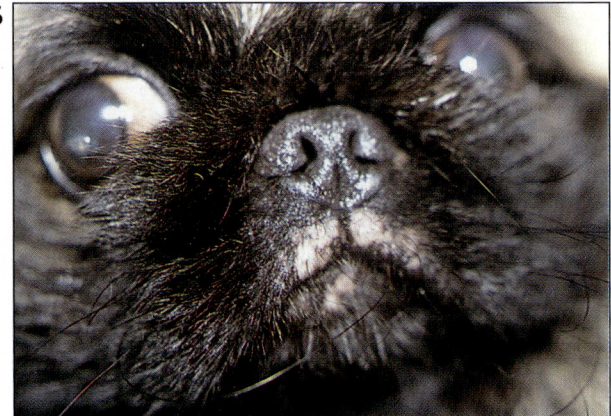

5   Patches. Symmetrical patches of hypopigmentation may be a feature of vitiligo.

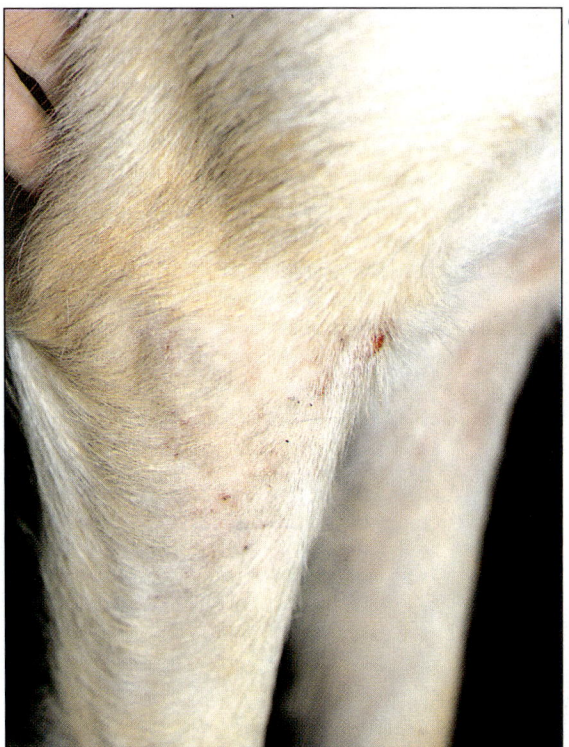

6   Papules. Superficial pyoderma is characterised by the presence of pustules. Most cases exhibit many more papules than pustules. In this case the pyoderma is secondary to atopy.

an endocrine dermatosis. In general, endocrine disorders are associated with widespread changes in pigmentation rather than macules or patches, but an exception is the patchy hyperpigmentation that may accompany Sertoli-cell tumour in the dog (**4**).

Hypopigmentation may also be post-inflammatory, particularly when the damage extends through the basement membrane and results in healing with scar formation. Non-inflammatory, possibly hereditary, acquired loss of pigmentation (vitiligo) may be seen in some breeds, notably the Belgian tervuren or the Rottweiler. Vitiligo frequently begins on the head, particularly the muzzle and lips and is often symmetrical (**5**).

Papules

A papule is a circumscribed, solid elevation of the skin up to 1cm in diameter. The elevation may be due to an accumulation of cells, fluid, debris or metabolic deposits and may be follicular in orientation or interfollicular. The cellular infiltrate will vary with the pathological process under way but in the commonest cause of papules, that of superficial pyoderma, the infiltrate will be neutrophilic in nature (**6–8**).

Follicular papules may be seen in cases of follicular dystrophy and defects in keratinisation. In these cases the accumulation of keratinaceous debris under the occluded follicular orifice produces the swelling (**9**). Papules resulting from metabolic deposits may contain

7 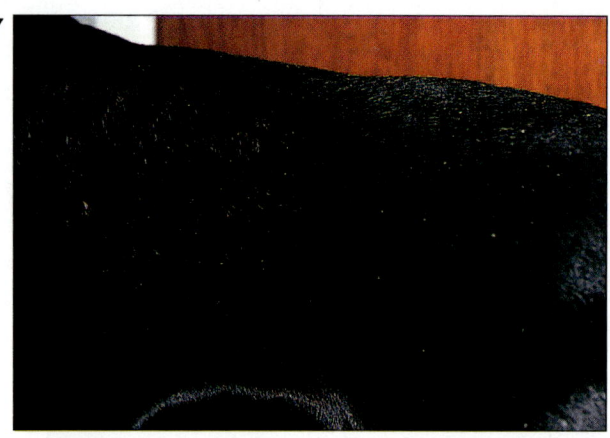 **8**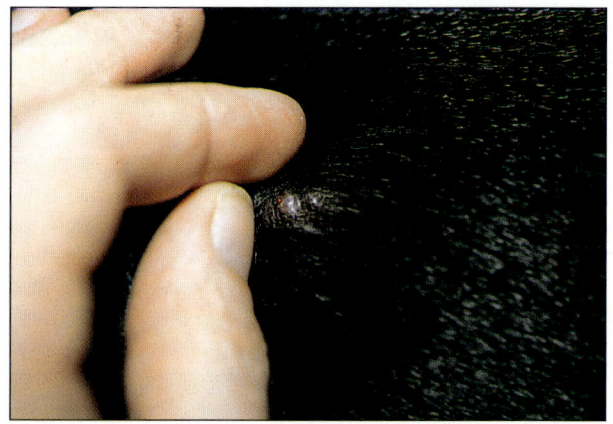

7 and 8   Papules. Some papules may be very difficult to see. The use of a hand lens will help. In this case (**8**) the papules are due to folliculitis on the flank of a Doberman pinscher and have been skylined by rolling the skin between finger and thumb.

9 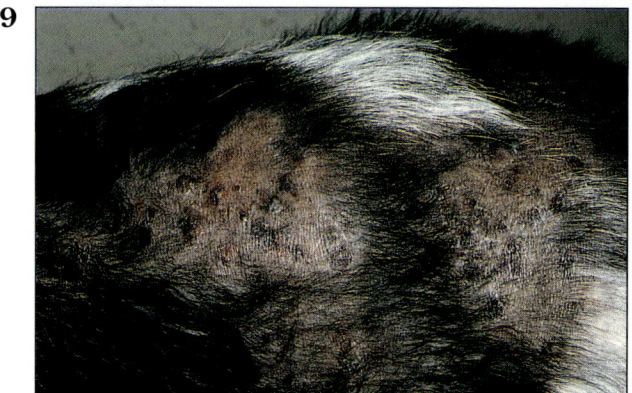 **10**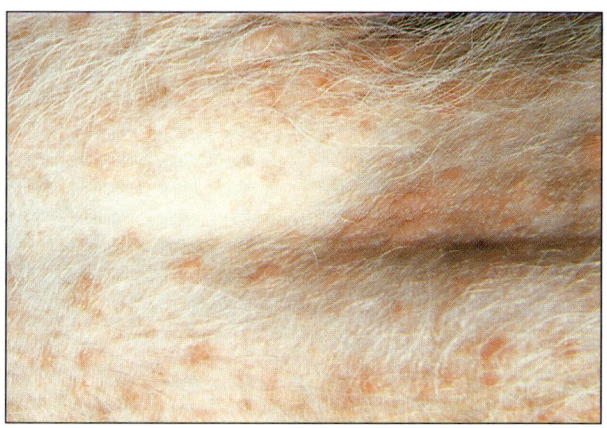

9   Papules. Papules are not always associated with infection. In this example they are due to an accumulation of keratinaceous debris in blocked follicles. In this case there was an idiopathic defect in keratinisation.

10   Papules. Erythematous papules are the primary lesions of allergic contact dermatitis. There is usually a well-defined margin between affected and unaffected skin.

calcium as in calcinosis circumscripta, or other products of metabolic origin such as mucin or lipid.

Papules often begin as erythematous macules, particularly in superficial pyoderma, where they may outnumber the pustules by 10 or 20 to one. They may also evolve into crusted papules as in miliary dermatitis in the cat or sarcoptic mange in the dog. In allergic contact dermatitis where the papule is the primary lesion then the progression to pustules does not occur and thus other lesions associated with pustules such as epidermal collarettes are also absent (**10**).

11

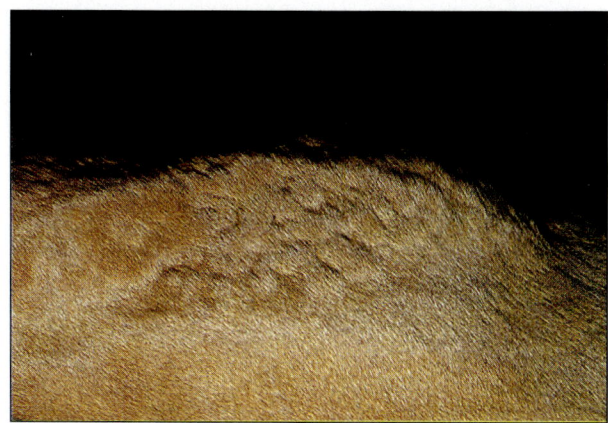
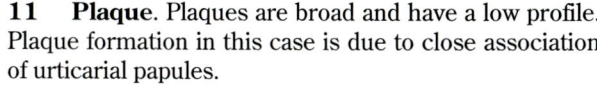

12

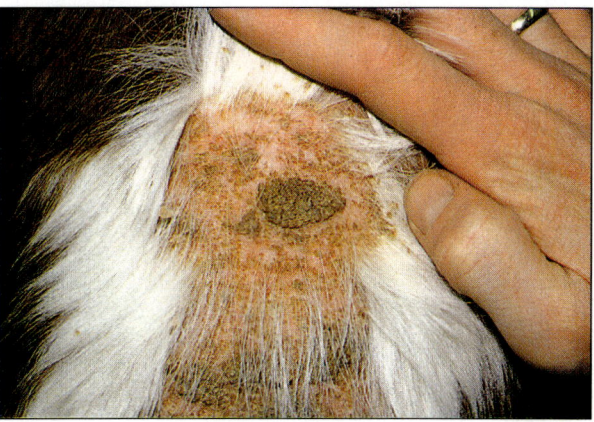

11   Plaque. Plaques are broad and have a low profile. Plaque formation in this case is due to close association of urticarial papules.

12   Vegetation. Plaques may also be due to accumulation of keratinaceous crust and scale when it is termed a vegetation. In this case of vitamin A–responsive dermatosis there is hyperproliferative follicular keratinisation and retention of the crust.

Plaques

A plaque is an elevation of the skin which is usually flat and is typically wide in relation to its height. Plaques may result from oedema (wheals), the coalescence of adjacent papules (**11**) or may be of neoplastic origin. Plaque-like accumulations of lipid scales or crust may occur in some of the dermatoses accompanied by a defect in keratinisation such as vitamin A–responsive dermatosis (**12**) or *Malassezia pachydermatis* infection.

13

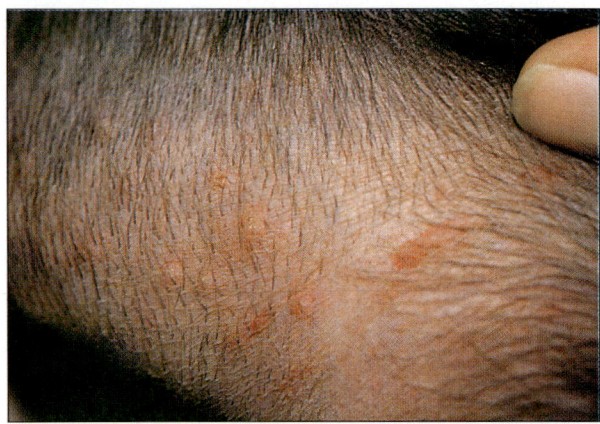

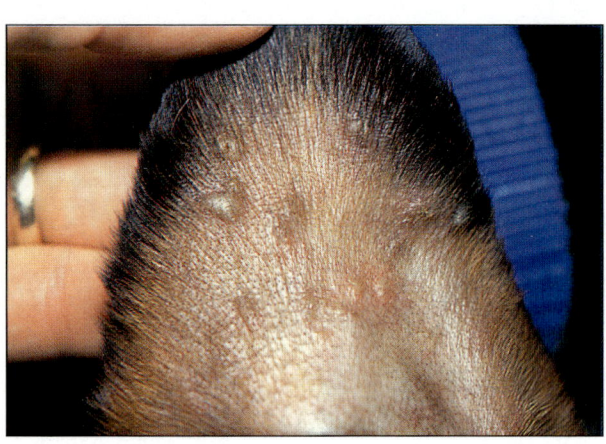

14

13 **Pustule**. Pustules are commonly found in bacterial infections. They may also be seen in demodicosis, dermatophytosis and autoimmune disorders. In this case the group of pustules is due to superficial folliculitis.

14 **Pustule**. A group of pustules on the pinna of a dog due to pemphigus foliaceus.

15

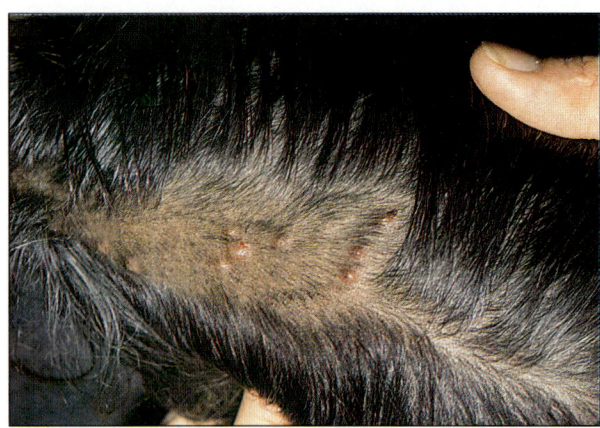

15 **Pustule**. A group of pustules in the interscapular region. Cytology revealed an eosinophilic infiltrate. Bacteriology failed to reveal organisms. The pustules coincided with the administration of ampicillin and resolved when it was withdrawn, suggesting drug reaction.

Pustules

Pustules are well-circumscribed elevations of the superficial layers of the epidermis. They may be follicular or interfollicular in distribution. The typical yellowish colour results from the stretching of the upper layer of the pustule by the gradual accumulation of infiltrate beneath, which becomes visible. In the case of the commonest cause, that of bacterial infection, the infiltrate will contain neutrophils, bacteria, debris and perhaps a few free keratinocytes (**13**). The keratinocytes are unattached owing to the action of bacterial and neutrophil toxins; in consequence they appear rounded in shape and are termed acanthocytes. In follicular infection the toxins may accumulate to sufficiently high levels that there are large number of acanthocytes.

Examination of the aspirated pustular contents in these cases may reveal sufficient numbers of acanthocytes to suggest the possibility of pemphigus foliaceus (**14**). In addition to pyoderma and pemphigus foliaceus pustules also may be a feature of demodicosis, dermatophytosis and sub-corneal pustular dermatosis and drug eruption (**15**).

Occasionally pustules may be unusually coloured, haemorrhagic (for example), very large or surrounded by a zone of erythema, and in these situations consideration should be given to staphylococcal hypersensitivity (**16** and **17**). These florid lesions are often found in cases where long-standing or recurrent bacterial infection is a feature of an underlying disease, particularly a hypersensitivity, such as atopy.

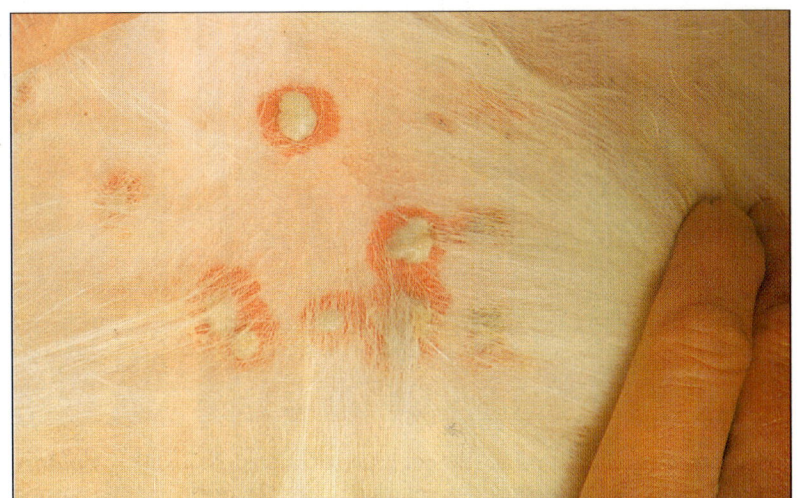

16 Pustules. A group of large pustules surrounded by zones of erythema. Staphylococcal hypersensitivity has been proposed as a mechanism for pathogenesis of these florid lesions.

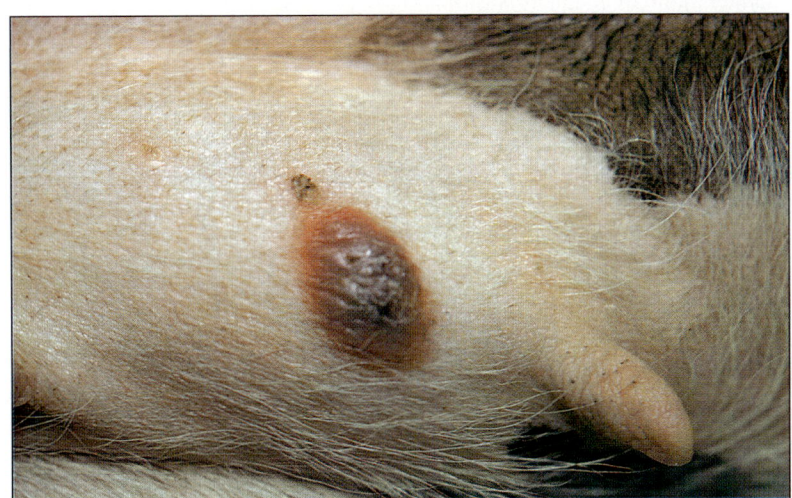

17 Pustule. A solitary haemorrhagic pustule. This dog was subject to repeated episodes of staphylococcal skin infection. Staphylococcal hypersensitivity.

In contrast, very large and flaccid pustules with minimal inflammation should prompt suspicion of immunosuppression, particularly hyperadrenocorticism.

Attention has already been drawn to the fact that lesions frequently undergo an identifiable evolution, and interfollicular pustules typically begin as macules which become papular and then pustular. Pustules are thin, fragile and transient. They rapidly rupture and become crusted.

Most cases of superficial pyoderma exhibit only a few frank pustules but many papules and secondary lesions such as crust and scale. Some cases will also exhibit epidermal collarettes and perhaps post-inflammatory hyperpigmentation. In addition, many animals exhibit a patchy alopecia as a consequence of the follicular damage and associated self trauma.

18

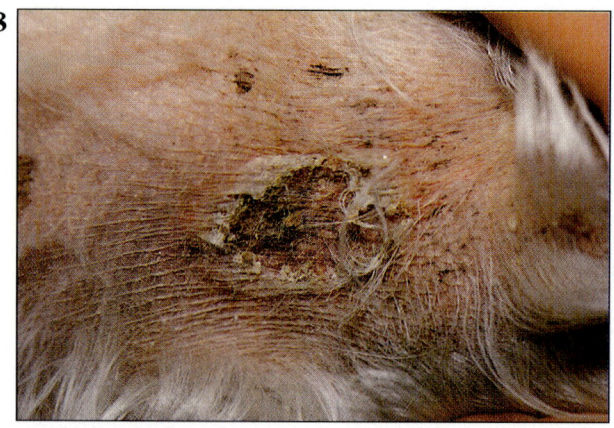

19

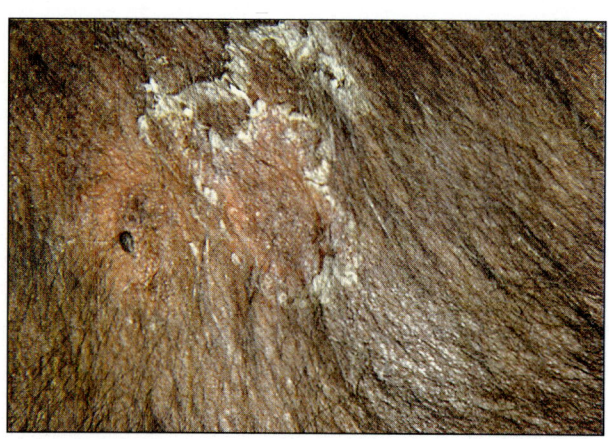

18 Epidermal collarette. Although these lesions are potential sequels to any pustular condition they are frequently found in association with superficial pyoderma.

19 Epidermal collarette. Coalescing epidermal collarettes forming polycyclic rings.

20

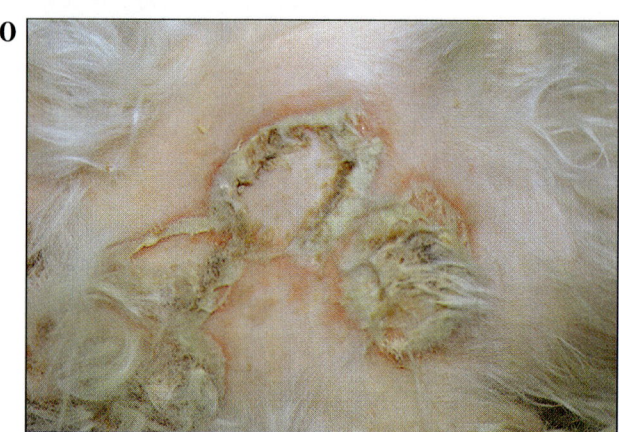

20 Epidermal collarette. A group of huge epidermal collarettes. This was a case of hepatocutaneous syndrome in a dog. The collarettes in this case are a sequel to large bullae.

Epidermal collarettes

Epidermal collarettes are regarded as secondary lesions by some authorities and as primary lesions by others. Epidermal collarettes are best conceived as decapitated pustules, vesicles or bullae which are spreading peripherally, giving the appearance of a ring of scale (**18**). Adjacent lesions may coalesce giving rise to large polycyclic rings of scale (**19**). There is often a peripherally spreading zone of accompanying erythema. Central healing with post-inflammatory hyper-pigmentation is common.

These lesions have the appearance of bull's eyes or targets. Epidermal collarettes are most commonly associated with superficial pyoderma but they may occur in any condition in which superficial pustules, vesicles or bullae are a feature, such as pemphigus foliaceus and sub-corneal pustular dermatosis (**20**). They are rarely seen in dermatophytosis.

21

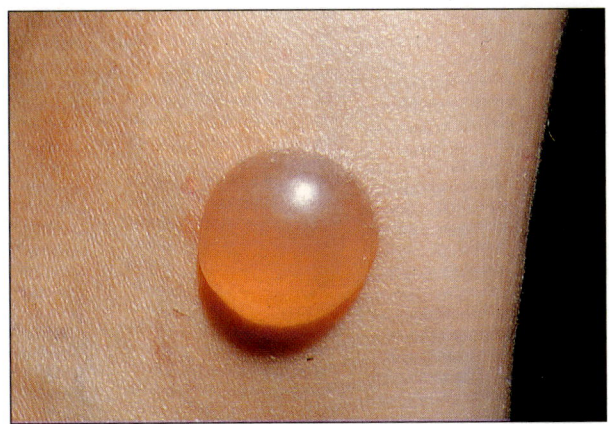

22

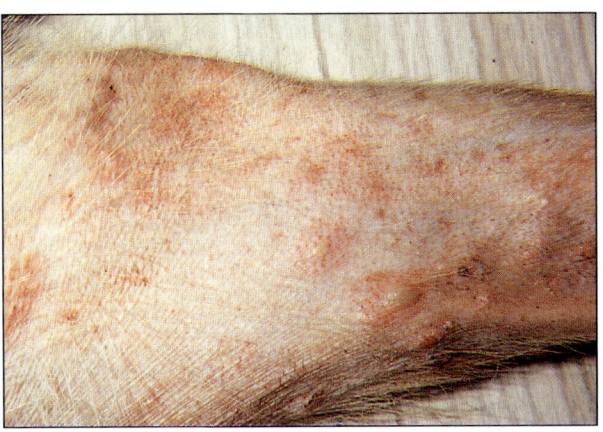

21 Vesicle. This vesicle is on human skin and follows a mosquito bite.

22 Bullae. Bullae are large, flaccid vesicles. In this case they are a consequence of cleft formation at the epidermal basement membrane. Bullous pemphigoid in a dog.

Vesicles and bullae

A vesicle is a well-demarcated elevation of the superficial layers of the skin less than 1cm in diameter (**21**). The elevation of the skin is due to the accumulation of intercellular fluid beneath the roof of the vesicle. The fluid is usually serum or an inflammatory exudate which imparts a pale, almost translucent nature to the vesicle. Compare this with the yellow, opaque nature of the pustule (e.g. **14**).

The depth of the lesion determines the thickness of the overlying roof of the vesicle and in most cases, such as viral diseases, irritant contact dermatitis and the vesicular autoimmune disorders (e.g. pemphigus foliaceus), the lesion is superficial. In consequence the roof is fragile and the vesicle usually of short duration. Secondary crust, exudate and erosions are common. In cases where the clinician is suspicious of an autoimmune disorder, it may be necessary to hospitalise the animal and perform repeated, regular examinations in order to observe the vesicles, obtain biopsies and make a definitive diagnosis.

Bullae are large vesicles, more than 1cm in diameter. They may occur as lesions in their own right, perhaps due to cleft formation in the epidermis (**22**), or they may arise due to coalescence of adjacent pockets of intercellular epidermal oedema. The depth of the bulla will affect the appearance of the lesions. Thus in deep lesions, such as occur with bullous pemphigoid (where the cleft is at the basement membrane), the intact bullae may be tense and well defined, whereas with the more superficial, suprabasal clefting of pemphigus vulgaris any intact bullae are rather flaccid with a tendency to enlarge at the edges.

This tendency to underun and cleft is exploited in a diagnostic test, the Nikolsky sign (see Chapter 3, Diagnostic tests and clinical pathology). Lateral pressure or a shearing force applied to the skin adjacent to a lesion in a case of pemphigus vulgaris may result in a vesicle being produced. This is not usually present in cases of bullous pemphigoid. As might be expected, the very size of these lesions imparts a degree of fragility, and they are rarely found intact.

23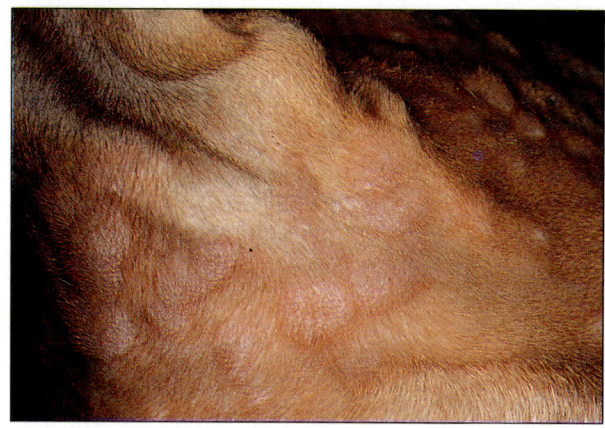

24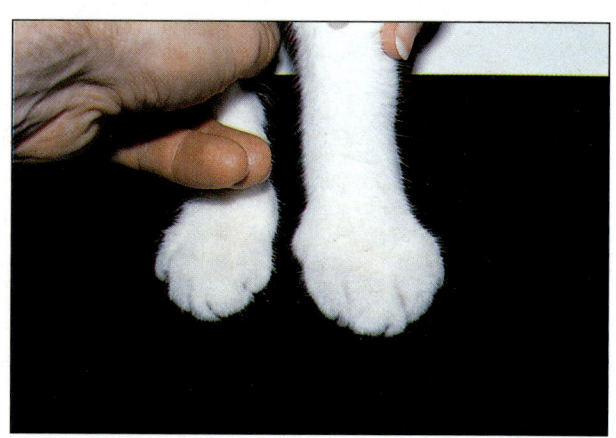

23 **Wheals**. Wheals usually are transient and are well-defined elevations of the skin due to local oedema. These lesions followed intravenous neostigmine.

24 **Angioedema**. Local accumulation of oedema may cause distension of large areas of skin, termed angioedema. This case illustrates angioedema in a cat's foot following a bee sting.

25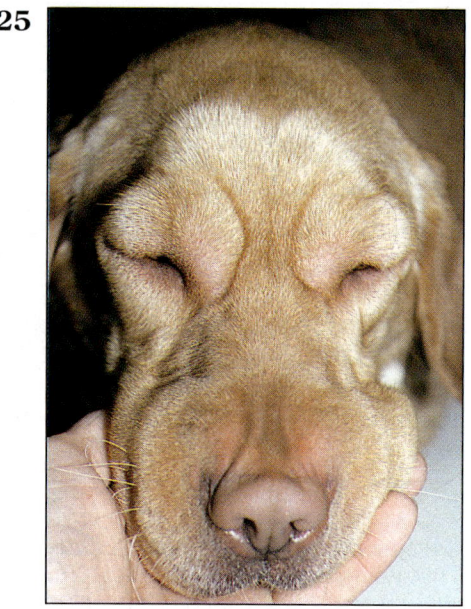

25 **Angioedema**. Acute facial angioedema in a dog. Probably a reaction to insect bite or sting.

Wheals and angioedema

Wheals are more or less well-defined elevations of the skin due to oedema. They may be round, oval or plaque-like and adjacent wheals may coalesce giving irregular shapes (**23**). They arise rapidly and frequently disappear within hours. Wheals are a consequence of oedema in the upper dermis and there is no accompanying pathological change to the cells of the epidermis. They may be colourless or pink-tinged and the colour blanches on diascopy (see Chapter 3). Occasionally oedema will cause distension of a region of the body such as an eyelid, the muzzle or a paw and this is termed angioedema (**24** and **25**).

In short-haired dogs the papules of superficial pyoderma may cause multiple elevations of groups of hairs which mimic wheals and may lead to an erroneous diagnosis of hives. Administration of glucocorticoids to these cases may make subsequent management of the pyoderma difficult. Careful examination and identification of lesions is of paramount importance.

26

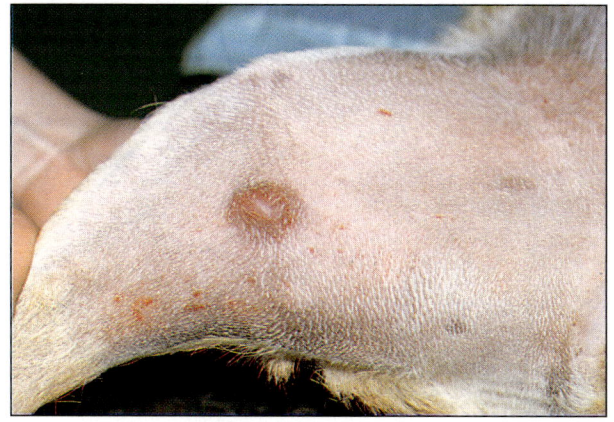

27

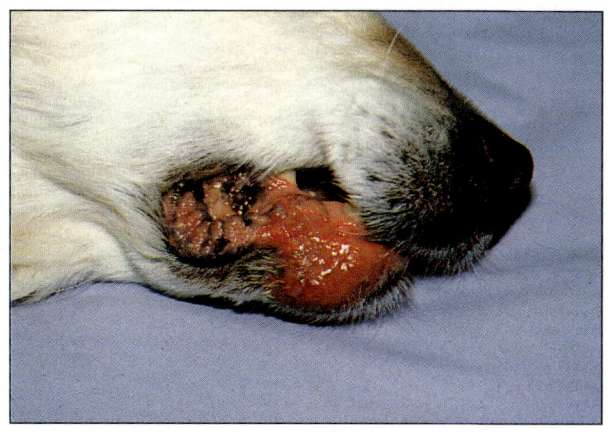

26   Nodule. A nodule is larger than 1 cm in diameter. The illustration is of a solitary, erythematous nodule. Mast cell tumour.

27   Mass. A large ulcerated mass on the lower lip of a golden retriever. Mycosis fungoides.

28

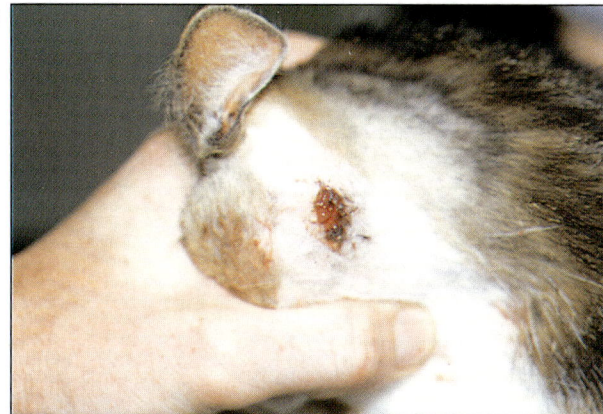

29

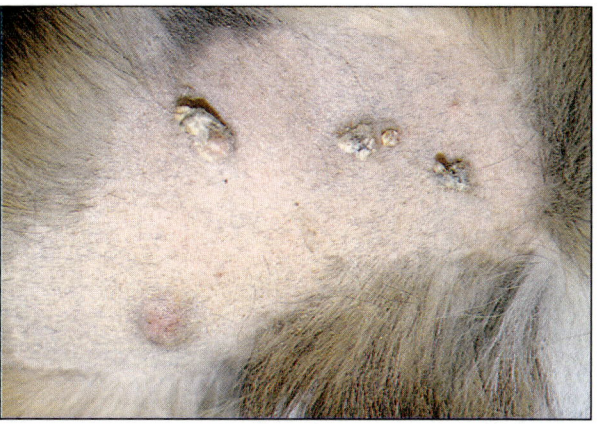

28   Mass. A very large ulcerated mass on the side of a cat's head. Cytology revealed the causal organisms of cryptococcosis (*Cryptococcus neoformans*).

29   Cysts. Epithelially-lined, usually of adnexal origin. Three sebaceous cysts on the flank of a dog.

Nodules, tumours and cysts

Nodules are circumscribed elevations of the skin that are larger (**26**) than the 1cm upper limit defined for papules. In addition to being larger they often extend into the dermis rather than remaining confined to the epidermis. As is the case with papules the infiltrate may be infectious, inflammatory, granulomatous, neoplastic or of metabolic origin.

Tumours are masses of neoplastic origin, whether benign or malignant. The term tumour is often applied to a large nodule. Tumours may be mobile or locally infiltrative, ulcerated or domed, plaque-like or pedunculated (**27** and **28**).

Cysts are cavities within the skin that are lined by epithelium, usually of adnexal origin rather than epidermal. The contents of the cyst reflects the epithelial lining, i.e. sebaceous cyst derived from the sebaceous gland or apocrine cyst derived from the epitrichial sweat gland (**29**). Cysts may burst or discharge to the surface via a fistula or sinus.

30

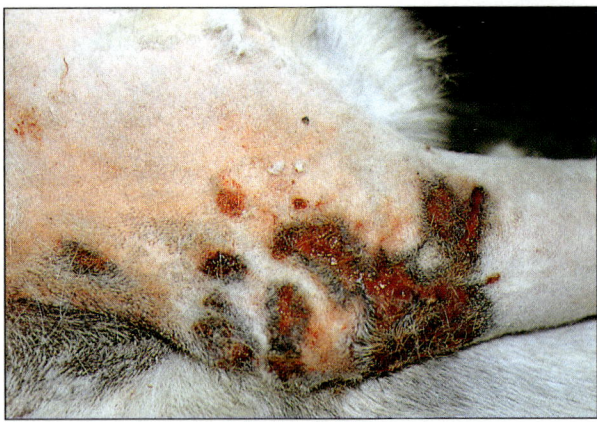

30   Fistula. Illustration depicts discharging fistulae on a German shepherd dog with deep pyoderma.

31

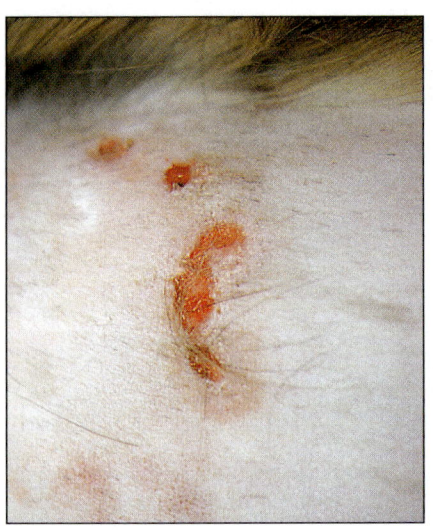

31   Fistula. Discharges are not always caused by infection. In this case there is a sterile panniculitis.

32

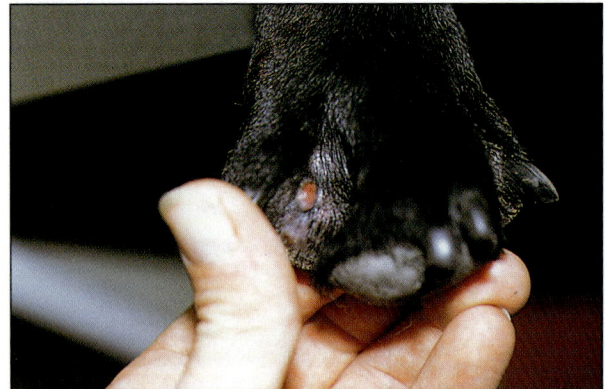

32   Sinus. A sinus is a tract with an epithelial lining. Deep interdigital pyoderma and sinus formation. Note that these lesions are not cysts.

33

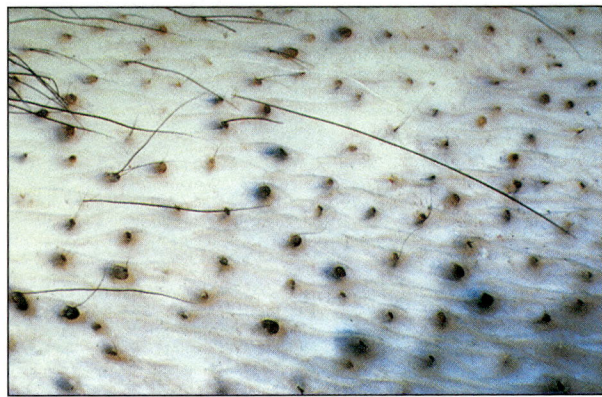

33   Comedo. A comedo is a blocked follicle. Defects in keratinisation are a common cause of these lesions. In particular they are associated with hyperadrenocorticism.

Fistula and sinus

A fistulous tract connects an area or focus of inflammation to the skin surface. These may be seen in cases of deep pyoderma, anal furunculosis, foreign body penetration, panniculitis or mycetoma for example (30–32). A sinus is an epithelially-lined channel connecting a deep lesion to the skin surface, as in dermoid cyst and sinus in the Rhodesian Ridgeback. Long-standing foci of deep pyoderma such as are seen in canine acne or pododermatitis may also be accompanied by sinus formation.

Comedones

A comedo is a dilated hair follicle which contains a pigmented impaction of lipid and keratinaceous debris occluding the orifice. The lesion is usually slightly elevated above the skin surface (33). The comedo is the primary lesion of acne in man but is not pathognomonic. Comedones are commonly found in animals suffering from defects in keratinisation, both primary and secondary: they are found in cases of demodicosis and are a frequent finding on the abdomen of dogs with hyperadrenocorticism.

34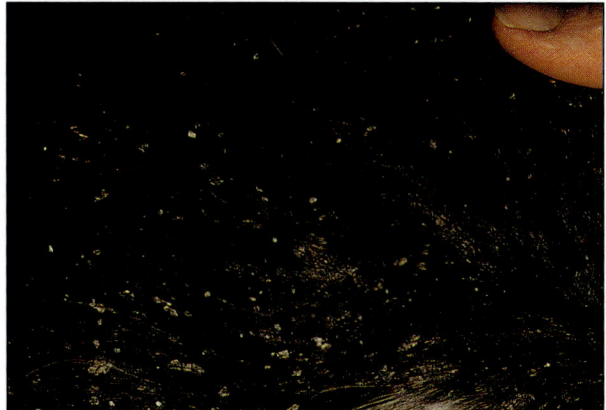

34 **Scale**. Scale is associated with the shedding of large rafts of keratinocytes, rather than the inapparent loss of individual squames. In this example there is an accumulation of heavy scale in the hair due to an idiopathic defect in keratinisation.

35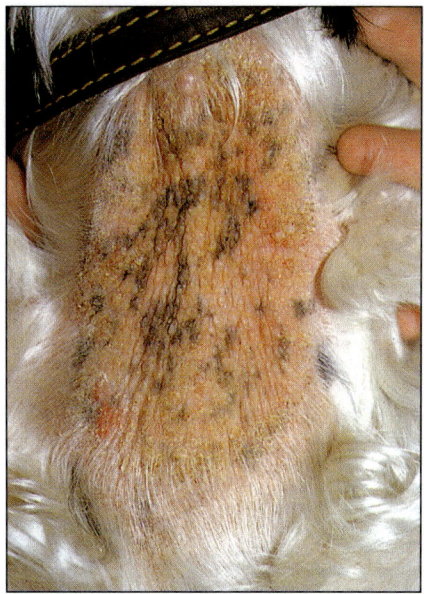

35 **Scale**. In some cases characterised by defects in keratinisation the defect in sebaceous gland function is severe enough to result in lipid-rich greasy scale adhering to the hair and skin. This is well-illustrated in this example of a dog with an idiopathic defect in keratinisation.

Scale

Under normal conditions in the dog the process of keratinisation ensures a steady replacement of the epidermis with cells derived from a dividing pool in the basal layer. It takes about 21 days for cells to reach the upper layer of viable epidermis, the stratum granulosum. In Cocker spaniels with defects in keratinisation this time is reduced to 3 or 4 days and, furthermore, there is a larger percentage of the basal cell population involved in the process. As a result there are increased numbers of poorly differentiated cells shed from the surface of the skin where aggregates of them are visible as scale (**34** and **35**).

Keratinisation also is aberrant in the adnexae and the production of sebum is therefore affected. The result is apparent as scale, smell, oiliness and crust and, although the clinical manifestation may vary from individual to individual, the underlying changes are similar. Keratinisation, however, is easily altered by numerous other internal factors and also by external factors, and thus scale and oiliness are secondary features of many diseases, particularly those caused by ectoparasites but also bacterial skin disease, endocrine dermatoses and dermatoses with a hypersensitive aetiology.

36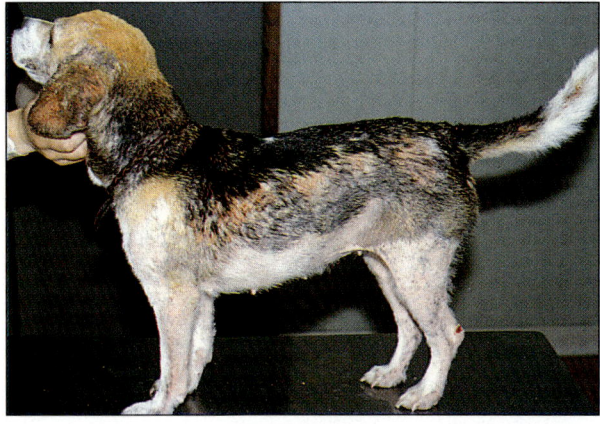

37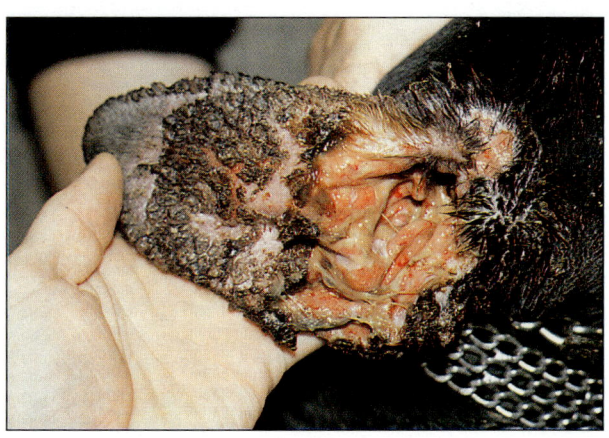

36   Crust. Crust is formed by accumulation of cutaneous debris and exudate, particularly serous exudate. This Beagle has severe sarcoptic mange and generalised pruritus.

37   Crust. The colour of any crust is influenced by the content. Accumulation of haemorrhagic crust on the ventral aspect of a pinna secondary to acute otitis externa.

38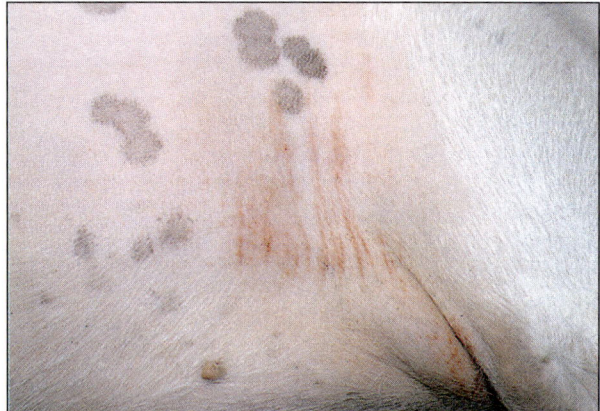

39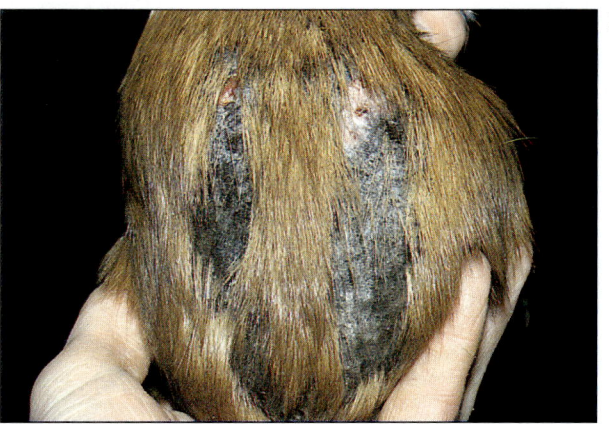

38   Excoriation. Cutaneous damage resulting from self trauma. Note the linear excoriations in the axilla of this English Bull terrier with atopy.

39   Excoriation. Lesions may be bilateral and accompanied by alopecia as in this case of *Trixacarus caviae* infection in a guinea-pig.

Crust

Crust is composed of dried exudate mixed with debris on the skin surface. In animals the amount of crust may be spectacular, mainly a consequence of the hair shafts which stabilise the crust and help to retain it. The exudate may be serum, blood or pus and the balance of each will determine the colour of the crust (**36** and **37**).

Excoriation

Excoriations are areas of epidermal damage. They are superficial and often linear, and are a result of self trauma (**38**). They are thus a feature of the pruritic dermatoses and in some individuals they can be very severe (**39**). Excoriations are prone to secondary infection, for example the per acute pyotraumatic dermatitis.

40

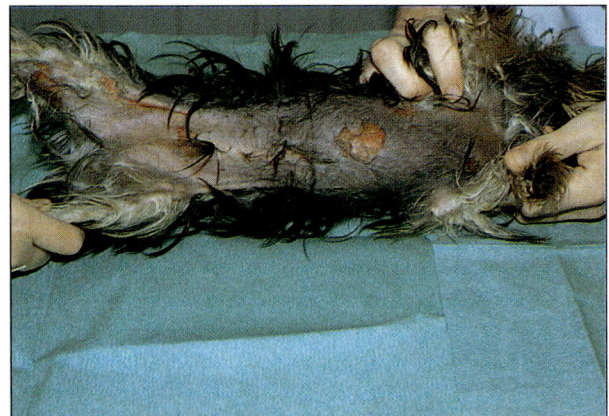

41

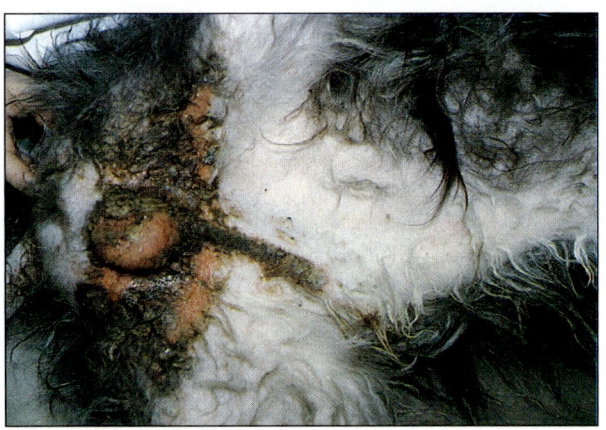

40 **Erosion**. Erosions occur when the epidermis is lost but the basement membrane is not. These erosions on the ventral body surface of this Yorkshire terrier resulted from scald; a consequence of being dropped into a hot bath.

41 **Ulcer**. In ulceration the epidermis and the basement membrane are lost. This bearded collie has an ulcerated scrotum associated with hepatocutaneous syndrome.

42

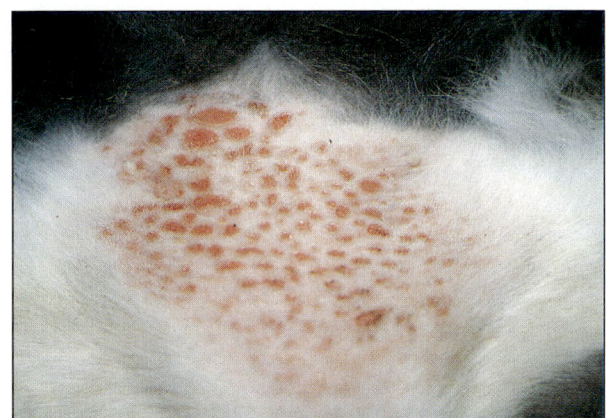

42 **Ulceration**. Multiple ulcerated papules characteristic of feline eosinophilic plaque.

Erosion

Erosions are a result of loss of the viable epidermis although the basal layer is intact. Erosions are formed when vesicles or bullae rupture to expose their base. They may be found in diseases characterised by vesicles or bullae (such as autoimmune disorders) and in cases due to exposure to physical or chemical agents (**40**). Healing occurs without scar formation.

Ulceration

In ulceration the integrity of the basal layer is destroyed, the dermis is involved and healing is often by scar formation. Ulceration may be a feature of a number of diseases, for example deep bacterial or fungal infection, self-trauma as in feline eosinophilic plaque, calcinosis cutis in canine hyperadrenocorticism, irritant contact dermatitis or neoplasia (**41** and **42**).

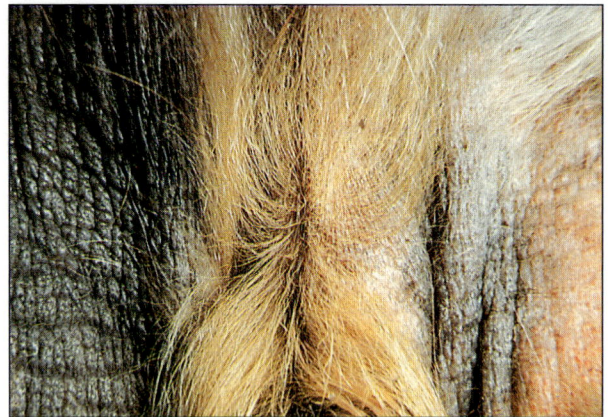

43

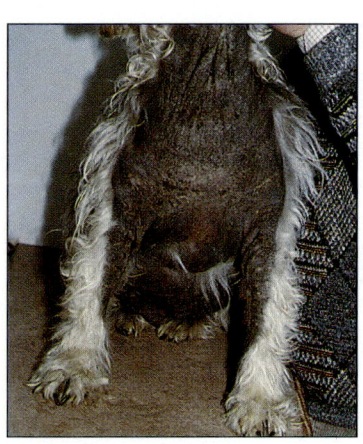

44

43   Lichenification. Thickening of the skin with exaggeration of the natural striae. Perineal lichenification due to flea-bite hypersensitivity.

44   Lichenification. Cutaneous changes often accompany endocrine dermatoses. This dog has extensive ventral lichenification associated with hypothyroidism.

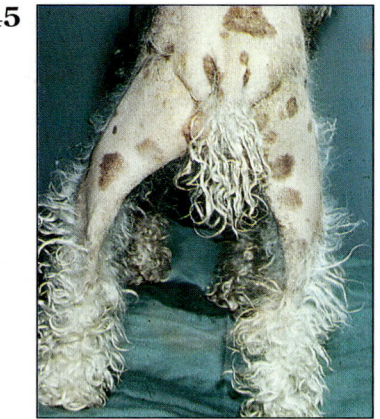

45

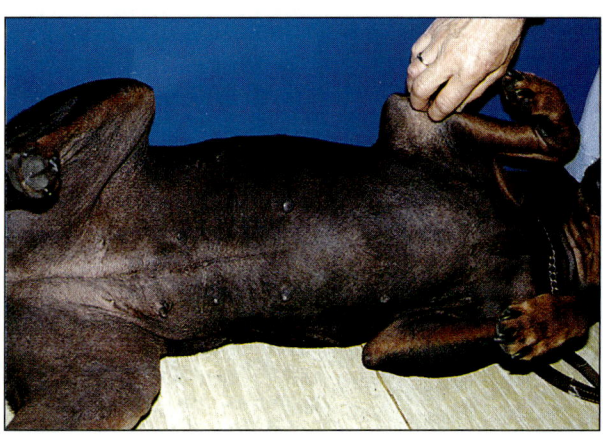

46

45   Hyperpigmentation. Hyperpigmentation in endocrine dermatoses is usually regular in distribution, at least in affected areas. In cases of elevated oestrogen such as Sertoli-cell tumour or, as in this case, cystic ovaries, then patchy hyperpigmentation is seen.

46   Hyperpigmentation. Chronic dermatoses, of whatever cause, tend to become hyperpigmented. There is extensive ventral hyperpigmentation, in this case due to allergic contact dermatitis.

Lichenification

Lichenification is a response to chronic trauma, particularly friction but also inflammation. There is a thickening of the epidermis with an accompanying hyperpigmentation in most instances. The gross thickening results in exaggeration of the folds and fissures and intertriginous maceration with secondary infection is common (**43** and **44**). The appearance of the skin is often dry.

Hyperpigmentation

Hyperpigmentation is usually a consequence of melanin excess. Melanin is synthesised within melanocytes and packaged within organelles called melanosomes. These melanosomes are passed from the melanocyte to the keratinocyte and account in large part for skin pigmentation. Other contributions to the normal colour of the skin are made by erythrocytes in the superficial dermal vessels, which may carry oxygenated or reduced haemoglobin, and from other pigments such as carotene.

47

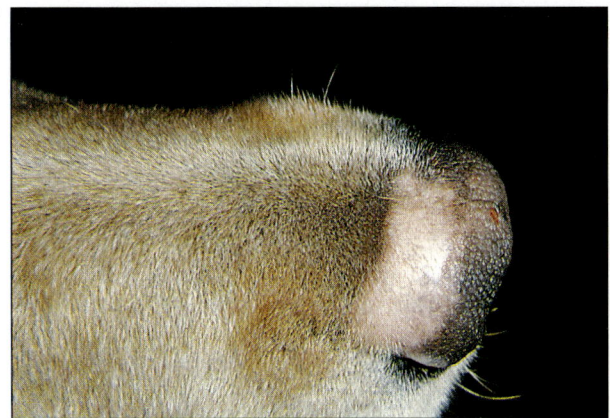

48

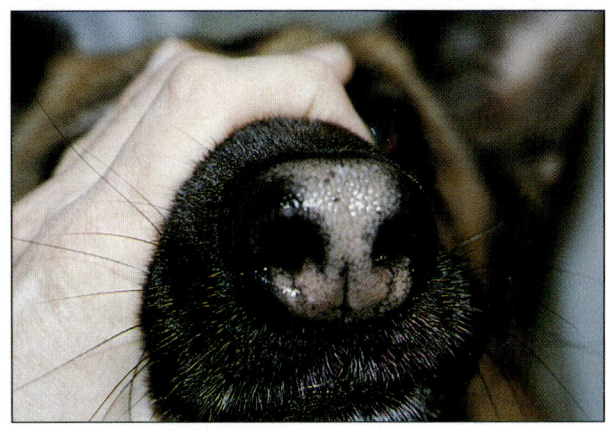

47 Hypopigmentation. Most often, inflammatory episodes are accompanied by hyperpigmentation. However, if melanocytes are destroyed, or their function impaired, then post-inflammatory hypopigmentation may be seen. This case of discoid lupus erythematosus features a loss of cutaneous pigment.

48 Vitiligo. Loss of pigment in the planum nasale is not uncommon in Doberman pinschers or German shepherd dogs.

49

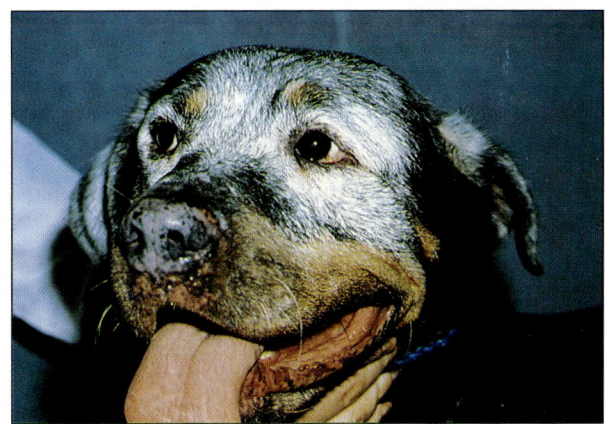

49 Vitiligo. In some cases there is very extensive loss of pigment.

Excess melanin may be due to increased numbers of melanocytes or an increased amount of melanosomes in the epidermis. Increased numbers of melanocytes are present in lentigo. In contrast, in post-inflammatory hyperpigmentation, hyperpigmentation due to chronic inflammation or an endocrine dermatosis there is increased melaninisation and melanin deposition (**45** and **46**). Occasionally, other pigments may be deposited in the skin and will give rise to different colouration—jaundice for example.

Hypopigmentation

Hypopigmentation may occur as a post-inflammatory phenomenon, for example after a bite wound or an episode of superficial pyoderma there may be localised leucotrichia (**47**). Loss of pigment may also be idiopathic. German shepherd dogs and Doberman pinschers may frequently be seen with loss of pigment on the planum nasale (**48**). An hereditary-acquired loss of pigment (vitiligo) has been reported in the Belgian tervuren and Rottweiler (**49**).

50

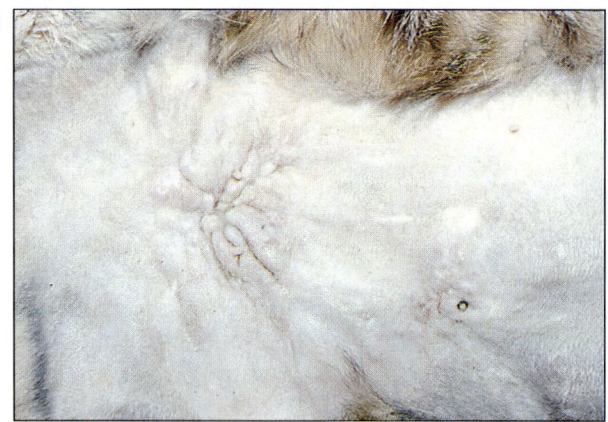

50 Scar. Atrophic, often pallid, hairless skin may follow severe cutaneous damage.

Scar

Healing by scar formation occurs when the basal layers of the epidermis have been breached and the underlying dermis is damaged and involved in the inflammatory reaction. The ensuing healing process involves fibrosis and often contraction. The resultant skin surface is often thin, devoid of hair and hypopigmented (**50**).

Chapter 3:

Diagnostic tests and clinical pathology

The purpose of sample collection and examination is to arrive at a definitive diagnosis, for example demodicosis, or, to rule out alternatives from the differential diagnosis. A knowledge of the history of the case and a complete physical examination will often suggest a limited differential diagnosis and this may dictate which diagnostic tests to apply. In other instances the case details may suggest no immediate diagnosis and many tests may be necessary.

Expertise in clinical sampling and the subsequent interpretation of specimens are essential skills for the practising dermatologist. Reliance on others to perform the basic tests is not to be recommended. Firstly, an immediate answer is available if the clinician performs them. Secondly, samples may deteriorate in the post and the incidence of false negative results will rise. Thirdly, only the clinician involved is sufficiently motivated to spend the time necessary to get an answer. Thus, in a suspected case of scabies it may take 20 minutes of concentrated microscopic examination to find a mite or an ovum.

The following description of diagnostic tests and clinical pathology is, in general, in the order in which they would be performed. There is no virtue in performing all tests on every case, but the clinician should understand the advantages and the limitations of each, and which are indicated in any particular instance.

Direct examination of the hair and skin

Direct examination is important. Do not race for the skin scrape! Examine the hair, feel its texture and look at the surface of the skin. In hypothyroidism it may feel dry and coarse, it is easily epilated and there may be mild scale. The colour of the hair may have changed; in protein deficiency for example there may be a loss of coat colour. In some instances coat colour may be associated with disease, as in colour dilute alopecia and follicular dystrophy.

The distribution and extent of any alopecia should be noted. Although classically associated with endocrinopathies, alopecia may accompany any disease in which there is follicular pathology or self trauma. There may be a loss of undercoat and retention of primary hairs in some conditions, particularly hypothyroidism and hyperadrenocorticism. Alopecia with a symmetrical distribution is strongly suggestive of an endocrine aetiology; hair loss on or around the dorsal midline or flanks is often found in hypothyroidism.

In contrast, hair loss associated with gonadal aberrations is more commonly found on the ventrum or around the neck. Patchy hair loss, particularly if associated with pruritus, suggests ectoparasites, pyoderma, dermatophytosis or hypersensitivity. Large parasites such as ticks, lice and fur mites may be easily seen, particularly with the use of a hand lens.

The skin surface should be examined. Look for primary lesions such as pustules, papules and patches of erythema. Use of a hand lens is recommended as some lesions are quite small. For example, superficial folliculitis in a Doberman pinscher may only be confirmed in some instances if the very small pustules can be identified. To the unaided eye they look like papules. It may be necessary to roll the skin between finger and thumb in order to 'sky line' the lesion.

> The clinician should be aware of the normal appearance of lesions. For example, pustules and epidermal collarettes are usually associated with inflammatory signs: large pustules and collarettes associated with minimal inflammation may be a feature of hyperadrenocorticism.

Although secondary lesions are in themselves non-diagnostic, consideration of their appearance and distribution may be helpful. Thus, in sarcoptic mange, the initial distribution of the lesions and their subsequent spread, is often characteristic. Similarly, cheyletiellosis in rabbits is frequently associated with the presence of large, soft flakes of scale in the interscapular region.

51

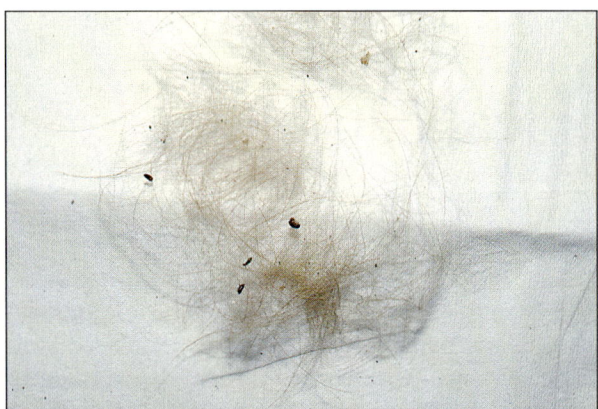

52

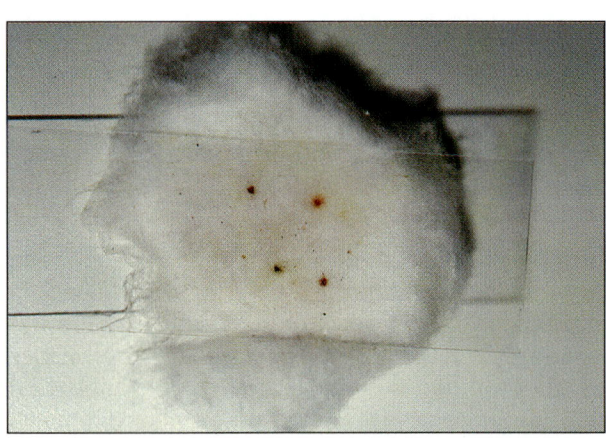

51   Examination of coat brushings. Hair and debris is brushed from the coat onto a white surface. Fleas and flea faeces may be seen in this illustration.

52   Examination of coat brushings. Suspicious particles are placed onto damp cotton wool. Haemoglobin diffuses from flea faeces and appears as staining around the faecal particles.

Diascopy

Diascopy is a procedure for differentiating erythematous changes in the skin. Erythema, particularly if patchy, may represent increased capillary permeability, due to inflammatory changes within the skin, or haemorrhage. Gentle pressure with a clean glass slide will cause blanching of the skin if the colour change is due to inflammatory changes. Patches of haemorrhage will not blanch.

Testing for the Nikolsky sign

In certain dermatoses characterised by cleft formation in the epidermis, it may be possible to cause further splitting of the skin by exerting lateral pressure. Using a dry finger or a rubber eraser, the skin adjacent to an erosion or ulcer is pushed. If further splitting occurs then a positive Nikolsky sign is present. The test is a useful indicator that there is a loss of cell-to-cell adhesion and suggests that an autoimmune or immune-mediated disorder may be present. It may be possible to obtain a positive Nikolsky sign on skin of normal appearance in affected animals. A positive Nikolsky sign may be suggestive of pemphigus diseases or toxic epidermal necrolysis.

Examination of coat brushings

The examination of coat brushings is a simple test and one that is ideal for detecting the presence of flea faeces in the coat. It may also allow identification of fleas and *Cheyletiella* spp. The animal is gently restrained on a white table top, or over white paper, and a fine-tooth comb is used to comb the coat rapidly. Small animals may be supported under the forelimbs, held in a vertical position and the coat ruffled with the hand. Hair and debris fall to the white surface (**51**) where they may be examined with a hand lens. Suspicious samples may be collected with damp cotton wool and examined under a hand lens: blood staining is positive for flea faeces (**52**).

Advantages
• The test is easy to perform and the result is available immediately.
• The examination of coat brushings is a useful technique for demonstrating the presence of fleas or flea faeces on dogs and cats.

Limitations
• Does not sample the skin surface.

53 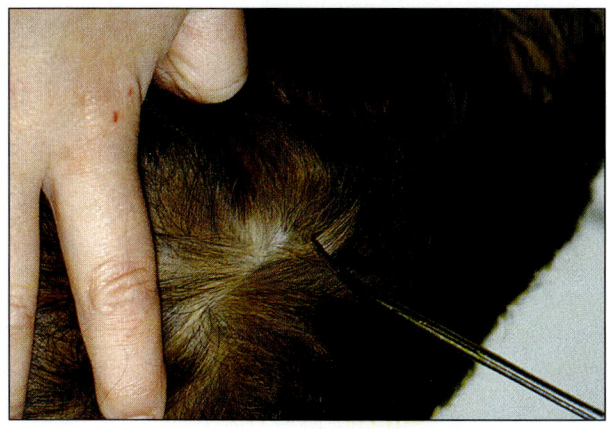 **54**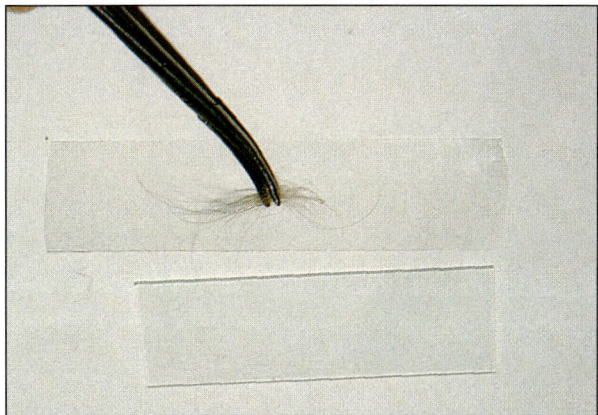

53–55 Trichogram preparation. A small tuft of hair is removed with forceps and laid onto transparent adhesive tape. This is then laid onto a glass slide and examined under a microscope.

55 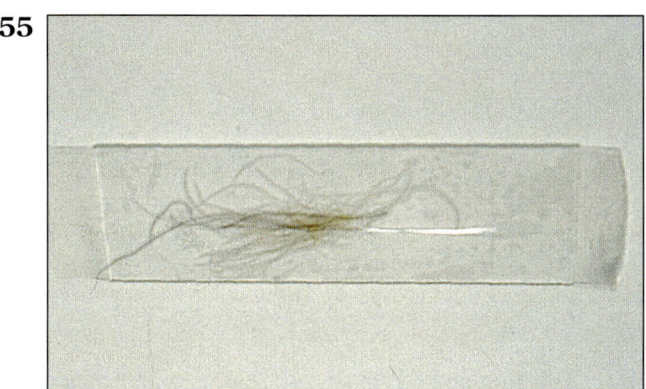 **56**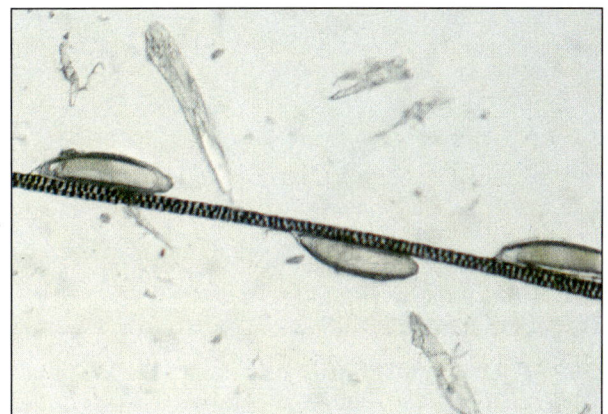

56 Trichogram. Parasites or their ova may be found attached to the hair shafts. The illustration shows ova of *Myobia musculi* on a hair from a mouse. This technique is a useful method of demonstrating ectoparasites in mice and other small mammals.

Trichogram preparation

This test yields information on the hair root, shaft and tip. A small sample of hair is plucked with fingers, forceps or haemostats. It is fixed to clear adhesive tape which is, in turn, affixed to a glass slide (**53–55**). Microscopic examination will allow identification of fur mites, adherent egg cases (pediculosis, cheyletiellosis, myobic mange, **56**), fractured ends to the hair shaft and assess-ment of anagen/telogen ratios. The clinical significance of the latter is debatable. However, the assessment of the morphology of the distal tip of the hair shaft may be of great value. For example, in some cases of feline alopecia it may prove difficult to assess whether the hair loss is as a result of self-epilation or follicular pathology.

In the former case the tip is often broken and

57

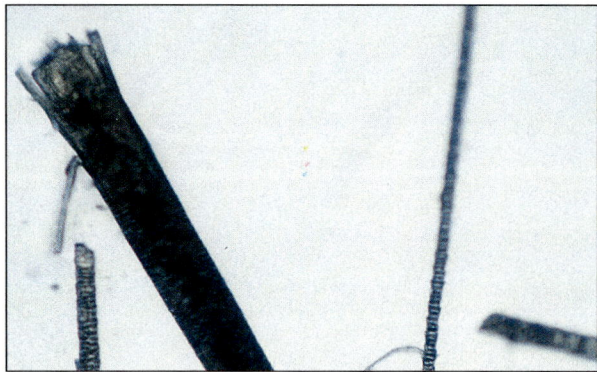

58

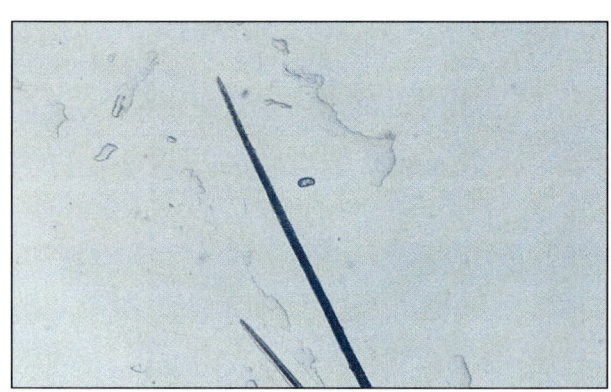

57   Trichogram. In cases of self epilation, as in this case, there may be obvious evidence of trauma to the shafts with fractured, bitten-off ends visible.

58   Trichogram. Examination of the tip should reveal gently tapering points as in this case from a cat with normal hair.

59

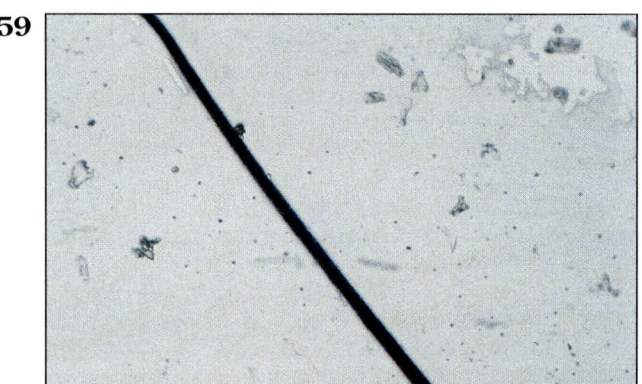

60

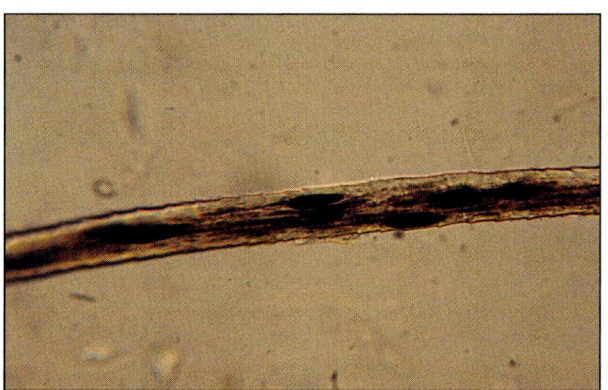

59   Trichogram. Primary hair from a black and tan Doberman pinscher. Note the regular dispersal of the small melanin granules which produce an even coloration in the shaft.

60   Trichogram. Primary hair from a colour dilute Doberman pinscher. Note the uneven distribution of the large melanin granules. (Illustration courtesy D. Bentley.)

61

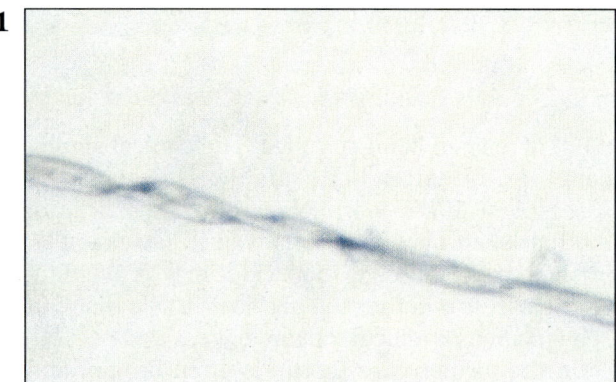

62

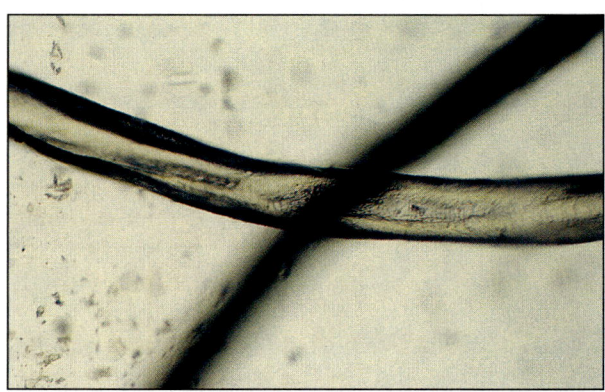

61   Trichogram. *Pili torti* (twisted hair) from a kitten with patchy alopecia.

62   Trichogram. Abnormal hair from a cross breed with congenital alopecia associated with follicular dystrophy.

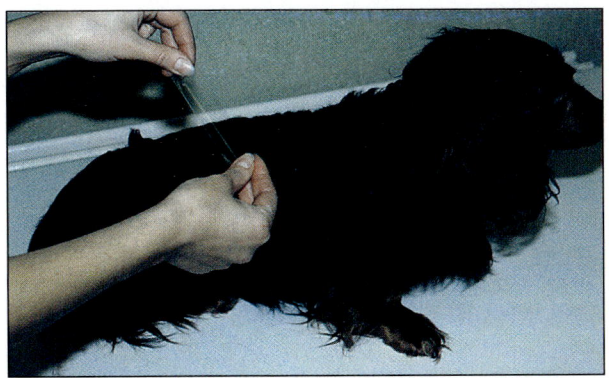 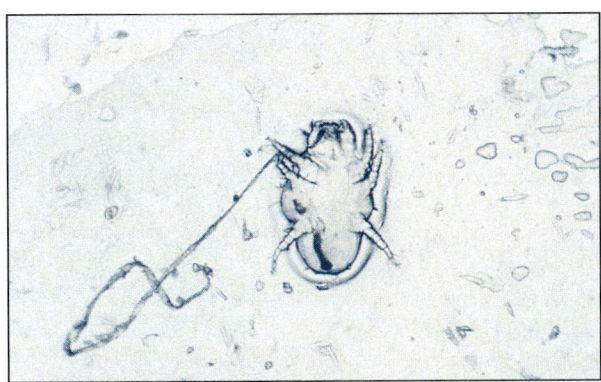

63 Tape stripping. Application of acetate tape to the hair and skin is a useful method of collecting samples. Hair, some ectoparasites, follicular casts, scale and debris are collected and examined under the microscope.

64 Tape strip of unclipped coat reveals identifiable *Cheyletiella* spp. mite. Tape stripping is not a good method by which to rule out ectoparasitism; it may, however, prove useful.

 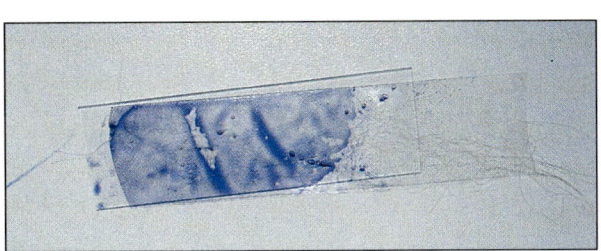

65 Tape stripping. Hair is clipped and a piece of clear adhesive tape is pressed onto the skin surface. It is then stained with Dif Quik, for example, laid across a glass slide and examined under the microscope.

fractured or possesses a squared-off end (**57**). If there is no self trauma then a smooth tapered end is found (**58**). Examination of the shaft may reveal evidence of follicular pathology. Thus, abnormally large and sparsely distributed melanin granules are found in cases of colour dilute follicular dysplasia (**59** and **60**). *Pili torti* and other defects in shaft morphology may also be identified (**61** and **62**).

> **Advantages**
> • Trichograms may be the only method of demonstrating that alopecia in a cat is a result of self epilation rather than follicular pathology.
> • Examination may reveal disorders of the hair shaft which may reflect follicular pathology.
>
> **Limitations**
> • Trichograms are not a reliable method of diagnosing, or ruling out, ectoparasite infections.

Adhesive tape stripping

This procedure allows direct sampling of the coat or skin surface; hair, squame morphology, ectoparasites and micro-organisms may be observed. Acetate stripping of the unclipped coat is a method of collecting hair and surface ectoparasites (**63** and **64**). It is particularly useful when examining small, mobile mammals such as mice which can be difficult to skin scrape. Tape strips can also be taken of the skin after the hair has been clipped. Semi-quantitative results are available as the area of sample is known.

A commercial, clear, adhesive tape (such as 3M) is gently pressed onto the clipped skin surface, removed, stained with Dif Quik and then laid across a glass slide (**65**). Microscopic examination of the stained strip will allow identification of normal squames, rafts of adherent parakeratotic keratinocytes, ectoparasites, bacteria and yeast (*Malassezia pachydermatis*) and follicular casts (**66–69**).

66

67

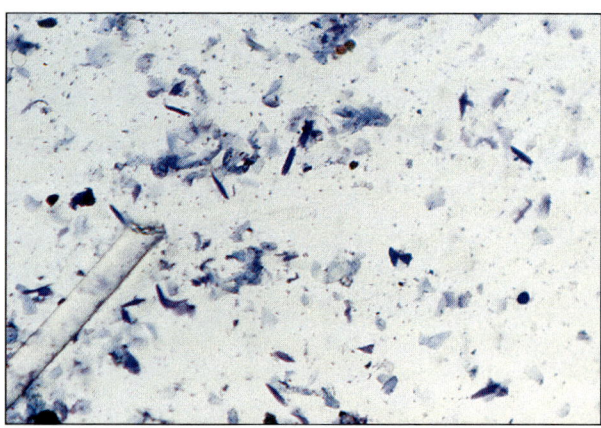

66 and 67   Tape stripping. Samples (under low power) from normal skin demonstrating fragments of hair shaft, squames and debris.

68

69

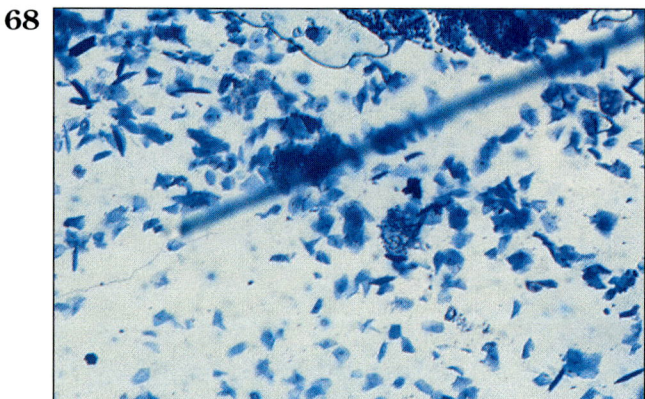

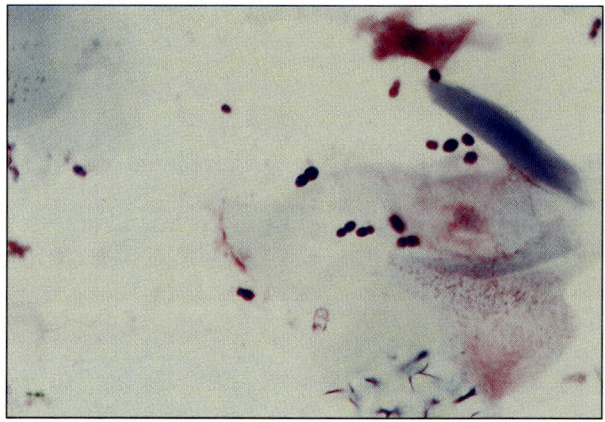

68   Tape stripping. Sample (under low power) from a dog with *Malassezia pachydermatis* infection. The small blue-black stained yeast may be seen in groups on the surface of the squames.

69   Tape stripping. High-power view of tape strip stained with Dif Quik demonstrating many *Malassezia pachydermatis* organisms. (Illustration courtesy R Bond.)

Advantages
• Useful diagnostic aid, particularly in the diagnosis of *Malassezia pachydermatis* infection. More than three or four yeasts per dry high power field may be significant.
• Useful in the diagnosis of myocoptic and myobic mange in rats and mice. These parasites may be difficult to recover by skin scrapings.

Limitations
• Requires the use of stains.
• Only samples the surface of the epidermis.

70
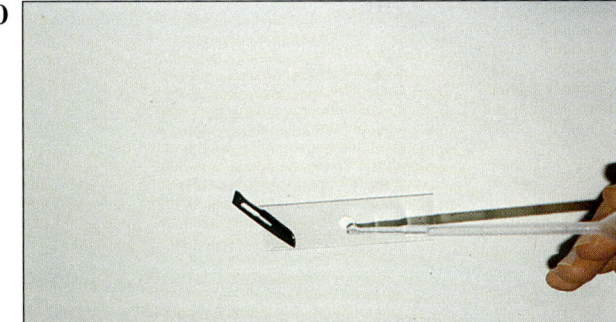

71
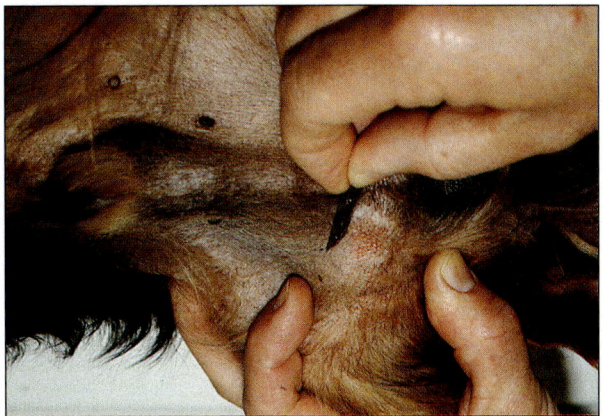

70 and 71   Skin scraping. A moistening agent, in this case liquid paraffin, is applied to the slide. Hair is clipped, some moistening agent applied to the skin and, for a right-handed operator, the skin is tensed between forefinger and thumb of the left hand. The blade is drawn across the tensed skin and the accumulated sample transferred to the slide.

72
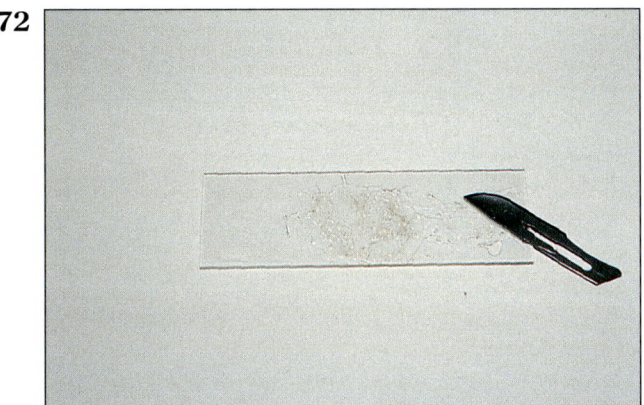

73
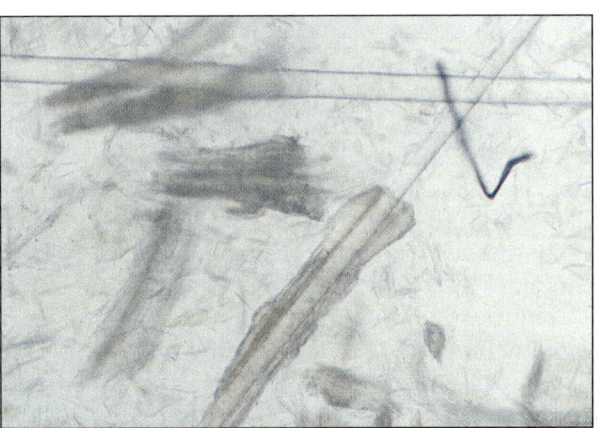

72   Skin scraping. The sample is gently mixed with the moistening agent. There should be a transparent mixture with no large lumps present.

73   Skin scraping. Microscopic examination under low power should reveal a thin smear with an even distribution of particles across the field of vision. Note the follicular cast on the central hair in this example.

Skin scraping

This procedure samples the surface, the epidermis and the upper dermis. Hair is clipped, some moistening agent is applied to the skin surface, the skin is tensed with forefinger and thumb of the left hand and the blade is dragged across the skin repeatedly (**70** and **71**). Areas of thick crust and exudate should be avoided since they will be impossible to examine in the final preparation.

The scraped sample and more moistening agent are gently mixed on the slide until a thin, transparent mixture is made (**72** and **73**). Superficial scrapes are indicated for *Cheyletiella* spp., deeper ones over large areas for *Sarcoptes scabiei* and deep ones for suspected *Demodex* spp. Thorough microscopical examination of properly-taken skin scrapes should allow elimination of demodicosis from the list of differential diagnoses in most cases. However, scabies and dermatophytosis, in

74

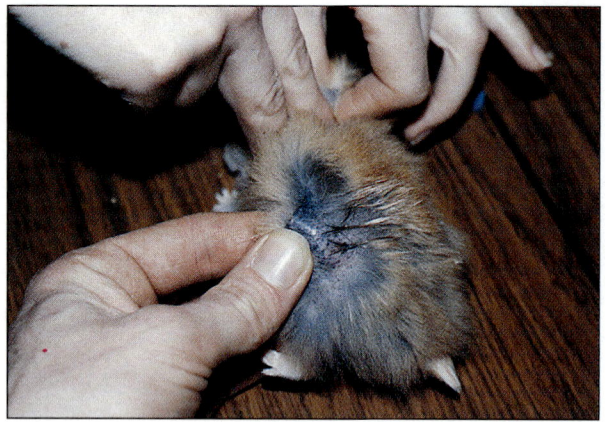

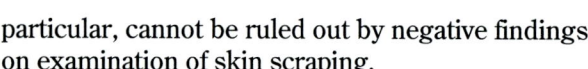

75

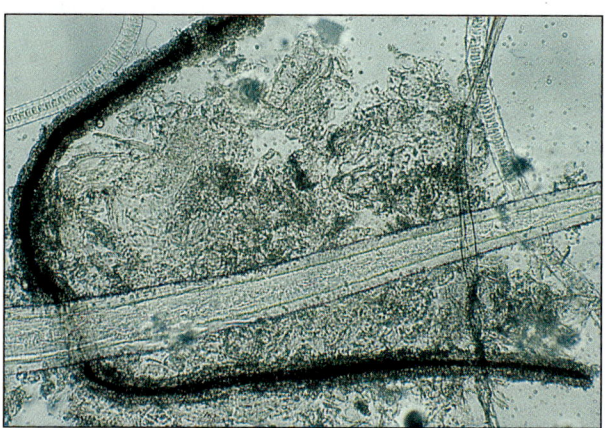

74 Skin scraping. When skin scraping small mammals with mobile skin it is easiest to tense and support it over the index finger.

75 Skin scraping. Dermatophytosis may be detected by the presence of spores on the hair shaft. This imparts a dark, thickened appearance to the affected shaft.

particular, cannot be ruled out by negative findings on examination of skin scraping.

Skin scraping of the very mobile skin of small, rapidly-moving mammals such as mice and gerbils may result in laceration of the skin unless great care is taken. Tensing of the skin in these species is best achieved by drawing a fold of skin over the tip of the index finger of the left hand with the left thumb (**74**). This stabilises and supports the skin.

Liquid paraffin is most commonly used as a moistening agent. It is less likely to run off the slide than aqueous agents and it is not caustic to skin or clothing. An alternative agent is 10% potassium hydroxide (10% KOH), which is useful as it will clear thick, heavy scale. The use of 10% KOH is advocated in diagnosis of dermatophytosis since spores may be identified on hair shafts. On low power microscopic examination the spores impart a thickened, dark appearance to affected hair shafts (**75**).

Examination under high power will reveal many small, refractile spores on the outer cortical surface of the hair shaft. Endothrix infection (on the inner, medullary surface) is not common in animal dermatophytosis. A common mistake is to misinterpret the brown melanin granules within the medullary cavity as fungal elements. The addition of blue-black ink to 10% KOH will improve contrast and allow easier identification of fungal elements. Skin scrapes of surface debris are also useful for detecting dermatophytosis. Dry skin scrapes stained with Dif Quik after heat fixing may be used to demonstrate *Malassezia pachydermatis*.

Advantages
• The skin scraping is the most useful diagnostic test to master since it samples all levels of the epidermis.
• No stains are required and an immediate result is available.

Limitations
• Cannot adequately sample heavily crusted or fibrosed skin. In particular, pododermatitis of any breed, and any suspect dermatosis of the Chinese Shar pei, should be subject to biopsy since skin scrapings will not penetrate deeply enough to rule out demodicosis.

Concentration techniques may be required at times if ectoparasites are suspected but cannot be found on microscopic examination of skin scrapings. Accumulated debris is placed in a test tube and 10% KOH added. The suspension is gently heated until the debris has dissolved. The mixture is then centrifuged at 1000 rpm for one minute, the supernatant removed and the tube half filled with water and then topped up with saturated sugar solution. Centrifuge again and transfer the surface film with a pipette to a microscope slide. Cover with a cover slip and examine.

76

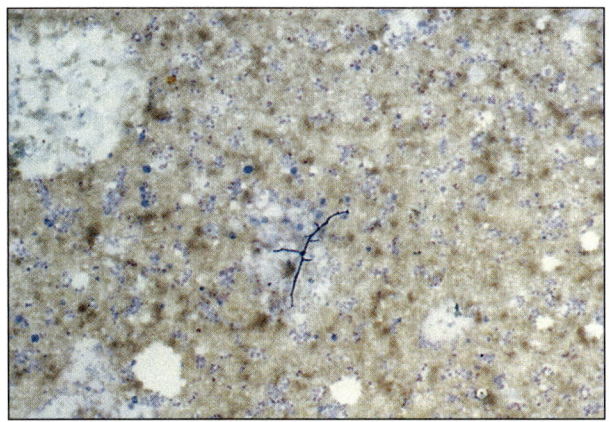

77

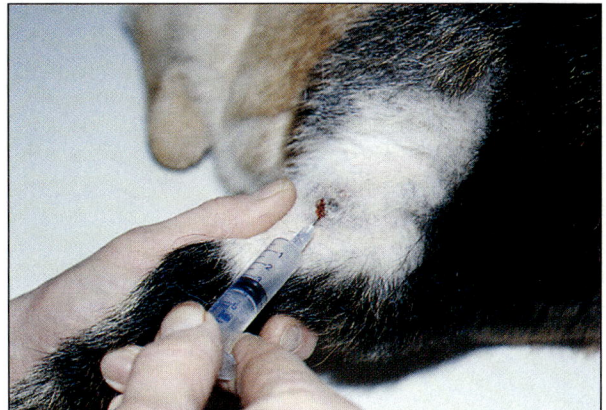

76   Impression smear. Fungal hyphae (subsequently identified as *Aspergillus* spp.) in a stained, air-dried smear from a discharging sinus.

78

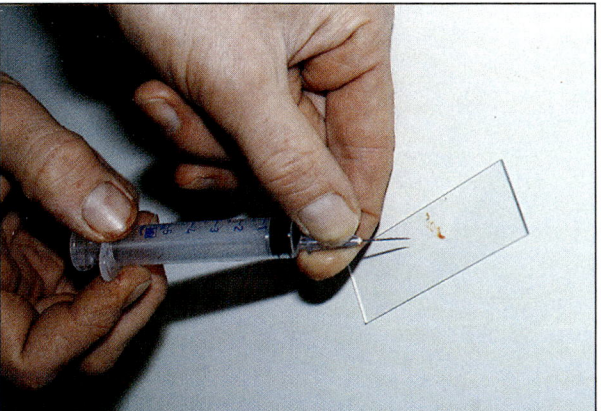

79

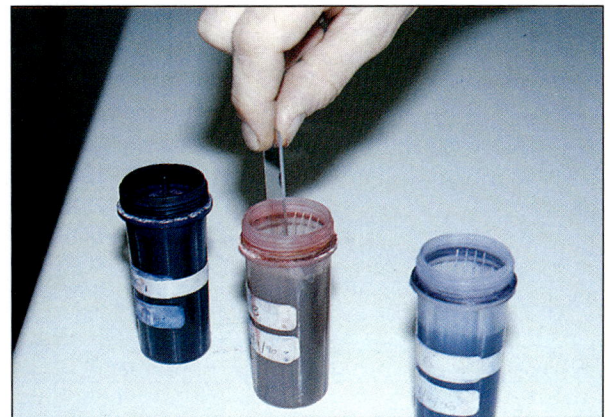

77–79   Fine-needle aspiration. The surface of the skin is cleansed with spirit. A 25g needle is introduced (**77**) and the plunger sharply withdrawn. The process is repeated in several directions. The syringe is removed, the needle detached from the syringe, the plunger withdrawn to the end of the barrel and the needle is then re-attached to the syringe. The plunger is pushed rapidly down the barrel to expel the aspirated sample from the needle onto a slide (**78**). It is smeared and air-dried before being stained (**79**).

Impression and aspiration cytology

Both techniques sample cells. Impression smears are used to sample cells from the surface of erosions and ulcers or from the orifices of discharging fistulae. Aspiration cytology samples from within pustules and vesicles or from within lymph nodes, nodules and neoplasms. An impression smear is taken by pressing a cleaned glass slide against the lesion, allowing the sample to air dry and staining with Dif Quik. The presence of micro-organisms such as bacteria, yeast or hyphae may be detected (**76**) and this may suggest an empirical choice of treatment, pending results from more definitive diagnostic tests. Cytological sampling of the mucosal lining of the preputial sheath may be of value in the diagnosis of Sertoli-cell tumour: the elevated oestrogen levels result in squamous metaplasia of the epithelium (anucleated, keratinised squames) similar to the changes in the vaginal epithelium which occur during oestrus.

80

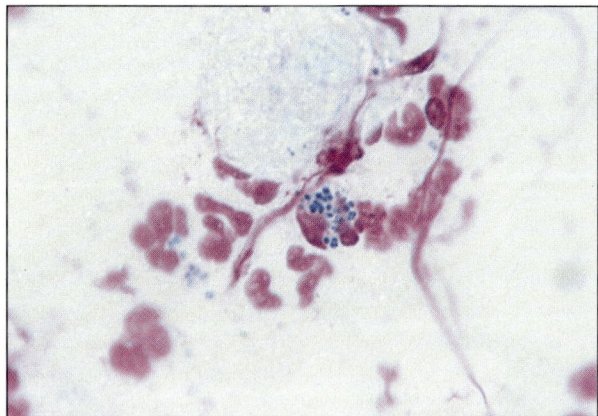

80   Fine-needle aspiration. Examination of samples from a pustule may reveal intraneutrophilic cocci.

81

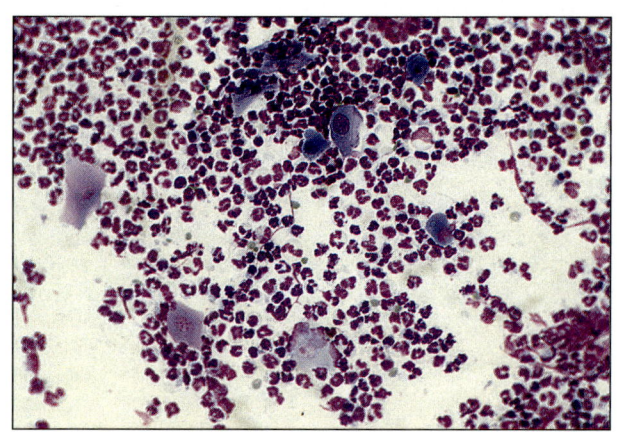

81   Fine-needle aspiration. Sample from a vesicle associated with pemphigus foliaceus demonstrates rounded epidermal cells (acanthocytes) surrounded by very 'clean' neutrophils in a manner similar to a cogwheel (Tzank test).

82

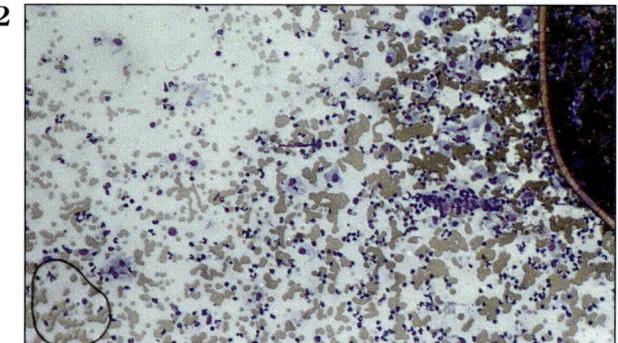

82   Fine-needle aspiration. Sample from a nodule on a cat's head reveals *Cryptococcus neoformans*.

83

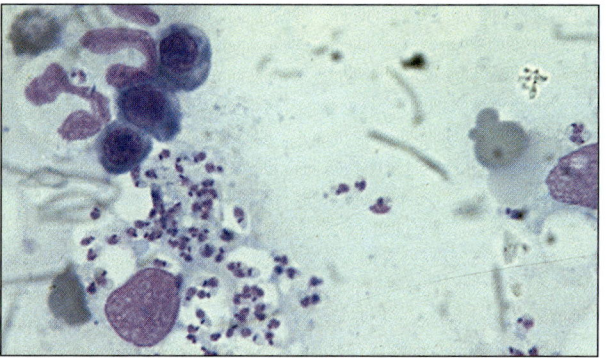

83   Fine-needle aspiration. Sample from a lymph node of a dog with Leishmaniasis reveals the causal organism.

Aspiration sampling is more complex[3]. A 25g needle, attached to a 2 or 5ml syringe, is gently introduced into the lesion of interest. The plunger on the syringe is sharply withdrawn and then allowed to fall back gently into the barrel. If sampling nodules, lymph nodes or neoplasms the procedure is repeated from different angles to allow a more representative sample to be collected.

The syringe and attached needle are then removed from the lesion. The syringe and needle are separated, the plunger withdrawn to the end of the barrel, the needle re-connected and the contents of the needle are expelled onto a glass slide by rapidly pushing the plunger down the barrel (**77** to **79**). After air drying the sample is stained with Dif Quik or a stain of choice. Identification of intraneutrophilic cocci from an aspirate of a pustule is diagnostic of superficial pyoderma (**80**).

Aspiration of pustules or vesicles (Tzank test) and identification of acanthocytes surrounded by adherent neutrophils may be highly suggestive of pemphigus foliaceus (**81**). Examination of a nodule or lymph node may reveal causal organisms in cases of infection by *Cryptococcus neoformans* or *Leishmania* spp. (**82** and **83**). Aspiration of a neoplasm may allow tentative identification of a mast cell tumour, and this information may be of value when contemplating surgery. Mast cell tumours require 2 to 3cm margins of excision whereas histiocytomas, for example, do not. However, aspirates sample very small volumes of tissue and are rarely representative. Histopathological examination of excised tissue is necessary for tumour identification and is essential if grading of malignancy is required.

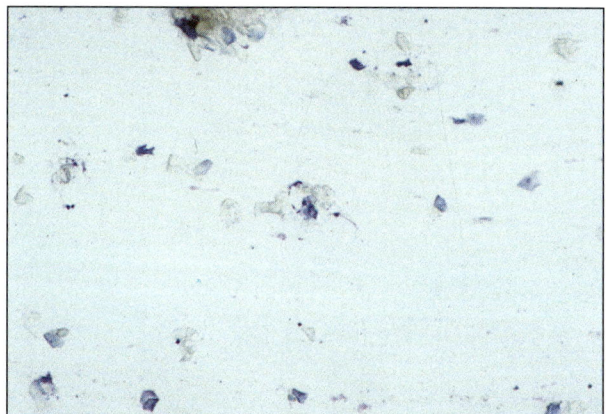

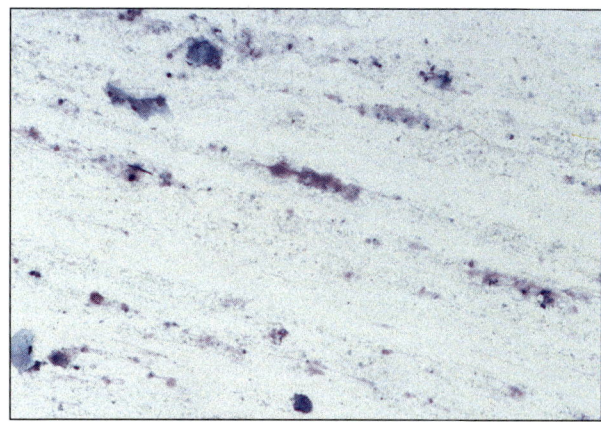

84 Otic cytology. A stained smear taken from a swab which was inserted into the normal external ear canal of a dog. Note the large areas previously occupied by lipid which has been removed by the fixative. There are no inflammatory cells and only a minimal amount of discharge.

85 Otic cytology. Sample from a dog with otitis externa demonstrates an increased amount of discharge and micro-organisms are apparent.

Advantages
• Impression smears yield useful, but usually not diagnostic, information.
• Aspiration of pustules and vesicles may be diagnostically useful, particularly in differentiating between bacterial infection and pemphigus foliaceus.
• Aspiration of nodules, neoplasms and lymph nodes may be diagnostic and should provide useful information, particularly if surgery is anticipated.
• An immediate result is available.

Limitations
• Because of the very small volumes of tissue sampled by fine-needle aspiration, the clinician should submit specimens for routine histopathological examination wherever the diagnosis of autoimmune or neoplastic disease is suspected.

Otic sampling

Cytological evaluation of samples from cases of otitis externa is often indicated and may be helpful in the selection of appropriate topical therapeutics.[1] Little diagnostic value should be placed on the colour of the otic discharge since discharges even from inflamed ears may not yield micro-organisms. Samples should be taken before any ceruminolytics are instilled into the external ear canal and before any cleaning of the canal takes place. The sample is collected with a cotton swab that is gently inserted into the vertical ear canal, rotated, and then withdrawn.

The swab is smeared onto a glass slide, and the smear is allowed to air dry before being stained (**84 and 85**). The presence of mites, bacteria and *Malassezia pachydermatis* may be detected by microscopic examination of this preparation. Bacteria will be principally of two types: cocci (coagulase positive and negative staphylococci) and rods (principally Gram-negative bacteria of enteric origin).

In cases where bacteriological culture is necessary it may be helpful to shield the swab from contact with the upper portions of the vertical canal. This may be achieved using a sterile plastic otic cone through which the swab is passed. The use of an ear curette will allow collection of shave biopsy samples from the deeper parts of the vertical ear canal and the horizontal ear canal. Samples are placed into 10% formal saline and submitted for histopathological interpretation.

Advantages
• Otic cytology is quick, easy and useful. Therapeutic decisions can be made on the basis of the identification of mites, cocci, rods and yeast.

Limitations
• No information on the antibacterial sensitivity patterns.

86 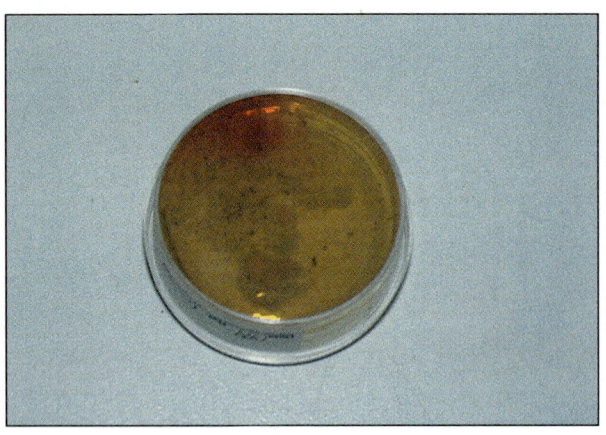 87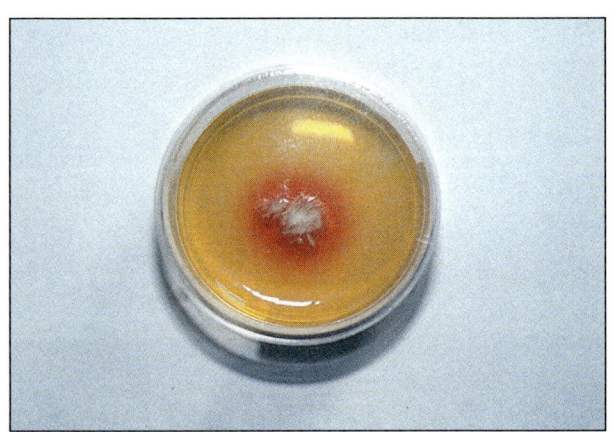

86 and 87   Fungal culture. Dermatophyte test medium (DTM) is a reliable medium for fungal culture. The medium is yellow. Positive cultures are associated with a red coloration appearing in the medium at the same time as the first signs of fungal growth are apparent.

88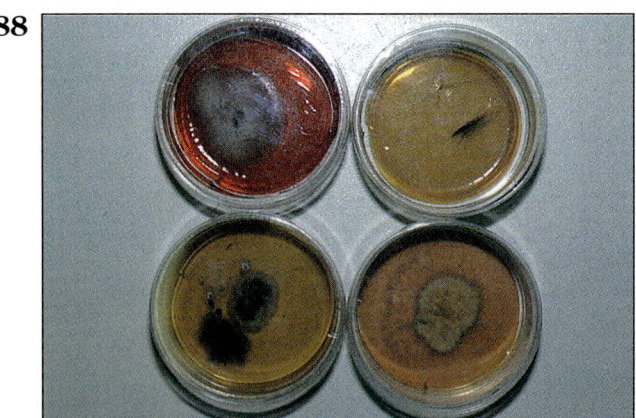

88   Fungal culture. Four negative cultures. In one there is no growth, in two there is growth but no colour change and in the fourth there is late colour change associated with a large colony.

Sampling for fungal culture

Excess hair should be removed from the periphery of the lesion to reduce the risk of contamination. Hair and scale are removed for culture with forceps or a scalpel blade. Contamination may be minimised by taking only small samples. The use of a Wood's light may be helpful if the dermatophyte is a strain of *Microsporum canis* which exhibits fluorescence. The Wood's light should be used in a dark room and allowed to warm up prior to use. Rarely, hairs will also require a minute or two under the light before they are observed to fluoresce.

In addition to *M. canis* a few other fungi may fluoresce (*M. distortum, M. adouinii* and *T. schoenlii*, for example). Selecting fluorescing hairs will increase the chance of a positive fungal culture. The scale and hair are inoculated onto a culture plate containing a medium such as Dermatophyte Test Medium (DTM). Sabouraud's medium allows identification of colony pigmentation and the characteristic macroaleurospores, and this is useful for definitive diagnosis of the species of dermatophyte (**Table 3**). However, DTM cultures will produce macroaleurospores which allow species identification. Culture plates must be examined daily for growth. On DTM plates, dermatophytes are indicated if colony growth is accompanied by an early colour change in the medium (**86–88**).

Table 3 *Summary of the cultural and anatomical features of macroaleurospores of the common dermatophytes*

Species	Pattern of spores on the hair shaft	Cultural characteristics	Anatomy of macroaleurospores
M. canis	Small spores in random array	White fluffy colony with yellow to orange/tan reverse pigment	Asymmetric, thick walled, more than 6 cells. Knob at one end
M. gypseum	Large spores arranged in chains	Flat, granular, cream-to-cinnamon brown. Reverse pigment is yellow or tan	Symmetric, thin walled and with less than 6 cells
T. menta-grophytes	Small spores in chains	Flat, powdery and cream in colour with brown reverse pigment	Cigar shaped. Often associated with spirals of hyphae and many round microaleurospores

Macroaleurospores are identified from 'Roth's flag preparations': a small square of clear adhesive tape is attached to the stem of a swab or to forceps and touched to the surface of a colony. The flag of tape is then placed onto a drop of methylene blue on a glass slide. Microscopic examination under high power will allow identification of macroaleurospores.

Samples from suspected cases of subcutaneous, intermediate or deep fungal infections should be taken under advisement from the receiving laboratory since specialised media or incubation may be required.

Advantages
- Dermatophyte culture is simple and is easily accomplished in practice with DTM plates.[5]
- Definitive diagnosis is possible.

Limitations
- Cultures must be examined daily as the critical changes occur over a short time course.

Sampling for bacteria

The use of a cotton swab and transport medium is the usual method for aerobic bacteria. Pustules should be opened with a sterile needle and pus collected. If only a very small amount of pus is present then ensure that the swab is not held vertical when sampling: bacteriologists will roll a swab across a plate and tiny samples on the tip may thus be missed. When sampling discharging fistulae or furuncles the skin surface is first cleansed with spirit and then allowed to air dry. The affected skin is then squeezed and the uncontaminated discharge collected with the swab. Punch biopsy specimens may also be used for culture and an uncontaminated sample may be obtained by removing the upper (epidermal) portion and submitting the deeper portion. Samples from cases of suspected mycobacterial infection, actinomycosis or nocardioisis should be taken under advisement from the receiving laboratory since specialised media and incubation may be required.

Sampling for anaerobic bacteria is more difficult. A swab which is rapidly placed into anaerobic transport medium should be delivered to the laboratory within a few hours if meaningful results are to be obtained. An alternative is to use a punch and to place the biopsy deep into anaerobic transport medium. The biopsy may be macerated to yield viable anaerobic organisms from within its depths and under these conditions anaerobes may remain viable for much longer periods.

- Coagulase-positive *Staphylococcus intermedius* should be isolated from nearly all cases of canine pyoderma.
- In cases of mixed infection with different bacteria exhibiting varying antibacterial resistance patterns, choose the antibacterial agent that is indicated for *Staphylococcus intermedius*.

Advantages
- Provides information on the antibacterial sensitivity pattern of the bacteria isolated.

Limitations
- Results are only as good as the sample submitted.

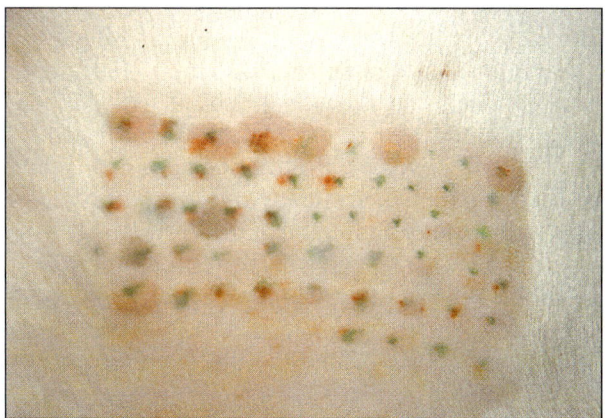 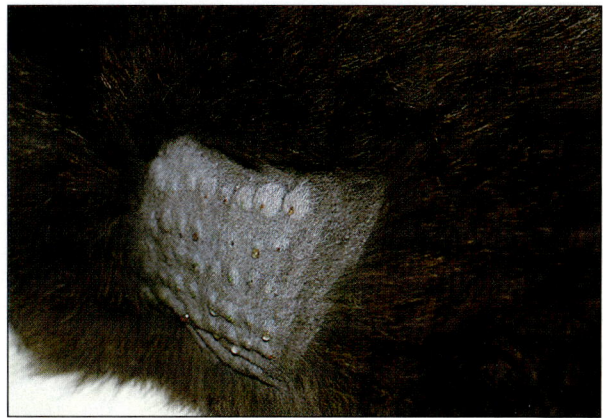

89 and 90   Intradermal skin testing. Positive reactions in a dog and a cat. These are identified by erythema, steep sided wheals and a size comparable to that of the positive control. In these cases the positive control was histamine, positioned at the upper left of the panel.

Intradermal skin testing

This procedure is used to demonstrate the presence of allergen-specific IgE on mast cells at the site of the intradermal injection. The inference is that Type I hypersensitivity exists to the epitopes of environmental dusts, insect extracts and pollens that were injected, i.e. the dog (or cat) has atopy. It is also of value in the diagnosis of flea bite hypersensitivity, although in this instance a limited series comprising positive and negative controls and aqueous flea extract only are used (see Chapter 9, **338**).

Intradermal injection is simple but demands practice and good restraint of the animal. Sedation may be used but premedicants such as acepromazine should be avoided: most clinicians use xylazine or detomidine for chemical restraint. Hair is gently clipped from the flank and injection sites are marked 1cm apart, avoiding the skin of the lower lateral thorax and ventral abdomen in which it is more difficult to place the injections. Care should be taken to avoid inflamed or infected skin.

A 0·5 or 1ml syringe with a 27g needle is used to inject 0·05ml of freshly-prepared aqueous solutions or suspensions of allergens and positive and negative controls, (diluted histamine and saline, respectively). The sites are inspected after 10 minutes and reactions are graded from 1 to 4, with 1 corresponding to the reaction at the site of the negative control and 4 to the site of the histamine (**89** and **90**).

An alternative scoring scheme relies on measuring the two greatest diameters of each wheal and taking the mean. These values are then compared to values at the sites of positive and negative control and interpreted in a similar manner to that described above. False-positive reactions may occur if irritant or overly strong dilutions are injected. Intradermal skin testing is much more difficult in cats: restraint is more difficult, injection technique is more demanding and reactions are difficult to read. The intradermal skin test is considered to be the most sensitive test currently available for the identification of the allergens implicated in an atopic individual.

Advantages
- An immediate result is available.
- Considered more accurate than RAST and ELISA.

Limitations
- Allergens should be fresh and stored in the refrigerator. Old or denatured allergen is a common reason for a false-negative result. Other common explanations for false-negative reactions are improper selection of sedative and poor technique.
- The test is extremely glucocorticosteroid-sensitive.
- Should only be considered as an **aid** to the diagnosis of atopy.

RAST and ELISA testing

These *in vitro* tests attempt to identify allergen-specific IgE in serum. This offers advantages to the patient in that a blood sample rather than an intradermal test is all that is required. However, in the normal dog there are high levels of circulating IgE as a consequence of exposure to endoparasites and these can interfere with, and hinder, the interpretation of the assay resulting in essentially subjective as opposed to objective results.[13] Another complication will arise if IgGd is involved because RAST and ELISA will not measure this. Agreement with results of intradermal skin testing is variable, but reasonable results with immunotherapy, based on results obtained with RAST or ELISA, have been obtained.

Advantages
- The tests are less glucocorticosteroid-sensitive than the intradermal skin test.
- A single blood sample is all that is required.

Limitations
- Should be regarded as a method of identifying allergens *vis à vis* immunotherapy and not of diagnosis alone.
- Results not available immediately.

Exclusion and provocative exposure and closed patch testing

These are techniques used in the diagnosis of allergic contact dermatitis. Exclusion from various areas of the domestic environment or from areas of vegetation out of doors may result in the amelioration of clinical signs. Controlled re-exposure (provocative) will result in the recurrence of clinical signs (usually within 2 to 5 days) when the allergen is contacted.

Closed patch testing is more complicated (see Chapter 8). Animals are hospitalised and suspect allergens from the animal's environment are held in close contact to the clipped skin under nickel cups (Finn chambers). The animal must be restrained from removing these patches. They are carefully removed after 48 hours and the sites examined for oedema, induration and erythema.

Punch biopsy

The principal aim of cutaneous punch biopsy is to obtain samples for histopathological examination. As mentioned above, the technique may also be used for microbiological samples. Commercial 4, 6 and 8mm punches are ideal and the 6mm size is most commonly indicated. Local analgesia with manual restraint is sufficient in most cases although nervous animals may require sedation. General anaesthesia is indicated for biopsy of the footpads and nasal planum and a 4mm punch is a useful size for these areas.

The skin surface is not prepared, apart from clipping, and local anaesthetic is injected into the subcutical tissues (**91**). When using a biopsy punch, care should be taken not to twist the punch too hard as this will exert a shearing force onto the tissues and deform them.[2] Care should be taken not to damage the tissue: punches should be sharp and ophthalmic instruments should be used to remove the sample from the skin and place it into 10% neutral buffered formal saline (**92–94**).

Advantages
- Punch biopsy is quick, simple and a cost effective diagnostic tool.
- Helps to rule out many of the potential differential diagnoses.
- May be the only diagnostic tool which effectively samples severely crusted or fibrosed skin.

Limitations
- Only samples a minute area of the skin (a 6mm punch samples 0·003 m²).
- Although a definitive diagnosis may not always be obtained, a knowledge of the histopathological details in the lesions will help the clinician toward a diagnosis.

91–94 Punch biopsy. The site is selected and marked. Local analgesia is induced with the subcutical injection of local anaesthetic. A biopsy punch is gently pushed through the skin, avoiding heavy pressure and severe twisting. The sample is gently removed and placed into neutral buffered 10% formal saline.

Immunofluorescence samples

Direct immunofluorescence has been used as a means of demonstrating the presence of immune components in epidermis and basement membrane in order to support a diagnosis of an immune-mediated or autoimmune disease. Samples deteriorate rapidly unless preserved in special media, such as Michels. Recently the use of peroxidase–antiperoxidase methodology has been successfully applied to routinely fixed formalin specimens.[8] This method has obvious advantages in sample collection and is more sensitive than direct immunofluorescence, although specificity is lowered as a result.

Basal and dynamic endocrine assay

Basal thyroid assays

Basal total tetraiodothyronine (T4, thyroxine) less than 10 nmol. l^{-1} may suggest hypothyroidism, particularly if there is an associated hypercholesterolaemia of greater than 7·0 mmol. l^{-1}. Greater accuracy has been claimed by application of a formula based on the concentration of free T4 (FT4) and cholesterol: $k = 0.7 \times FT4 (pmol. l^{-1}) - cholesterol (mmol. l^{-1})$. Interpretation is based on bands, where $k < -4$ confirms hypothyroid, $k > 1$ confirms euthyroid status and values between require dynamic testing.[7]

Advantages
- Require a single sample.

Limitations
- Both tests incur significant errors.

TSH, ACTH and low dose dexamethasone testing may be carried out on the same day, if desired.

Although oral prednisolone at 1·1 mg kg^{-1} decreases serum T3, T4 and FT4 it has no effect on the response to TSH.

Aberrations of thyroid, adrenal and gonadal hormones will cause abnormal responses in growth hormone assay.

Canine serum hormone concentrations are relatively unaffected by haemolysis if serum is removed and the sample stored at 4°C.

Dynamic testing

Thyrotropin stimulation test (TSH test): two protocols have recently been validated.[6,9]

---

1. Take a basal blood.
2. Inject 0·1 IU kg^{-1} thyrotropin intravenously.
3. Take a second blood after 6 hours.
4. Submit bloods for total T4.

Interpretation: In normal dogs the post-TSH sample is at least 1·5 the basal and should be a minimum of 35 nmol. l^{-1}.

---

1. Take a basal blood.
2. Inject 2·0 IU thyrotropin intravenously.
3. Take a second blood after 4 hours.
4. Submit bloods for total T4.

Interpretation: In normal dogs the post-TSH sample is at least 24 nmol. l^{-1} greater than the pre-TSH and should be a minimum of 45 nmol. l^{-1}.

Thyrotropin releasing hormone (TRH test)[6]

---

1. Take a basal blood.
2. Inject 0·02 mg kg^{-1} TRH, by *slow* intravenous injection.
3. Take a second blood after 4 hours.
4. Submit bloods for total T4.

Interpretation: In normal dogs the basal T4 should increase by 1·2 times and usually reaches a post-stimulation value of 30 nmol. l^{-1}.

The presence of circulating autoantibodies to iodothyronines and thyroid gland antigens have been associated with clinical signs of thyroid disease in variable percentages of affected dogs. This method of diagnosis may become more practical in the future. Autoantibodies interfere with assay of T4 and T3 and may cause spuriously high results.

Adrenal assay[10]

Single cortisol assay is of no value; dynamic testing is used.

Adrenocorticotrophin hormone test (ACTH) tests adrenocortical reserve capacity and is particularly useful when iatrogenic hyperadrenocorticism is suspected.

1 Take a basal blood.
2 Inject 1 vial (0.25mg) of synthetic ACTH intravenously.
3 Take a second sample after 90 minutes.
4 Submit for cortisol.
Interpretation: Irrespective of the basal sample the second sample should rise to 270–690 nmol. l^{-1}. Elevated levels suggest either adrenal hyperplasia or neoplasia but there is overlap with normal dogs.

Advantages
• Requires only two samples and can be completed within 90 minutes.
• Documents hypofunctioning adrenal glands.

Limitations
• Not as reliable as the low dose dexamethasone test in detecting hyperadrenocorticism.

Low dose dexamethasone test

1 Take a basal blood.
2 Inject 0·01mg kg^{-1} dexamethasone intravenously.
3 Take second and third samples at 3 and 8 hours.
4 Submit for cortisol.
Interpretation: In normal dogs the extraneous administration of dexamethasone suppresses the output of cortisol and at the 8 hour sample the cortisol will be less than 40 nmol. l^{-1}. In dogs with hyperadrenocorticism, levels do not depress to 40 nmol. l^{-1} at 8 hours. Dogs with pituitary-dependent hyperadrenocorticism may show some suppression at the 3 hour sample, only to escape at the 8 hour point.

High dose dexamethasone test

1 Take a basal blood.
2 Inject 0.1mg kg^{-1} dexamethasone intravenously.
3 Take second and third samples at 3 and 8 hours.
4 Submit for cortisol.
Interpretation: Normal dogs suppress to less than half the basal level at both sample times. Dogs with pituitary-dependent adrenocortical hyperplasia will suppress to less than half the basal at either one of, or both the sample times. Dogs with adrenal neoplasia do not suppress at either sample time.

Urinary corticoid/creatinine ratio

Non-invasive, accurate and useful for clients a long distance from the clinic. Urine is assayed for urinary corticoid and creatinine.[10] Some animals with polyuria and polydipsia not attributable to hyperadrenocorticism may also have elevated urinary corticoid/creatinine ratios and thus full urinalysis should be performed in order to minimise false positives.

1 Two consecutive morning urine samples are collected.
2 Immediately after the second urine sample the owner administers 0·1mg kg^{-1} dexamethasone by mouth at 8 hour intervals and collects a third sample after 24 hours.
3 Submit all three samples for determination of urinary corticoid and creatinine.
Interpretation: Normal dogs yield a urinary corticoid/creatinine ratio of less than 10×10^{-6} nmol. mol^{-1}. If the ratio of the third sample is less than 50% of the mean of the first two then, assuming that the ratio is abnormally high, a diagnosis of pituitary-dependent hyperadrenocorticism is made.

Advantages
• Easy sampling that does not require blood samples.
• Better diagnostic accuracy than the low dose dexamethasone test.

Limitations
• False positives may occur in some animals.[4]

Gonadal and growth hormone assay[11,12]
Growth hormone, like other hormones, is best assessed by dynamic testing. There are no dynamic testing protocols for assessment of gonadal hormones, thus basal assay must be used. Although gross abnormalities in one or other gonadal hormone may be documented, as in the case of the hyperoestrogenaemia that may occur in cases of Sertoli-cell tumour, the tests are frequently of little value. This situation may change as more is understood of their control and metabolism.

For assessment of growth hormone status:
1 Take a basal blood sample.
2 Inject either 10 µg. kg^{-1} clonidine hydrochloride or 100–300 µg. kg^{-1} xylazine intravenously.
3 Sample after 15, 30, 45 and 60 minutes.
4 Centrifuge and keep plasma at –20°C until required.
5 Assay for canine growth hormone or somatomedin, the concentration of which appears to parallel growth hormone.
Interpretation: Levels of growth hormone should peak after 15 to 30 minutes. Too few protocols have been published to give expected levels and clinicians are advised to contact a laboratory offering the test for their interpretation.

Advantages
• Dynamic testing of growth hormone is documented.

Limitations
• Very few laboratories offer the test.
• Some normal animals, particularly Pomeranians, may have abnormal growth hormone responses.

References

1. Chickering, W. R. (1988). Cytologic evaluation of otic discharges. In: August, J. R. (Ed.) *Veterinary Clinics of North America,* **18**: 773–782. W. B. Saunders, Philadelphia.

2. Dunstan, R. W. (1990). A user's guide to veterinary surgical pathology laboratories; or, why do I still get a diagnosis of chronic dermatitis even when I take a perfect biopsy? In: DeBoer, D. J. (Ed.) *The Veterinary Clinics of North America,* **20**: 1419–1427. W. B. Saunders, Philadelphia.

3. Evans, R. J. (1986). Cytology in diagnosis and assessment of neoplastic conditions. In: Gorman, N. T. (Ed.) *Contemporary Issues in Small Animal Practice, 6. Oncology,* pp. 25–44. Churchill Livingstone, New York.

4. Feldman, E. C. and Mack, R. E. (1992). Urine cortisol:creatinine ratio as a screening test for hyperadrenocorticism in dogs. *Journal of the American Veterinary Medical Association,* **200**: 1637–1641.

5. Harvey, R. G. (1990). Fungal culture in small animal practice. *In Practice, (Journal of Veterinary Postgraduate Clinical Study),* **12**: 11–16.

6. Henfrey, J. I. and Thoday, K. L. (1991). Optimisation of TSH and TRH stimulation tests in the diagnosis of canine hypothyroidism. *Proceedings of the 34th annual BSAVA Congress.* Paper synopses, p. 121

7. Larsson, M. G. (1988). Determination of free thyroxine and cholesterol as a new screening test for canine hypothyroidism. *Journal of the American Animal Hospital Association,* **24**: 209–217.

8. Moore, F. M., White, S. D., Carpenter, J. L. and Torchon, E. (1987). Localization of immunoglobulins and complement by the peroxidase antiperoxidase method in autoimmune and non-autoimmune canine dermatopathies. *Veterinary Immunology and Immunopathology,* **14**: 1–9.

9. Paradis, M., Lepine, S., Lemay, S. and Fontaine, M. (1991). Studies of various diagnostic methods for canine hypothyroidism. *Veterinary Dermatology,* **2**: 125–132.

10. Rijnberk, A. and Mol, J. A. (1989). Adrenocortical function. In: Kaneko, J. J. (Ed.) *Clinical Biochemistry of Domestic Animals,* pp. 610–629. Academic Press, San Diego.

11. Schmeitzel, L. P. and Lothrop, C. D. (1990). Hormonal abnormalities in Pomeranians with normal coat and in Pomeranians with growth hormone-responsive dermatosis. *Journal of the American Veterinary Medical Association,* **197**: 1333–1341.

12. Schmeitzel, L. P. (1990). Sex-hormone-related and growth hormone-related alopecias. In: DeBoer, D. J. (Ed.) *The Veterinary Clinics of North America,* **20**: 1579–1601. W. B. Saunders, Philadelphia.

13. Sousa, C. A. and Norton, A. L. (1990). Advances in methodology for diagnosis of allergic skin disease. In: DeBoer, D. J. (Ed.) *The Veterinary Clinics of North America,* **20**: 1579–1601. W. B. Saunders, Philadelphia.

Chapter 4:

Parasitic disease

Introduction

Parasitic infections of the skin account for the major part of small animal skin disease. Flea bite hypersensitivity is by far the commonest allergic skin disease seen in dogs and cats. Ectoparasitic conditions are the main reason for the presentation of guinea pigs, hamsters and mice to veterinary surgeons and they are a common problem in the rabbit. The most frequent clinical sign associated with the presence of an ectoparasite is pruritus, although there are exceptions. For example localised demodicosis and some case of cheyletiellosis may not be pruritic.

Ectoparasites should be always be suspected in any dermatoses but two parasites in particular, *Ctenocephalides felis* and *Demodex canis*, are so common and so multifaceted in their clinical presentation that they should always be considered. The initial examination of the animal should include a careful examination of the coat for fleas or flea faeces and all dermatological cases should be subject to skin scrapings which are examined microscopically for *Demodex canis*.

The diagnosis of a parasitic infection may be suggested by consideration of the history, particularly sarcoptic mange which typically begins on the elbows, hocks or pinnae and then generalises. *Sarcoptes scabiei*, *Ctenocephalides felis* and *Cheyletiella* spp. may be associated with zoonotic lesions and a knowledge of the distribution of the bites on the humans in immediate contact with the affected dog cat or rabbit may aid diagnosis (see Chapter 19).

In view of the potential for serious consequences, both for host and owner, prompt and accurate diagnosis is essential. Ectoparasitic diseases are easy to identify and most conditions respond well to control measures. The prognosis is generally good once the diagnosis is made except, perhaps, in the case of generalised demodicosis where bacteraemia is a possible complication of infection.

The treatment of ectoparasite infestations must take into account the life cycle of the parasite, its potential for contagion and the capacity of the parasite to survive in the environment.

The capacity to survive off the host can make control difficult unless environmental insecticides and acaricides are used. An added complication is that hypersensitivity to the parasite or its secretions may be a major component in the production of the clinical signs in many instances. Even if the parasite is killed the presence of its body may well provoke continued pruritus until it is removed from the skin. In the case of parasites killed whilst within the stratum corneum, particularly the sarcoptid mites, it may take one or two weeks for the epidermal tide to wash out the remains and for pruritus to reduce.

Flea infestation

Fleas are small, brown, laterally compressed, wingless insects which may clearly be seen running actively through the coat in some cases (**95**). Although lesions are most common on the caudodorsal trunk, the fleas themselves are best observed on the ventral abdomen and in the inguinal region where the hair coat is sparse. In some cases, especially in long-haired cats and dogs, they may be hard to find and it may be difficult to persuade the owner that flea infestation is the cause of the complaint. In these instances the presence of flea faeces will provide evidence of infestation (**96** and **97**). In some animals, notably giant breeds, fleas may be found on the head and around the hocks rather than on the preferred sites outlined above.

There are two species of fleas commonly involved in canine and feline infestations: *Ctenocephalides felis* , the cat flea, and *Ct. canis*, the dog flea (**98** and **99**). *Ct. felis* is the most common flea infesting dogs and cats in most parts of the world and it will also bite humans whereas *Ct. canis* is confined to dogs, although it too will bite humans. Other species of flea that may be found on dogs and cats include *Pulex irritans* (the human flea) *Xenopsylla cheopis* (the rat flea), *Echidnophagia gallinacea* (the sticktight poultry flea), *Spilopsyllus cuniculi* (the rabbit flea) and *Archeopsylla erinacei* (the hedgehog flea).[3,4] The saliva of the latter cross-reacts with that of *Ct. felis* and may thus be a cause of apparent failure in flea control programmes, particularly in suburban areas where the hedgehogs may come into contact with domestic pets.

The adult female flea requires a blood meal before being able to reproduce. Eggs are laid on the host and, being non-sticky, fall to the ground to complete their development. They appear as tiny, glistening, white spheres and are often to be found on window sills, chairs etc., where infected cats and dogs have been lying. The larvae that hatch from the eggs resemble tiny, bristly caterpillars although they may be distinguished by the presence of two prominent posterior projections, the anal struts.

They are quite active but avoid both light and low humidity by remaining in crevices, under vegetation or in the underlay of carpets. It is in these areas that the pupae form. The pre-emerged adult within the cocoon is highly resistant to low humidity and temperature and remains within the cocoon until the presence of a potential host is indicated by vibration, warmth and CO_2. Heavy infestation can build up in the house or garden without the owner becoming aware.[9,14,26]

Although any animal has the potential to develop a hypersensitivity to components in the flea saliva it has been demonstrated that both intermittent exposure and initial exposure in later life predispose dogs to the development of flea bite hypersensitivity. It has been proposed that all dermatological signs associated with the presence of fleas are manifestations of hypersensitivity. Types I, II, IV and cutaneous basophil hypersensitivity reactions may all be involved in the pathogenesis of the clinical signs in the dog and cat.[15]

In dogs the presence of infection is characterised by pruritus and associated clinical signs such as erythema, crusted papules and alopecia, particularly in the dorsal lumbosacral region (see Chapter 8). In severe cases, hyperpigmentation and lichenification may result. Pyotraumatic dermatitis may accompany some infections.[25]

In cats the signs may be more variable with a number of clinical pictures being recognised. There may be dorsal hyperaesthesia, characterised by episodic twitching of the skin of the back, accompanied by frenetic grooming and vocalisation. Other cases may exhibit crusted papules (miliary dermatitis), stubbled, patchy, alopecia over the base of the tail or varying degrees of symmetrical alopecia (see Chapter 8). Some cases of eosinophilic plaque have been associated with flea-allergic dermatitis.

Support for the diagnosis may be inferred by the presence of *Dipylidium caninum* (of which the flea is an intermediate host), the presence of zoonotic lesions and the presence of fleas on in-contact animals.

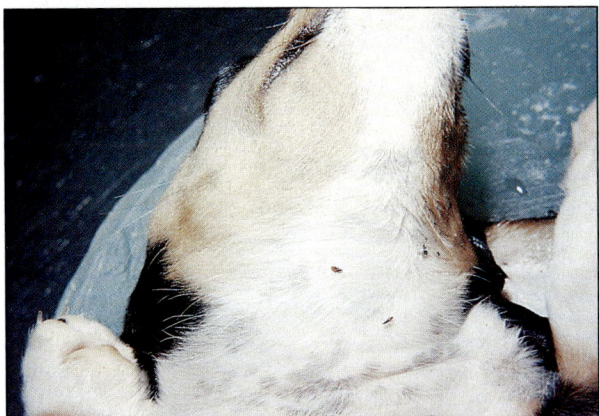

95 **Flea infestation.** Fleas on the ventral neck of a beagle dog. In many cases, particularly where there is flea-bite sensitivity, it is unusual to find fleas. Inspection of asymptomatic, in-contact animals, if available, is more rewarding.

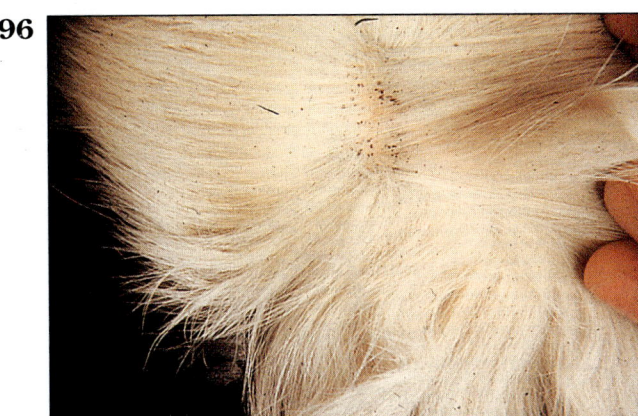

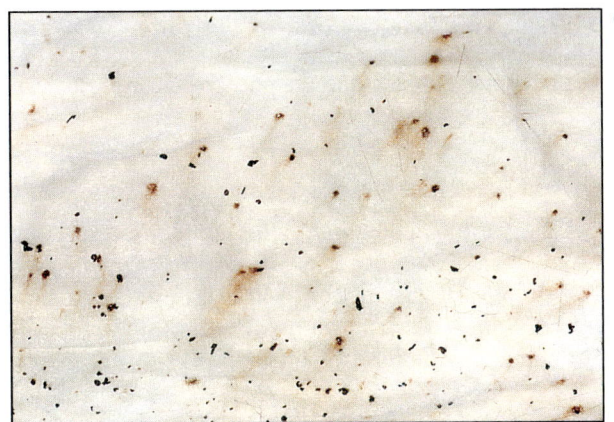

96 and 97 **Flea infestation.** Flea faeces in the coat of a long-haired cat. The presence of flea faeces implies the presence of fleas, even if none can be demonstrated. Flea faeces placed on damp white blotting paper or cotton wool (**97**) develop a red halo due to haemoglobin leaching out into the damp surrounding medium. This is a useful test to perform on debris produced by combing out the coat.

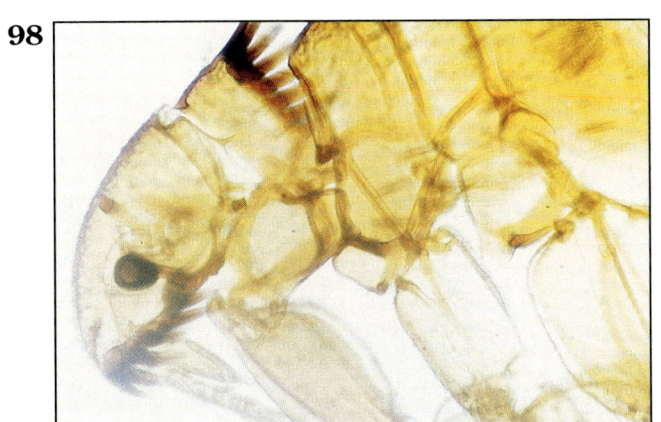

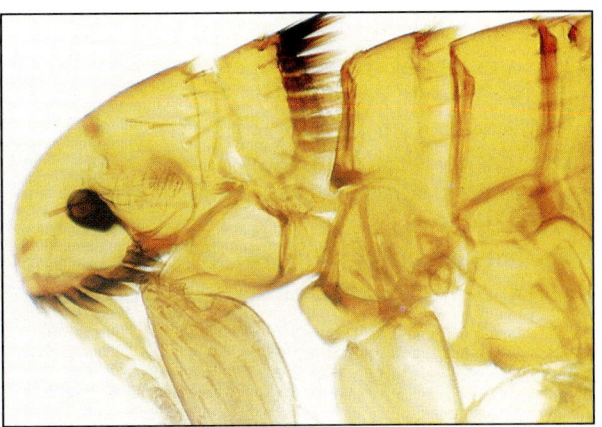

98 and 99 *Ctenocephalides felis* **and** *Ctenocephalides canis.* Note the prominent genal and pronatal combs and the shape of the rostral aspect of the head. In *C. felis* the first tooth on the pronatal comb is the same length as the second and the head is longer than deep. (Illustrations courtesy of M. R. Geary.)

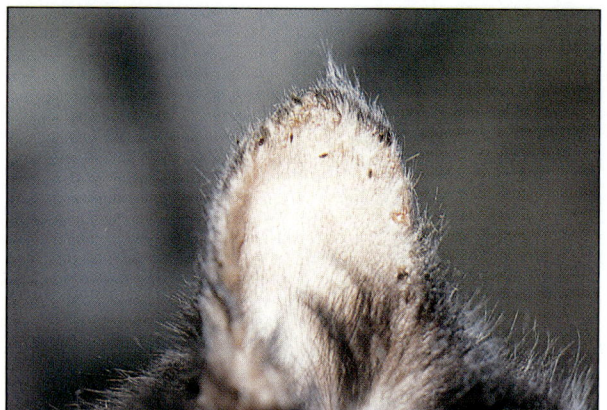

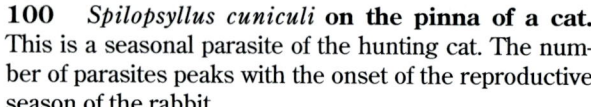

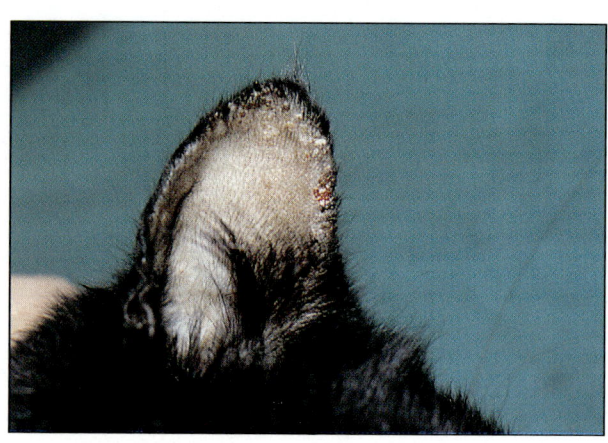

100 *Spilopsyllus cuniculi* **on the pinna of a cat.** This is a seasonal parasite of the hunting cat. The number of parasites peaks with the onset of the reproductive season of the rabbit.

101 *Spilopsyllus cuniculi* **infestation of a cat.** Note the crusting and alopecia on the pinnae.

The rabbit flea, *Spilopsyllus cuniculi,* causes a characteristic and occasionally severe dermatitis of the pinnae in cats.[16] There is erythema, crusting and self-inflicted trauma on the dorsal surface of the pinna and along the periphery (**100** and **101**).

The fleas may be seen as small black insects with their mouth parts embedded in the skin of the pinnae, giving rise to their colloquial name of 'stick fast fleas'. The condition is a seasonal threat to cats which hunt and kill rabbits.

Flea infestation is characterised by:
- No clinical signs.
- Pruritus and self-trauma.
- Zoonotic lesions.

The differential diagnoses include:
- All causes of pruritus.

The diagnosis can be made by:
- Demonstration of the presence of fleas or flea faeces.
- Compatible clinical signs.

102

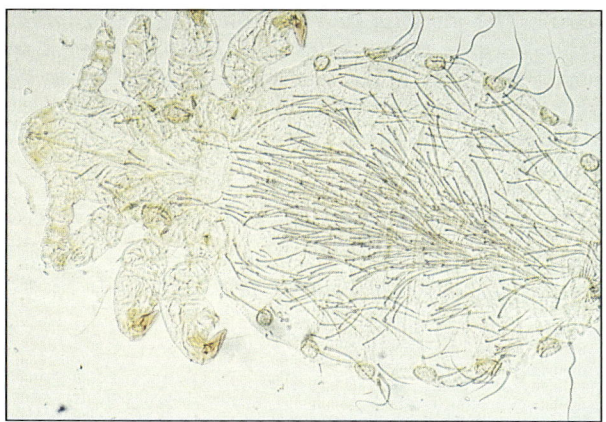

102 Pediculosis. *Linognathus setosus.* Photomicrograph.

103

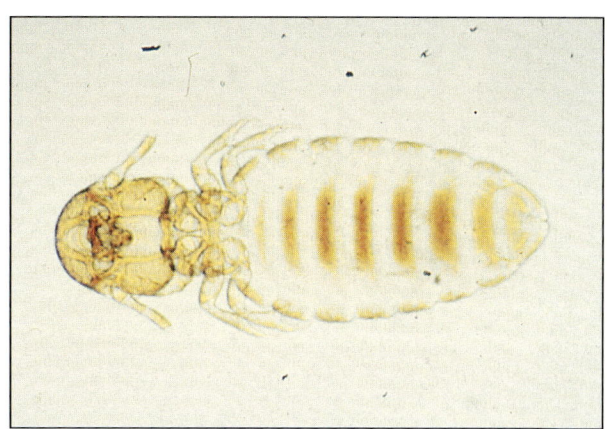

103 Pediculosis. *Trichodectes canis.* Photomicrograph.

104

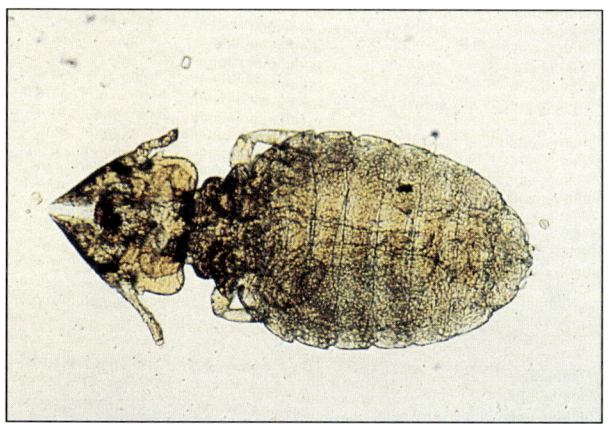

104 Pediculosis. *Felicola subrostratus.* This is a biting louse and is the only species of louse affecting the cat. Photomicrograph.

105

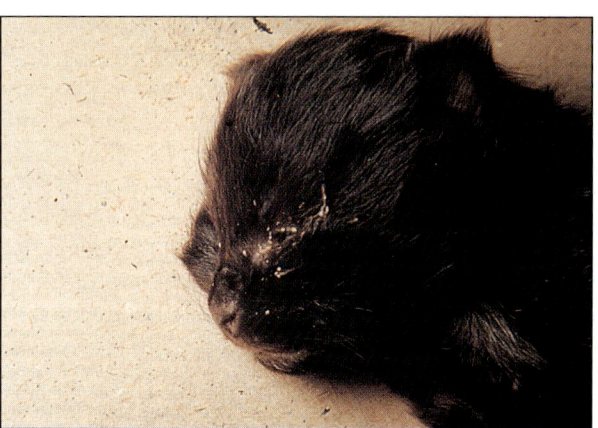

105 Pediculosis. Lice and ova of *Felicola subrostratus* affixed to the hairs on the head of a kitten.

Louse infestation (pediculosis)

Lice most commonly affect young animals, but elderly dogs and cats and those in a debilitated state may also be heavily infested. They are host-specific, obligate parasites and cannot live away from the host for more than a few days. The dog is host to two biting lice, *Trichodectes canis* and *Heterodoxus spiniger*, and one sucking louse, *Linognathus setosus*, while the cat is host only to the biting louse,

Felicola subrostratus (**102** to **104**).

The lifecycle of the louse is spent entirely on the host. The eggs are laid firmly attached to the hair shafts (nits) and hatch in seven to 10 days (**105**). The emergent larvae must feed within 24 hours and proceed to moult three times within about three weeks. Transmission of the infestation is usually by direct contact but may be via fomites, especially rugs and bedding.

106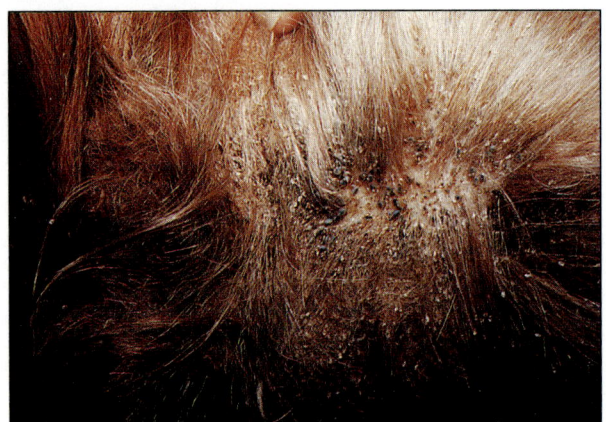

106 The sucking louse of the dog, *Linognathus setosus,* **on a Irish setter.** The parasites appear as small, blue, oval bodies with darker heads which move sluggishly. Note the ova attached to the hair shafts and the moderate scaling. (Illustration courtesy G. H. Muller.)

The presence of the insect (**106**), its bites and saliva produces variable pruritus which may lead to self trauma and, in dogs, may result in pyotraumatic dermatitis. Pale mucosae and weakness may be seen, reflecting the anaemia produced in heavy infestations with sucking lice in the dog (**107–110**). Predilection sites are the head (especially on the long-haired ears of spaniels), the axillae, the flexure of the elbow and the inguinal and perineal areas, although the whole body may be involved in generalised infestations. Excess scaling may occur which, together with the numerous whitish ova, gives rise to a heavy dandruff. Sucking lice tend to remain fairly stationary but biting lice are much more mobile and consequently can be difficult to find.

Guinea pigs are host to two biting lice, *Gliricola porcelli* and *Gyropus ovali*. Although they are usually an incidental finding[20], they may be the cause of a mildly pruritic dermatosis (**111** and **112**). Rats and mice may occasionally be encountered with louse infestations, *Polyplax spinulosa* and *P. serrata* respectively. *Polyplax* spp. are sucking lice and clinical signs of pruritus are common.

Pediculosis is characterised by:
- Scale.
- Variable pruritus.
- Anaemia and weakness in severe cases.

Differential diagnoses include:
- Other ectoparasitic infestations.
- Seborrhoeic disorders.

Diagnosis can be made by:
- Observation of the presence of lice and their ova.

107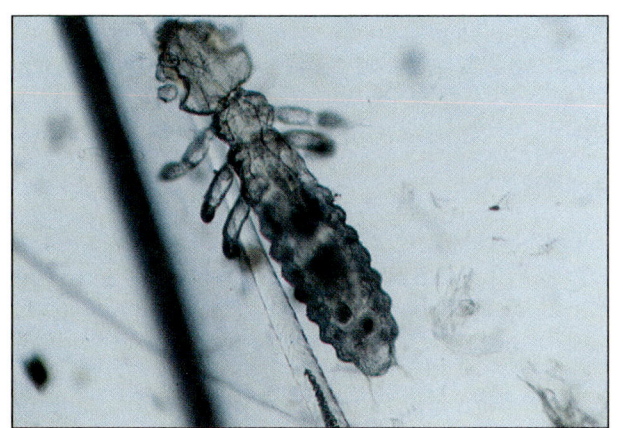

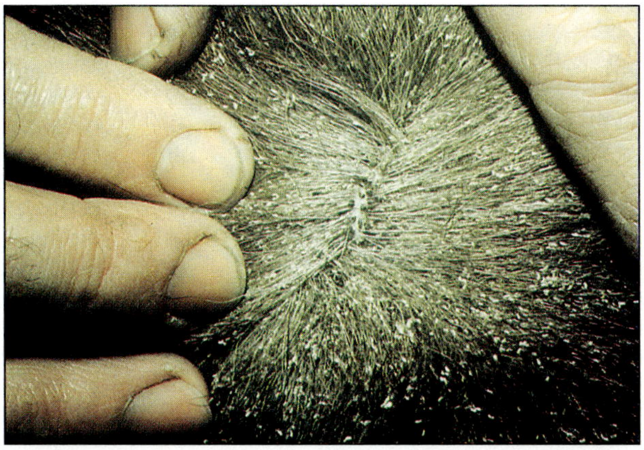

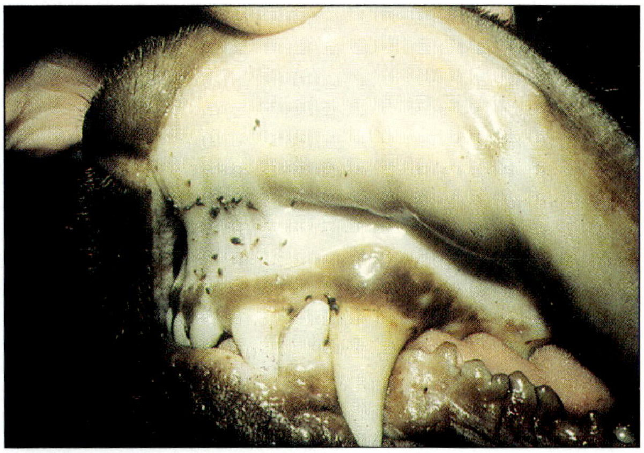

108

109

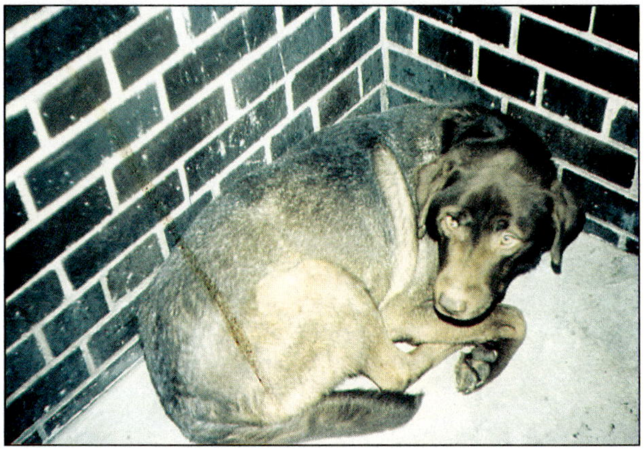

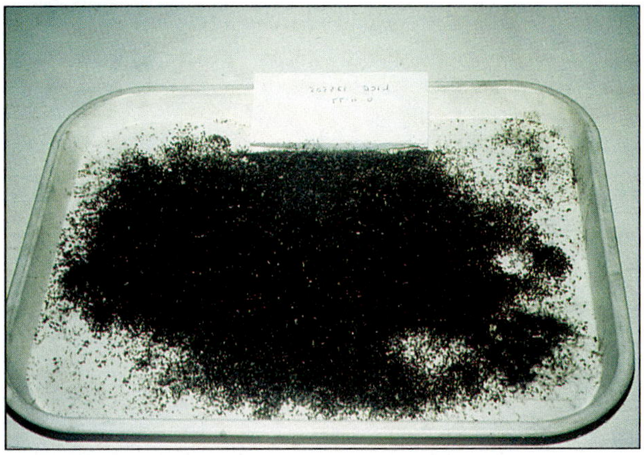

110

107–110 **Pediculosis in a cross-bred dog.** Very heavy infestation with *L. setosus* (**107**) has resulted in anaemia. Note the pallid mucosae (**108**) and depressed attitude (**109**). The final illustration (**110**) depicts the enormous numbers of lice removed from the dog. (Illustrations courtesy C. P. Mackenzie.)

111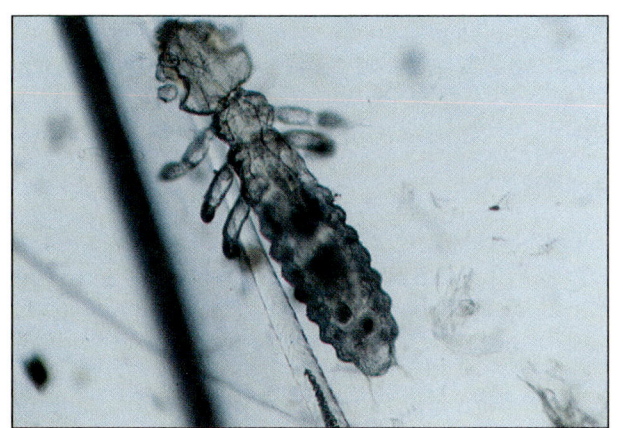

112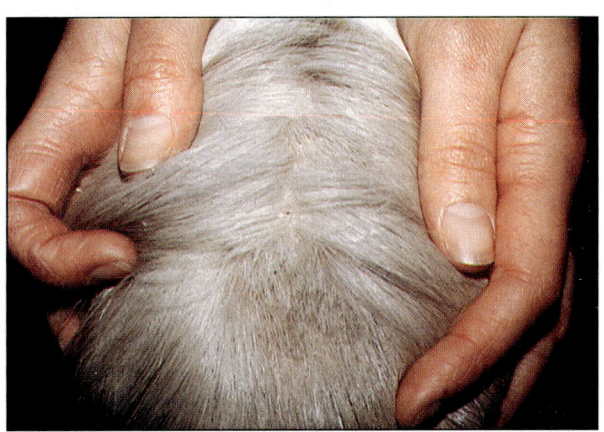

111 **Pediculosis in Guinea pigs** is caused by two species of biting lice, *Gliricola porcelli* and *Gyropus ovalis*. *G. porcelli* is illustrated.

112 **Pediculosis in a Guinea pig** causing mild pruritus and scale. (Illustration courtesy R. Bond.)

113

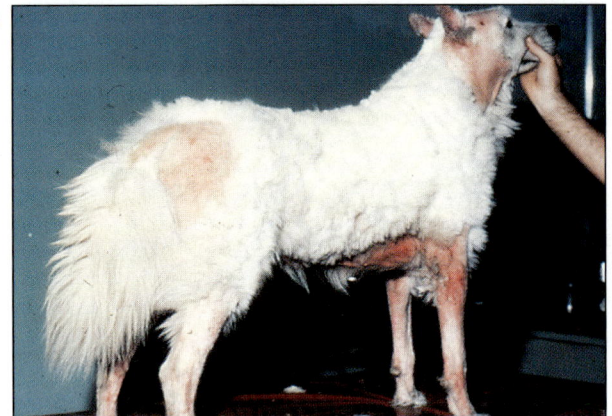

113 **Scabies.** Generalised infestation in a crossbred dog showing the predilection sites viz: the head, particularly the pinnae, lateral aspects of the elbows and hocks and the ventral trunk.

114

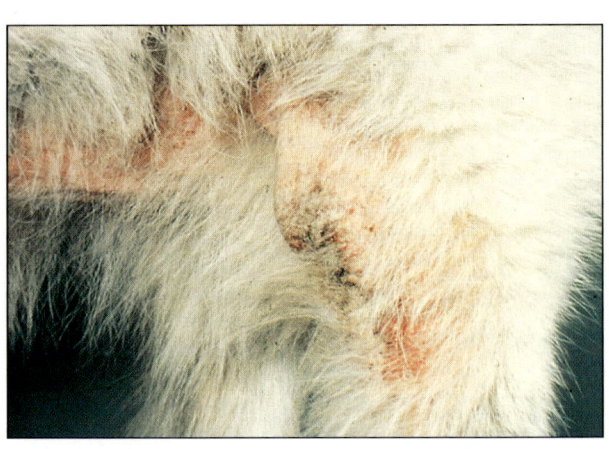

114 **Scabies.** Close up of the elbow of the dog illustrated in **113**. Note the erythema, crusting and alopecia.

115

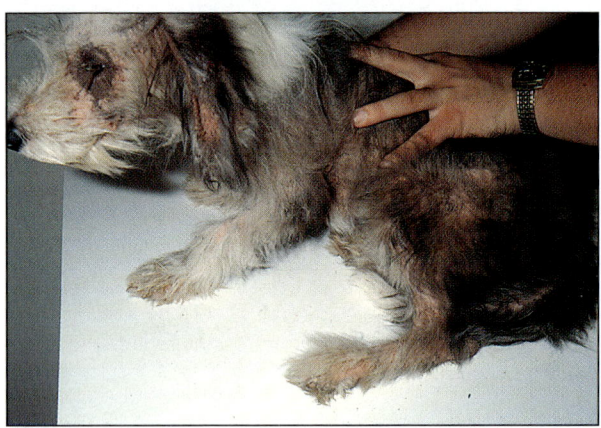

115 **Scabies.** Generalised disease in a young bearded collie illustrating the characteristic distribution of lesions.

116

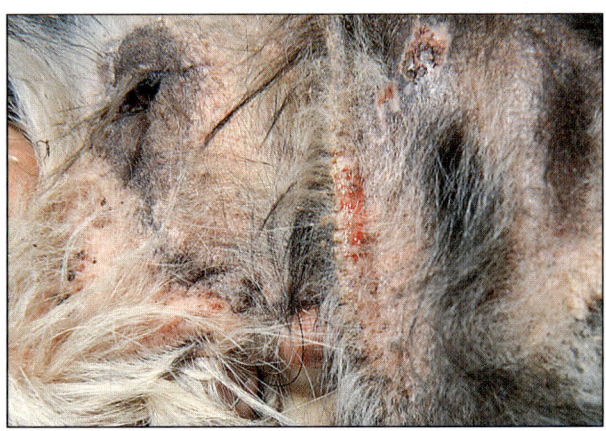

116 **Scabies.** Close up of the head of the dog depicted in **115** illustrating lesions along the edge of the pinna.

Sarcoptic mange (scabies)

Sarcoptes scabiei is a parasitic mite. The female burrows into the epidermis forming tunnels in which she lays her eggs. The presence of the mite and a hypersensitivity reaction to it causes a highly pruritic dermatitis—sarcoptic mange (scabies). Transmission is by direct contact or via fomites, such as bedding and rugs. People are often transiently infected from their animals.

Sarcoptic mange affects dogs regardless of age, sex, or breed and the disease is highly contagious. The mites will parasitise all areas of skin (**113**) but show a decided preference for certain regions. These areas, termed launch points, include the pinnae, axillae, elbows and the lateral aspect of the hock (**114–118**). Infection usually begins at these launch points and then spreads to adjacent areas on the head and ventral trunk before generalising.

The dermatitis produced by the presence of the mites is characterised by erythema, papule formation, hair loss and the formation of small, haemorrhagic crusts.[2,5] The intense pruritus leads to excoriations produced by self-inflicted trauma: secondary bacterial infection often occurs. In chronic cases the skin becomes thickened, corrugated and often hyperpigmented and

117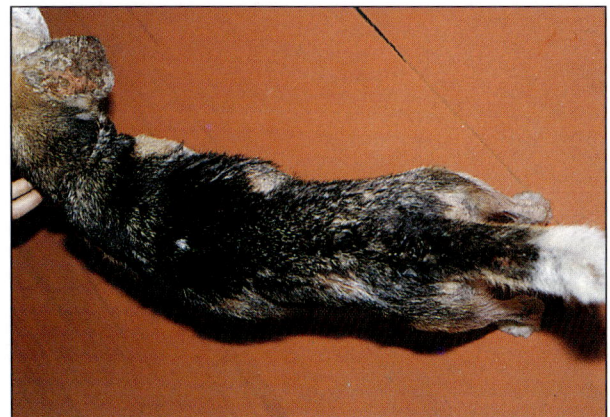

117 Scabies. Severe pruritus and extensive self trauma as a consequence of scabies in a Beagle.

118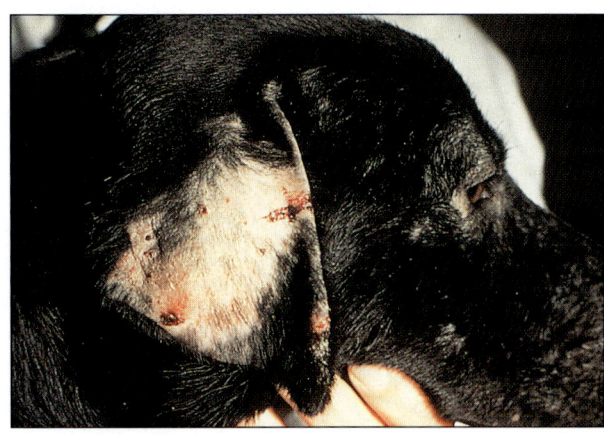

118 Scabies. Extensive lesions on the pinna of a Labrador retriever.

119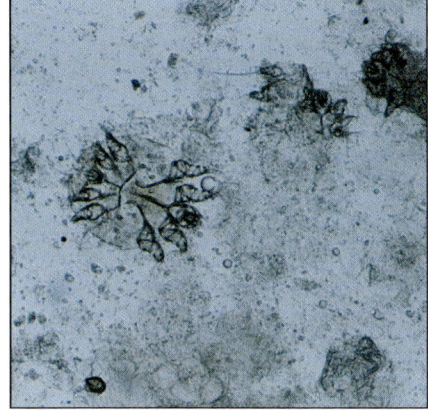

119 Scabies. Photomicrograph from a clinical case showing several mites.

120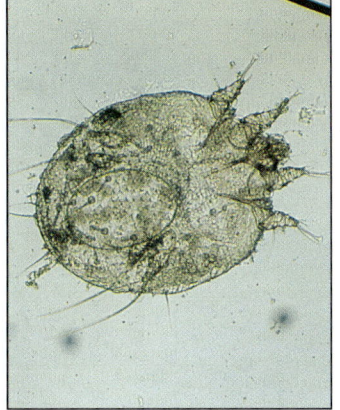

120 Scabies. Photomicrograph of an ovum-bearing female *Sarcoptes scabiei*. (Illustration courtesy K. V. Mason.)

121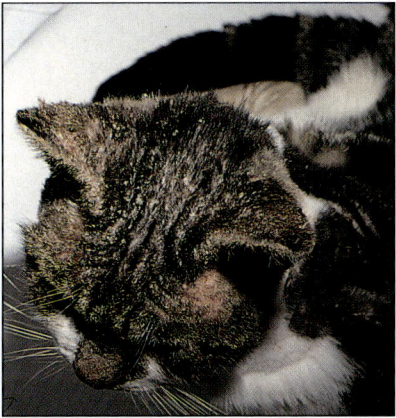

121 Feline scabies. A very rare case of sarcoptic mange in the cat. This cat was infected with Feline Immunosuppressive Virus and exhibits generalised thick crusting and minimal pruritus. (Illustration courtesy of E. A. Ferguson.)

there is often polylymphadenopathy. A mousy odour may be noted. The dog may become quite emaciated in advanced cases. Definitive diagnosis can be difficult and may require patient searching of every field of several skin scrapings (**119** and **120**). Concentration techniques may be useful (Chapter 3). The mite may be found in faecal flotations[2], a result of being ingested during grooming.

Scabies occurs in all the domestic animals but is very rare in the cat (**121**). Sarcoptic mange may cause disease in ferrets; either a generalised pruritus or, more rarely, a pododermatitis.

Scabies is characterised by:
- Intense pruritus and self trauma.
- Contagion.
- Zoonotic lesions.

Differential diagnoses include:
- Any pruritic condition.

Diagnosis is difficult but is made by:
- Demonstration of the mite or ova in skin scrapings.
- Characteristic zoonotic lesions.

122

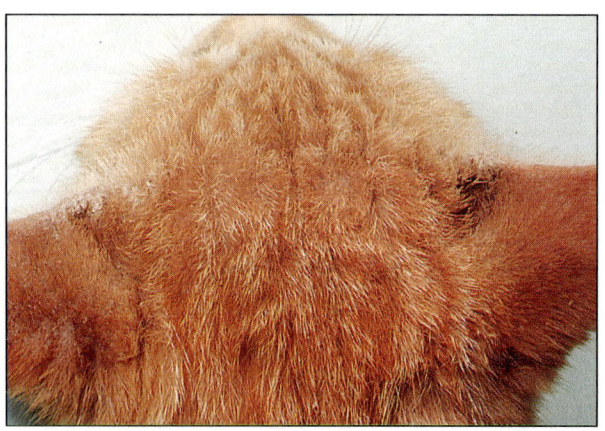

122   Notoedric mange. Early infestation showing the usual bilateral nature of the lesions at the prime predilection site, the rostral margin of the pinna.

123

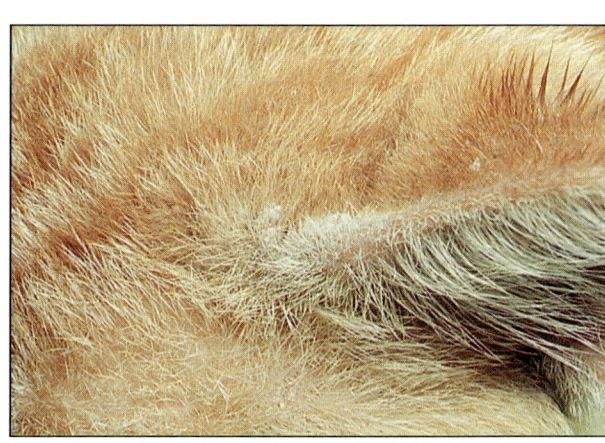

123   Notoedric mange. Close-up of the ear of the cat in **122**. Note the scale.

124

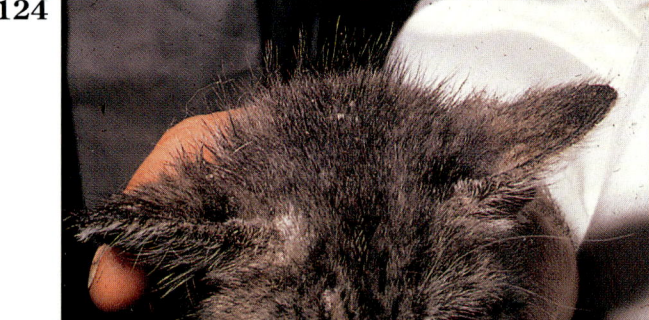

124   Notoedric mange. More advanced case with lesions apparent over the entire pinnae, the head and forehead.

125

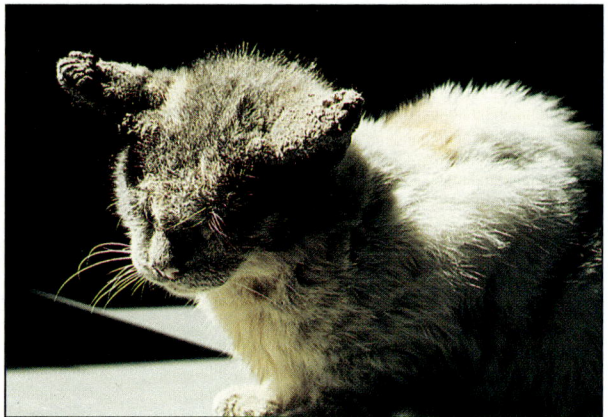

125   Notoedric mange. Severe case with extensive lesions over the entire head. Note the poor body condition of the cat. (Illustration courtesy of W. R. Kelly.)

Notoedric mange

Notoedres cati is the sarcoptid mite of the cat and is the cause of notoedric or head mange in this species. The condition is highly contagious, transmission occurring by direct contact or via fomites. Very occasionally, the infestation may be transmitted transiently to in-contact dogs and people. It is an intensely pruritic disease. The condition is now rare in temperate climates although it remains not uncommon in tropical and subtropical regions.

The female mite burrows into the epidermis between the hair follicles to lay her eggs and these burrows appear on the skin surface as the centres of minute papules. The skin becomes hairless, thickened, wrinkled and folded, and later is covered with dense, tightly adherent, grey crusts. Intense pruritus develops and the excoriations produced by scratching and rubbing often become secondarily infected.

126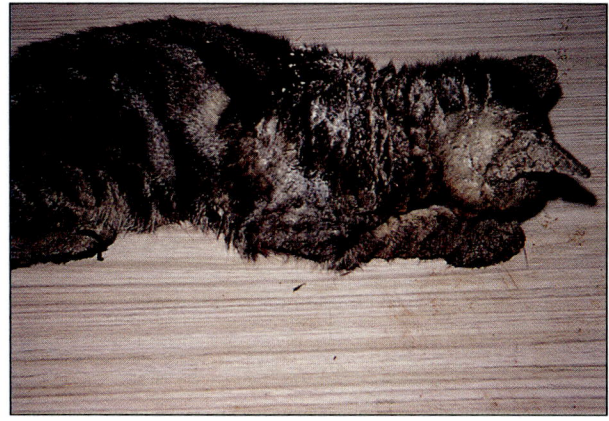

127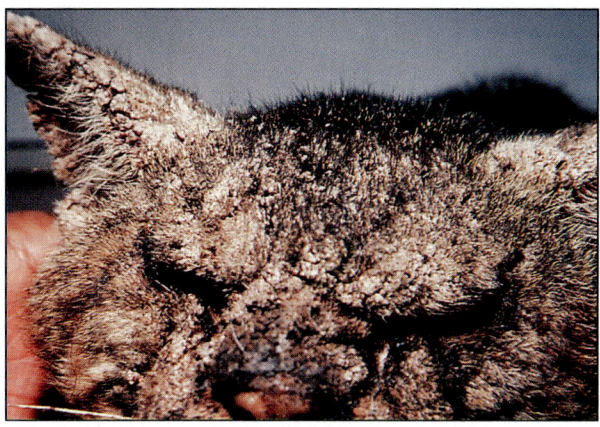

126   Notoedric mange. Rare case of generalised lesions in a moribund cat.

127   Notoedric mange. Close-up of the head of the-cat in **126**.

128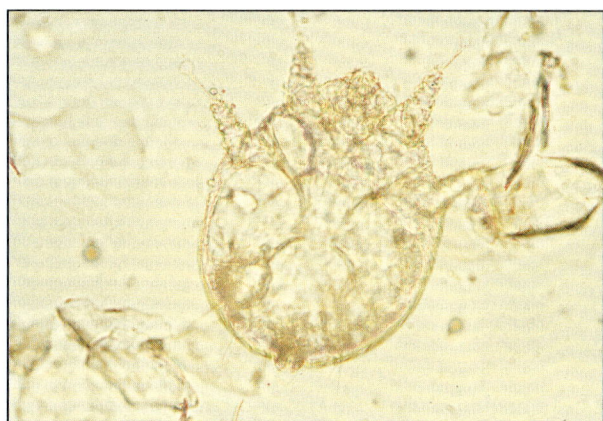

129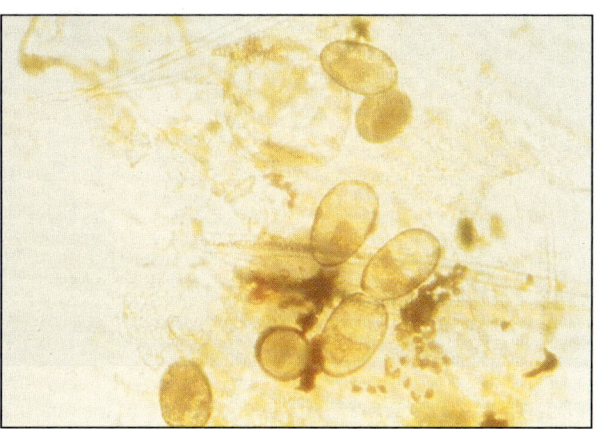

128   Notoedric mange. Photomicrograph of an adult *Notoedres cati*.

129   Notoedric mange. Photomicrograph of the scybala (the eggs and faecal pellets).

Distribution is characteristic with lesions, often bilateral, first appearing at the base of the leading edge of the pinna, then extending over the rest of the ear followed by the top of the head (**122–125**). There may also be extension to the feet and perineum, probably the result of the cat's grooming activities and its habit of sleeping in a curled up position. Very occasionally the condition may spread to involve the whole of the skin surface if the cat is debilitated or immunocompromised (**126** and **127**). In contrast to canine scabies, the mites are plentiful and usually are easy to demonstrate (**128** and **129**).

Notoedric mange is characterised by:
- Very pruritic, crusted and scaly lesions on the head and pinnae.

The differential diagnosis includes:
- Feline demodicosis.
- Food intolerance.
- Dermatophytosis.
- Fly-bite dermatitis.
- Actinic dermatitis.

The diagnosis can be made by:
- Demonstration of mites, ova and faecal pellets in skin scrapes.

130

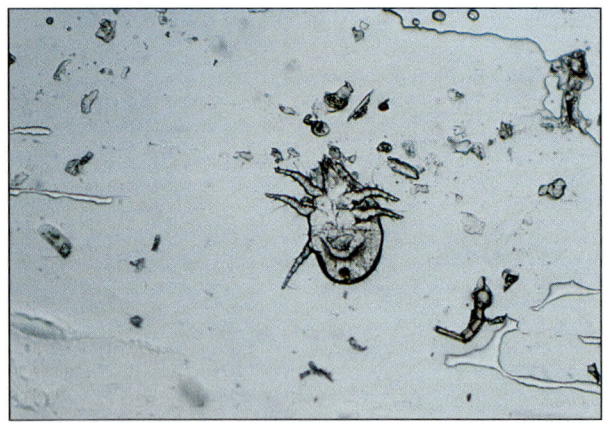

131

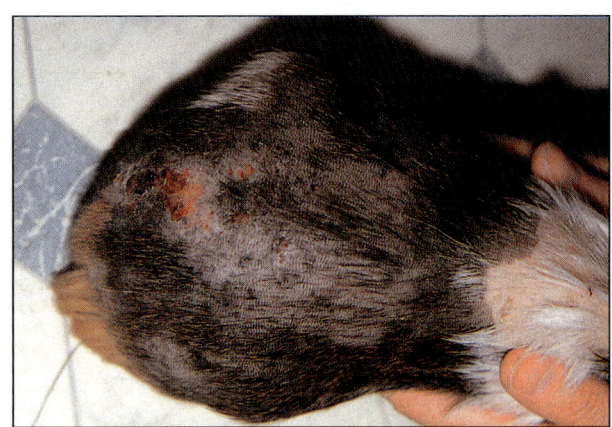

130   Trixacarid mange. Photomicrograph of *Trixacarus caviae*. A small, sarcoptic mite.

132

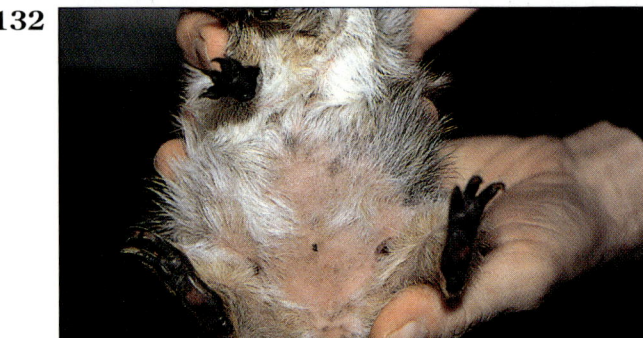

133

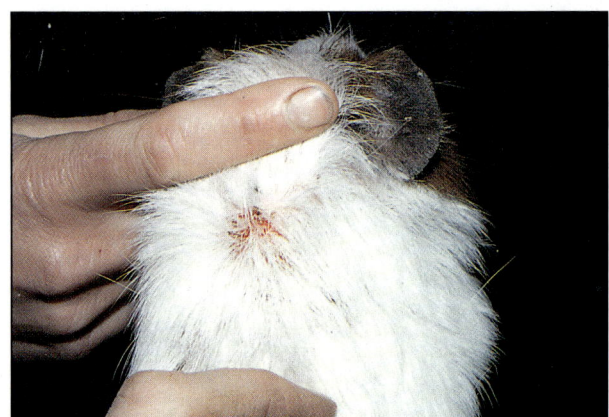

131–133   Trixacarid mange. A variety of lesions may be seen in guinea pigs with trixacarid mange: self-excoriation, crusting and alopecia (**131**), extensive ventral erythema, alopecia and crusting (**132**) and erythema in the interscapular region (**133**).

Trixacarid mange

Trixacarus caviae is a small sarcoptid parasite of guinea pigs (**130**). The disease is very common. Latent infection is a feature of trixacarid mange and disease may occur in animals months after contact with an infected individual. Trixacarid mange is often precipitated by stresses such as poor nutrition, malocclusion, bullying and poor management. The clinical signs vary but pruritus is a constant feature.[29] Animals may exhibit a highly pruritic dermatosis characterised by mild scale and minimal alopecia, a dermatosis characterised solely by severe self trauma to the dorsum or a dermatosis characterised by pruritic erythroderma (**131–133**).

Trixacarid mange is characterised by:
- Severe pruritus which may be accompanied by self trauma.

The differential diagnosis is:
- Dermatophytosis.

Diagnosis is made by:
- Demonstration of the parasite.

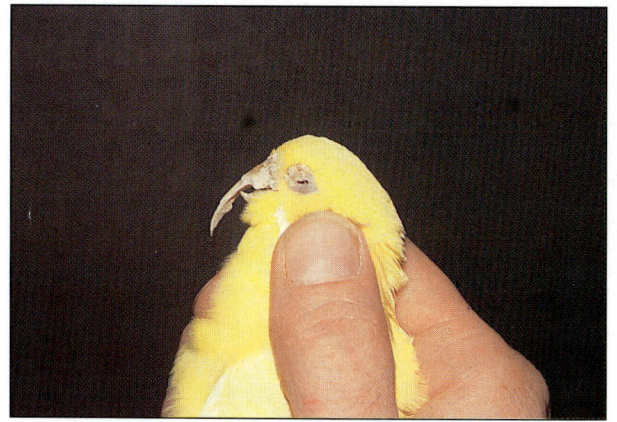

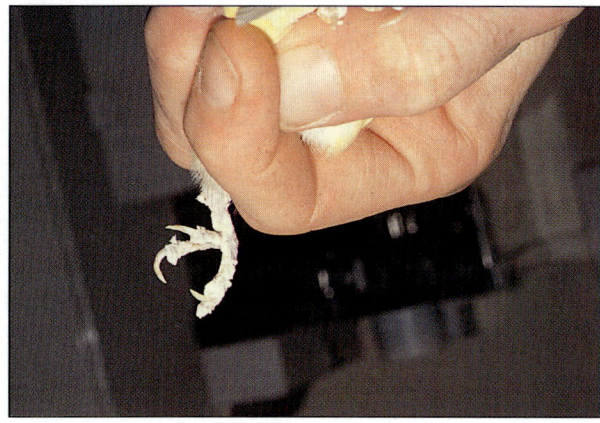

134 and 135   Cnemidocoptic mange in a budgerigar. The presence of the small sarcoptid mite *Cnemidocoptes piliae* results in hyperkeratosis of the cere and legs. The aberrant growth of the beak may be permanent.

Cnemidocoptic mange

Cere mites and depluming mites of the genus *Cnemidocoptes* are commonly the cause of disease in birds. Scaly leg and facial dermatitis are quite common in budgerigars and are caused by *C. piliae*. The latter condition may be accompanied by deformation of the beak which may be permanent (**134 and 135**). *C. laevis* (the depluming mite) is responsible for feather loss in parrots. It is found within the feather follicle. *Cnemidocoptes* spp. may also be responsible for loss of feathers in Psittacines, particularly around the head, neck and legs.

Cnemidocoptic mange in budgerigars is characterised by:
• Hyperkeratosis of the cere, legs or feet.

The differential diagnosis includes:
• Brown hypertrophy of the cere.

The diagnosis is made by:
• Demonstration of the mite in skin scrapings.

Otodectic mange

Otodectes cynotis is a surface-living mite inhabiting the external ear canals and adjacent skin of the head of dogs and cats where it feeds on epidermal debris (**136**). The lifecycle is spent entirely on the host although adult mites have a limited capacity to survive in the environment. The presence of the mite induces an accumulation of crumbly, brownish black discharge (**137**). In the dog the infection is usually accompanied by pruritus. There may not be any associated clinical signs in the adult cat although kittens are often markedly pruritic (**138 and 139**).

Immediate hypersensitivity toward the mite is thought to account for the severe pruritus that results in many cases.[28] Subsequent self-inflicted trauma may result in excoriations, especially to the dorsal surface of the pinnae and on the adjacent surfaces of the head. In dogs pyotraumatic dermatitis often occurs on adjacent areas of the head and aural haemotomas may form in both dogs and cats. There may be secondary bacterial otitis accompanying chronic otitis externa (**140** and **141**).

136

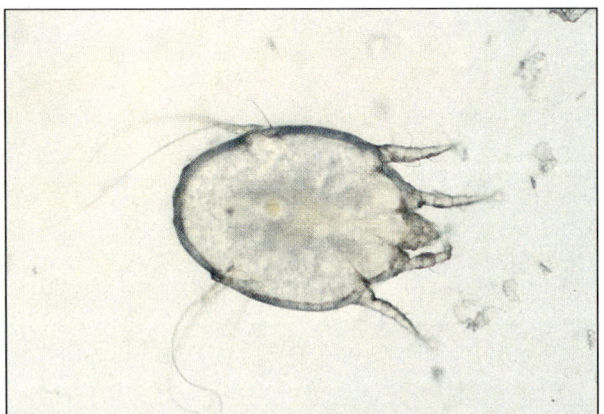

136   Otodectic mange. Photomicrograph of an adult male *Otodectes cynotis*.

137

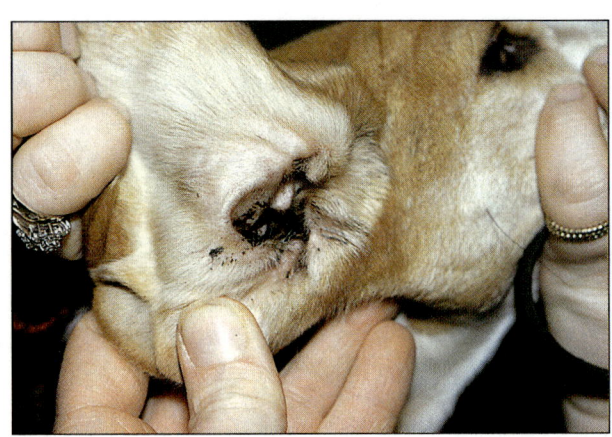

137   Otodectic mange. The presence of a black granular discharge within the external ear canal is often associated with the mite. In this pup there is, as yet, no significant inflammation.

138

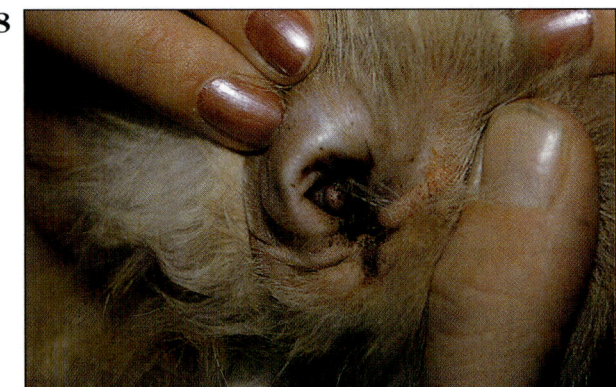

138   Otodectic mange. *Otodectes cynotis* is the major cause of otitis externa in the cat.

139

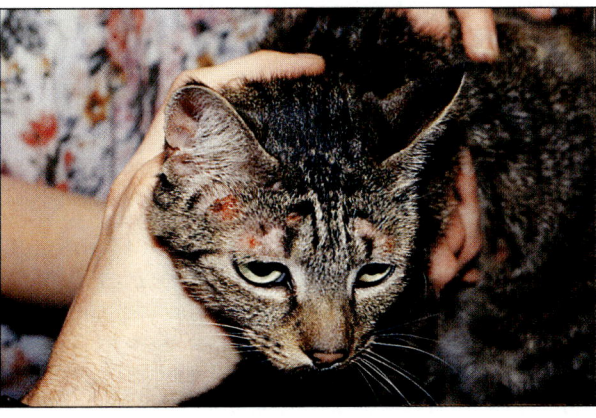

139   Otodectic mange. The presence of the mite may be a cause of facial pruritus and resultant self-excoriation.

Surprisingly, the most heavily infected animals, often adult cats, do not exhibit clinical signs. Although usually confined to the external ear canal the mite may cause a pruritic dermatitis in other sites, ectopic otodectic mange. In the cat lesions may be found around the base of the tail and sometimes on the tip of the tail, the latter probably due to transmission when the cat is curled up asleep. *Otodectes cynotis* may cause otitis externa in ferrets.

Otodectic mange is characterised by:
- Pruritus originating within the ear canal.
- Accumulation of characteristic discharge within the external ear canal.

Differential diagnoses include:
- Otitis externa due to other causes.
- Notoedric mange in cats and sarcoptic mange in dogs.
- Feline demodicosis.
- Atopy.
- Food allergy.

Diagnosis is made by
- Demonstration of mites by auroscopic examination of the external ear canals or in skin scrapings.

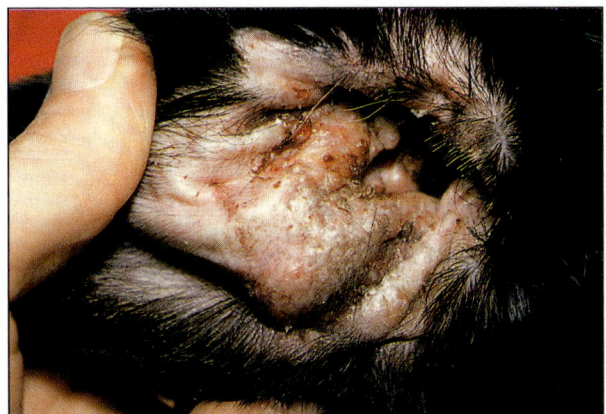

140 Otodectic mange. Mild erythema in the external ear canal of a dog.

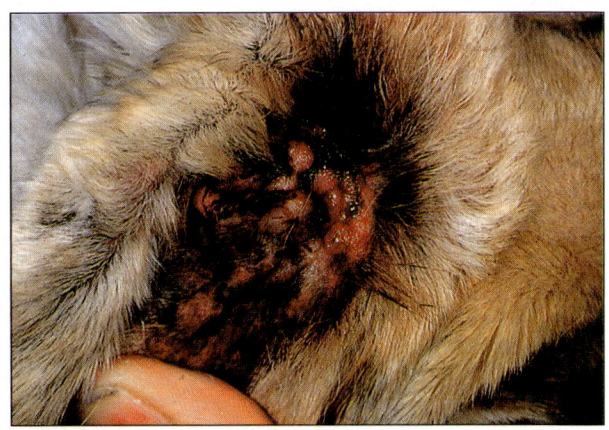

141 Otodectic mange. Chronic otitis secondary to long-standing mite infection.

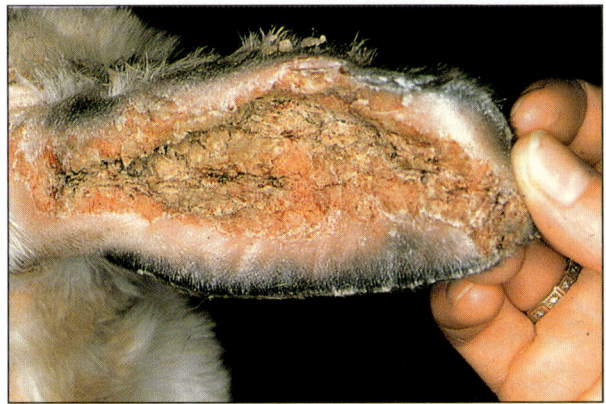

142 Psoroptic mange in rabbits may result in a massive accumulation of crust and scale in the external ear canal.

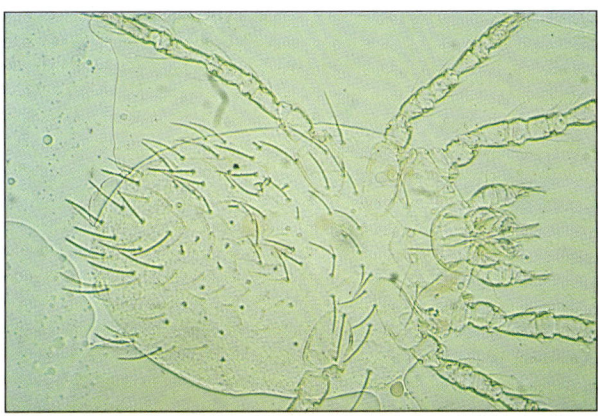

143 Trombiculidiasis. Photomicrograph of the six-legged larva.

Psoroptic mange of rabbits

Psoroptes cuniculi is an inhabitant of the external ear canal of rabbits. The clinical signs of infection are otic pruritus and discharge. Sometimes the production of scale within the external ear canal is sufficient to completely occlude the orifice (**142**).

> **Psoroptic mange is characterised by:**
> - Otitis externa and scale production.
>
> **There are few differential diagnoses.**
>
> **The condition is diagnosed by:**
> - Clinical signs and demonstration of the parasite.

Chigger, harvester or trombiculid mite infestation

A large number of different species are included in this group of mites, only the larval stages of which are parasitic (**143**). The natural hosts are rodents and other small animals. The most common species in the UK is *Neotrombicula autumnalis*; other species reported from various countries include *Leeuwenhoekia* spp., *Schongastia* spp. and *Eutrombicula alfreddugesi*. Infection occurs most commonly around harvest time, early autumn or fall, hence the name harvester mite.

The larvae climb low vegetation and attach themselves to passing animals, including people.

144

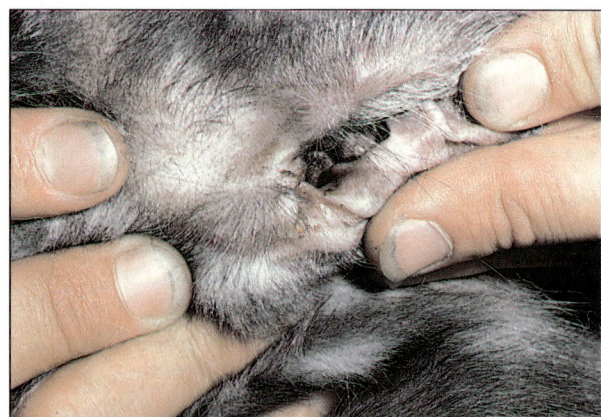

145

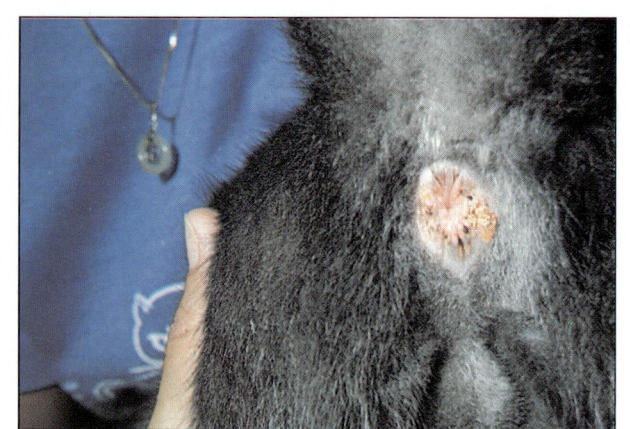

146

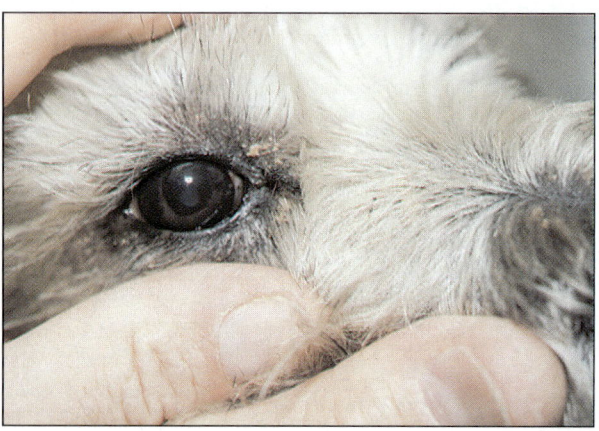

147

144–146 Trombiculidiasis. Many different species of mite are included in this group, although only the larva is parasitic. They are orange-red in colour and present as similarly-coloured spots which are composed of hundreds of larvae. Predilection sites are between the toes, within the folds at the base of the pinna (**144**), the perineum (**145**) and the medial canthi of the eyes (**146**).

147 Trombiculidiasis. Infestation is not limited to dogs and cats: infestation on a bandicoot.

In dogs and cats the larvae fix themselves to the skin by inserting their mouth parts and, in contrast to ticks, there are usually tens or hundreds of larvae in any one site. The bites causes variable pruritus with scaling and hair loss.

Predilection sites are between the toes, the inside of the pinnae, the perineum and the medial canthus of the eye (**144–146**). Repeated exposure over successive years can induce a state of hypersensitivity and thus pruritus may be intense in a number of cases. Infection is not limited to dogs and cats and may also occur in exotic animals (**147**).

Trombiculidiasis is characterised by:
- Pruritic lesions in predilection sites.

Differential diagnoses include:
- Seasonal dermatoses such as atopy.

Diagnosis can be made by:
- Observation of typical red/orange coloured larval mites.

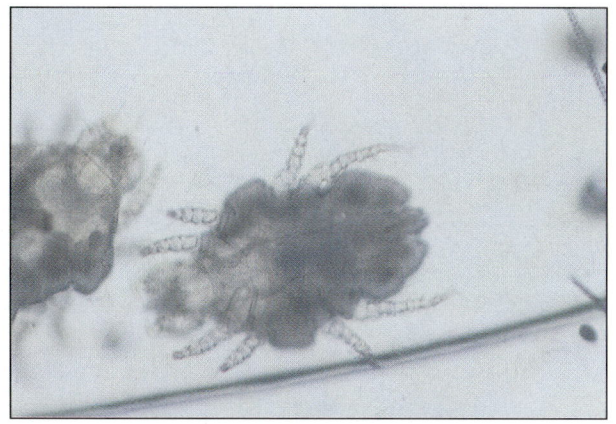

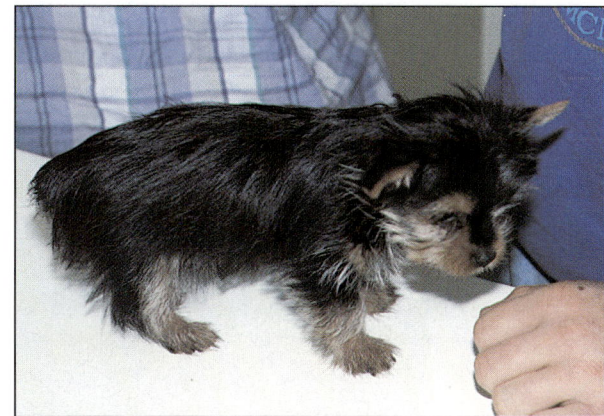

148 **Cheyletiellosis.** Photomicrograph of two adult mites.

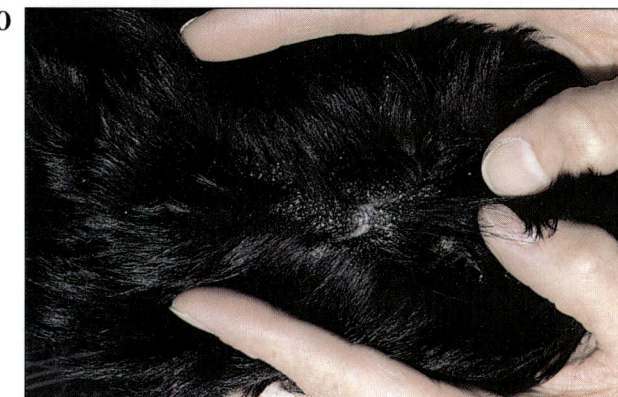

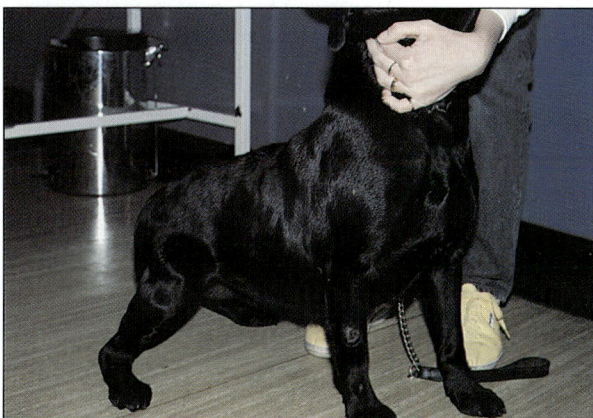

149 and 150 **Cheyletiellosis.** Typical presentation. A young dog with a mildly pruritic dermatosis associated with scale production and a close-up (**150**) illustrating the fine scale.

151 **Cheyletiellosis.** Patchy alopecia in an adult Labrador retriever as a consequence of chronic infection.

Cheyletiellosis

Cheyletiellid mites are relatively large, surface-living fur mites of dogs, cats and rabbits (**148**). Three species have been implicated, namely *Cheyletiella yasguri*, *C. blakei*, and *C. parasitivorax*. Although *C. yasguri* is thought to be confined to the dog there is some doubt as to the host specificity of the other two species. The mites can be transmitted to human contacts and zoonotic lesions occur in about 30% of cases. In both the dog and the cat, cheyletiellosis may be a difficult disease to diagnose because of the phenomenon of latency.

The diagnosis may be particularly difficult in multi-animal households because only one or two individuals may be affected at any one time and this may reduce the suspicion of a contagious dermatosis. Lesions in the dog vary (**149–151**) from dorsal scale with few associated clinical signs to moderate pruritus and patchy loss of hair.[1] In the cat the clinical signs may be even more variable with asymptomatic carriers being common, particularly in long-haired breeds (**152–154**). Clinical signs may include a papulocrustous dermatitis, mild, dry, scaling skin, severe pruritus or widespread alopecia.[22,27] In the rabbit the signs are usually confined to mild pruritus associated with large, soft white flakes of scale in the interscapular region (**155**).

152

153

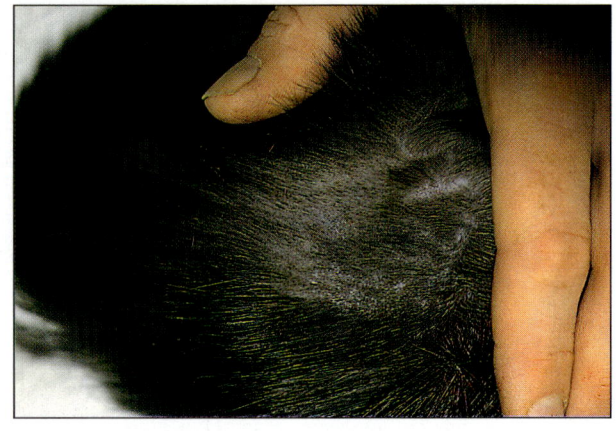

152–154   Cheyletiellosis. Infestation in a group of dogs or cats may produce a variety of clinical signs. In this colony of British long-haired cats there was focal alopecia (**152**), scale and papules (**153**) and patchy alopecia (**154**).

154

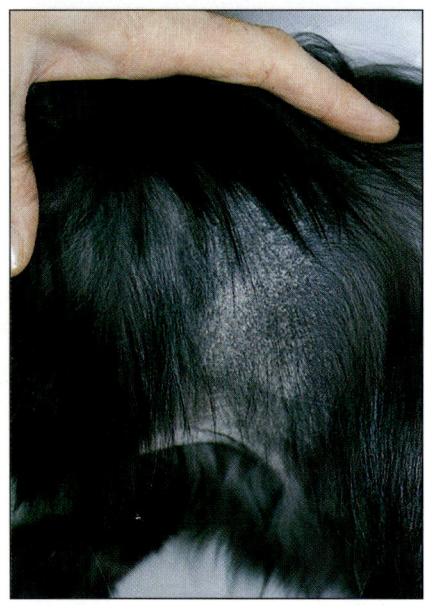

155

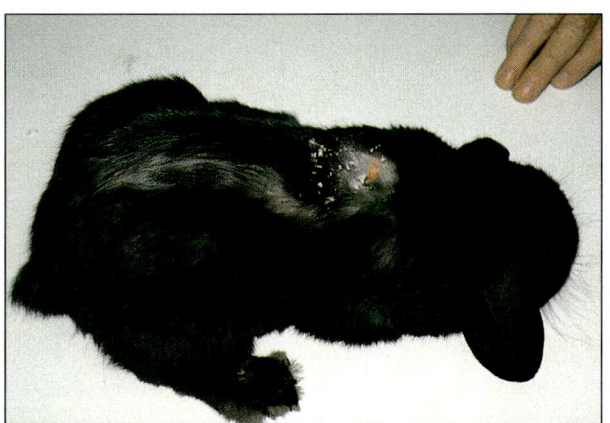

155   Cheyletiellosis. Infection in the rabbit typically presents as dorsal pruritus with large flakes of soft scale.

The mites create pseudo-tunnels in the scales and debris on the skin surface along which they move quite actively. This activity imparts a movement to the debris which has given rise to the term 'living or walking dandruff' to describe the condition. The entire lifecycle is spent on the host although the mites may survive off the host for a number of weeks if conditions are favourable. The ova, which unlike those of lice are non-operculate, are attached to the hair shafts by fine threads. Larvae hatching from the ova pass through two nymphal stages to become adults. Transmission is by close contact.

Cheyletiellosis is characterised by:
- Variable pruritus with scale formation in some instances.
- Zoonotic lesions.

Differential diagnoses include:
- Pediculosis.
- Seborrhoeic disorders.
- Dermatophytosis.

Diagnosis can be made by:
- Demonstration of the mites in skin scrapings or tape strip preparations.

156

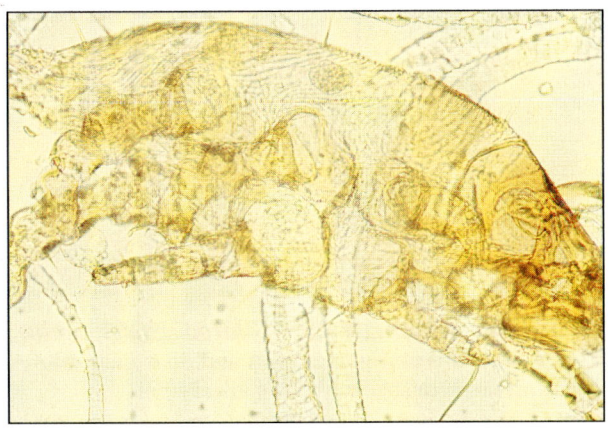

157

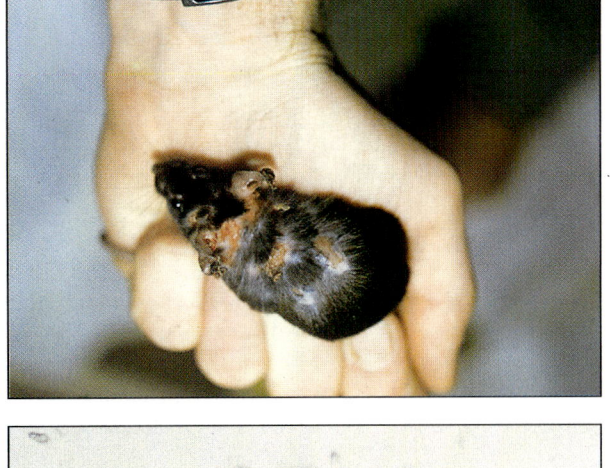

158

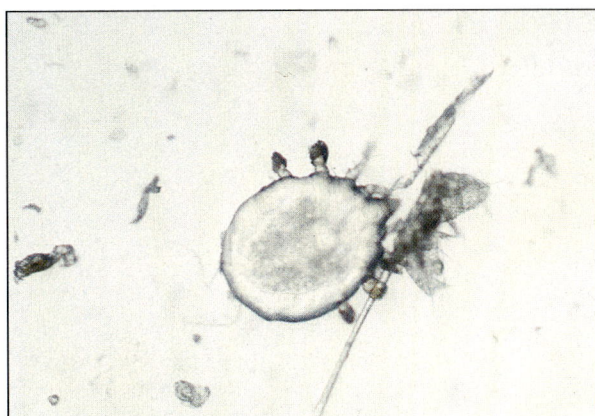

156 *Lynxacarus radovskyi* **infestation.** Skin scrapings showing an adult mite.

Lynxacarus radovskyi infestation

Lynxacarus radovskyi, the cat fur mite, has been reported to infest cats in Hawaii, Fiji, Australia and Florida. The mite clings to the outer third of the hair shaft imparting a 'pepper and salt' appearance to the ragged, unkempt-looking coat. Many infestations are subclinical but there may be a mild pruritus and some cats show widespread papulocrustous rashes. The predilection site is on the top line of the body but the mites may be found anywhere. The mite has an unusual elongated shape, somewhat reminiscent of a turtle when viewed in profile, with two flap-like sternal extensions which it uses in combination with the first pair of legs to grasp the hair shaft (**156**). The fur mite of the rabbit *Lystrophorus gibbus* is very similar both in shape and in habit (see **160** and **161**).

Lynxacarus radovskyi infection is characterised by:
- The presence of the characteristic mite.

Differential diagnoses include:
- Pediculosis.
- Cheyletiellosis.

Diagnosis can be made by:
- Demonstration of the characteristic mites.

157 and 158 *Myobia musculi* **and** *Myocoptes musculinus* are the principal ectoparasites of mice. Mouse mites can cause intense pruritus which results in severe self-excoriation, particularly on the neck and interscapular region. Photomicrograph (**158**) of *Myobia musculi* found on the mouse.

Fur mites of small mammals

These ectoparasites are a common cause of dermatological disease in mice and rats where infestation may be associated with severe pruritus and self trauma, particularly in mice. *Myobia musculi*, *Myocoptes musculinus* and *Radfordia affinis* are found on mice (**157** and **158**). *Myobia musculini* typically causes a pruritic dermatitis associated with crusts and ulcerations on the head, neck and dorsum.[30] Mixed infections are common and in these situations *Mycoptes musculinus* will be found in the groin and perineum whilst the other two will be on the dorsum and head. *Radfordia ensifera* causes a pruritic dermatitis on the dorsum of rats.

159

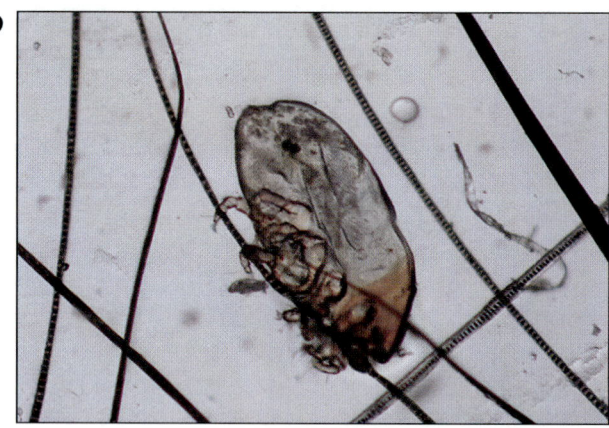

159 **Photomicrograph of** *Chirodiscoides caviae.* This is a fur mite of guinea pigs and, like *Lystrophorus gibbus*, is rarely associated with clinical signs.

160

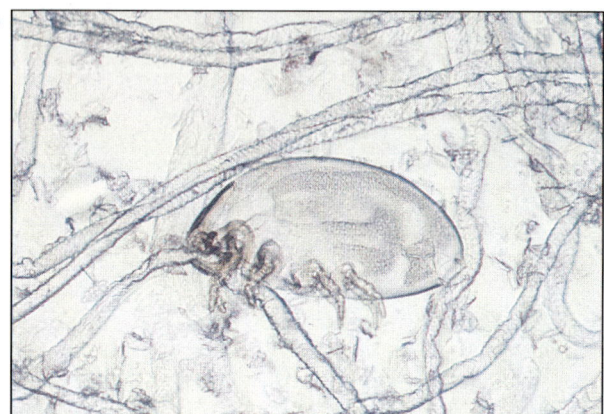

161

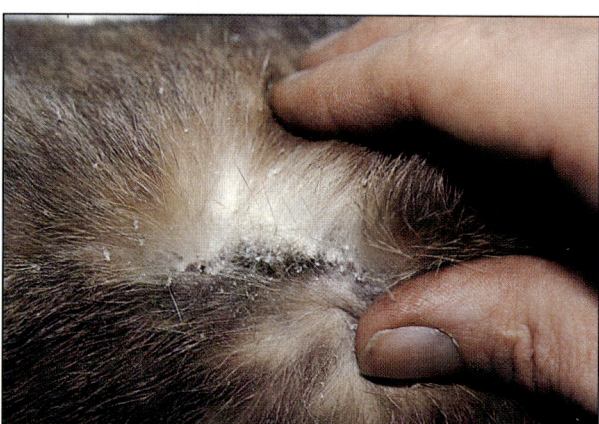

160 and 161 *Lystrophorus gibbus* **infestation** is often an incidental finding since clinical signs are rarely apparent. The mites cluster on the hair shafts (**161**).

Chirodiscoides caviae (**159**) is frequently found on guinea pigs as an incidental finding.[20] The mites cling to the lower portions of the hair shaft. *Lystrophorus gibbus* of rabbits is similarly an incidental finding in most instances (**160 and 161**). The mites of mice and rats are very mobile and this compounds the obvious technical difficulties of performing skin scrapings on the head and neck of a mouse. These infestations are best diagnosed by tape stripping or direct examination with illuminated magnification.

Fur mite infestations are characterised by:
- Pruritus and self trauma in mice and rats.
- Few clinical signs in guinea pigs and rabbits.

The differential diagnoses are few in these species.

The diagnoses are made by:
- Demonstration of the mites or their eggs on skin scrapings or tape strips or by direct examination.

162
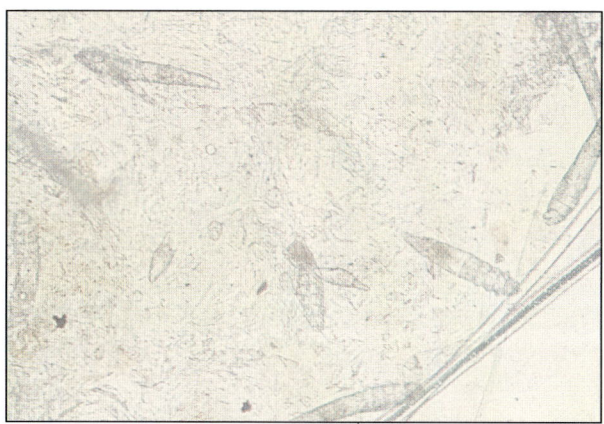

163
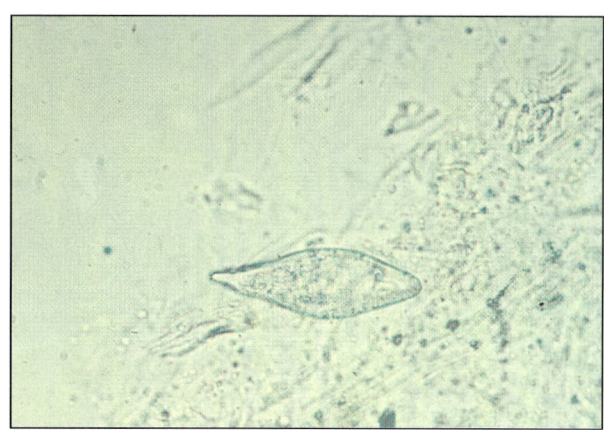

162   Demodicosis. Photomicrograph illustrating several adult *Demodex canis* mites, a nymph and two ova.

163–165   Photomicrographs of the various stages of the lifecycle of *Demodex canis:* spindle-shaped ovum (**163**), larva bearing three pairs of rudimentary legs (**164**) and nymph bearing four pairs of rudimentary legs (**165**).

164
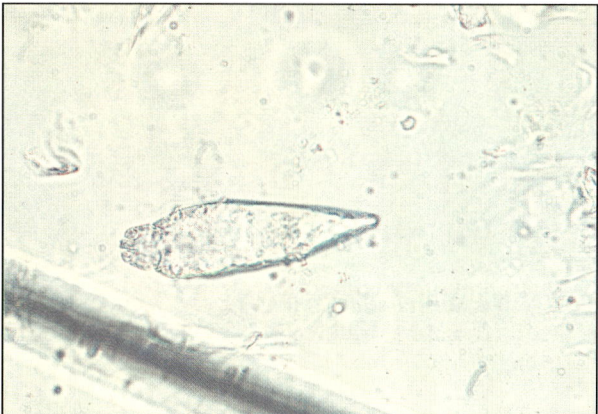

165
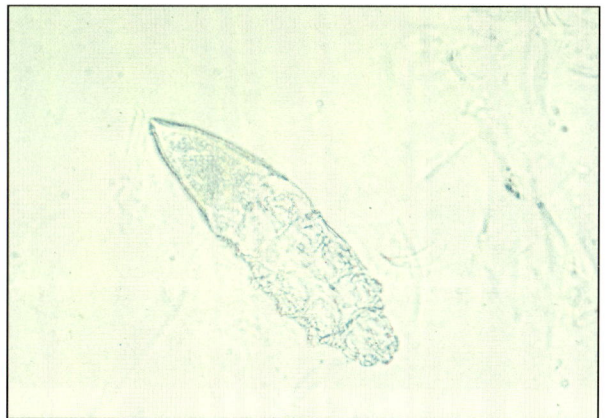

Demodicosis

Canine demodicosis

The mite *Demodex canis* (**162–165**) can be found in the hair follicles of most dogs where it feeds on sebum and the contents of the epithelial cells of the hair follicle. It is regarded as part of the normal skin fauna. Transmission of the mites is thought to occur within the immediate post-natal period during episodes of close contact, such as suckling.[13] This probably accounts for the fact that the predilection sites for the localised form of the disease are around the eyes and muzzle.

The presence of increasing numbers of mites causes damage to, and loosening of, the hair shaft with eventual loss of the hair from the follicle. This results in the classic lesions of localised demodicosis, an area of mild erythema associated with loss of hair. Whilst localised demodicosis is particularly seen in short-haired breeds of dog it may be that these minimally-pruritic lesions are not apparent in long-haired animals. In severe infestations the mites so crowd and distend the hair follicle that it ruptures, liberating mites, sebum, cellular debris and bacteria into the surrounding dermis. Here they induce a foreign body type reaction which, in the presence of staphylococci, results in the formation of an inflamed pustular lesion, abscessation, furunculosis and fistula formation.

Demodicosis is more common in tropical and subtropical regions where it tends to take a more aggressive course. Another feature of demodicosis in tropical and subtropical areas of the world is

166

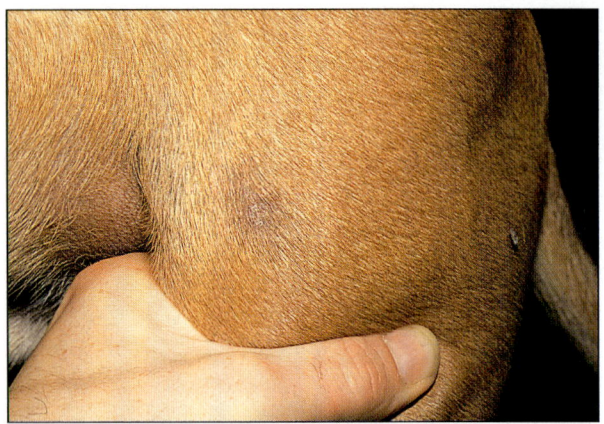

166 Demodicosis. Localised demodicosis on the leg of a Staffordshire Bull terrier pup. Note the loss of hair and the minimal inflammation.

167

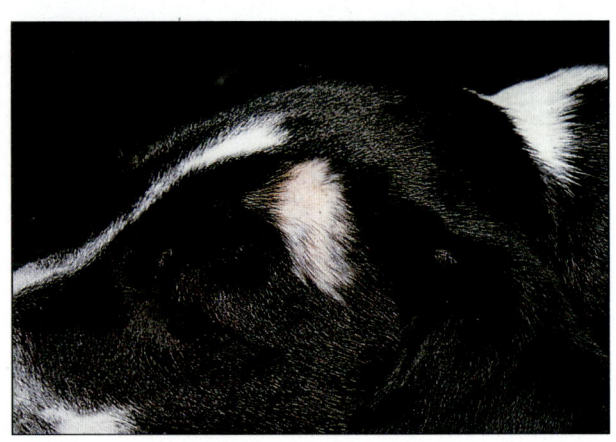

167 Demodicosis. Localised demodicosis on the head of a Border collie showing more obvious alopecia but, again, no inflammation.

168

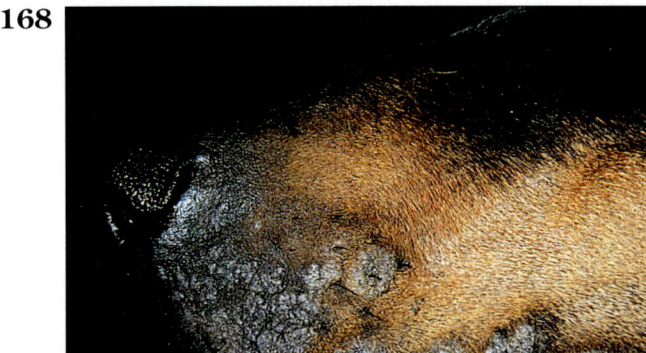

168 Demodicosis. Lesions of erythema, alopecia and scale associated with more severe localised demodicosis on the muzzle of a Doberman pinscher.

that it occurs with equal frequency in both long- and short-haired dogs. Demodicosis occurs almost exclusively in dogs less than 12 months of age. Infection which arises in adult animals is typically due to immunoincompetence, often iatrogenic. Most cases of canine demodicosis are classified into two forms, localised and generalised.

Localised demodicosis is the commonest form of the disease, often occurring as the dog is approaching puberty. It may be that changes in the cutaneous environment at this time render it more favourable to the mite. One or more patches of skin develop mild erythema and partial alopecia (**166–168**). The lesions are non-pruritic and affected areas may be covered with fine silvery scales.[18,19] Predilection sites are around the eyes and the muzzle and on the forelegs although lesions may be found on the trunk and on the rear

legs in some instances. Most cases of localised demodicosis will resolve spontaneously, presumably because of an immune response by the host. It has been postulated that the generalised disease occurs due to an hereditary, specific T-cell defect on the part of the host which allows mite populations to multiply. The follicular damage is frequently accompanied by a severe pyoderma and immunosuppressive products associated with the latter allow the disease to progress.

Generalised demodicosis is one of the most severe canine skin diseases and a very guarded prognosis should always be given. The disease commences either *de novo* or as an extension of localised demodicosis which generalises as numerous discrete lesions enlarge and coalesce to form plaque-like areas (**169–176**). Sometimes the condition does not become secondarily infect-

169

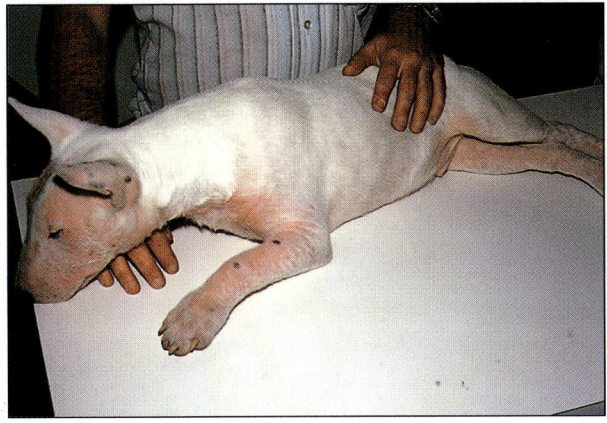

170

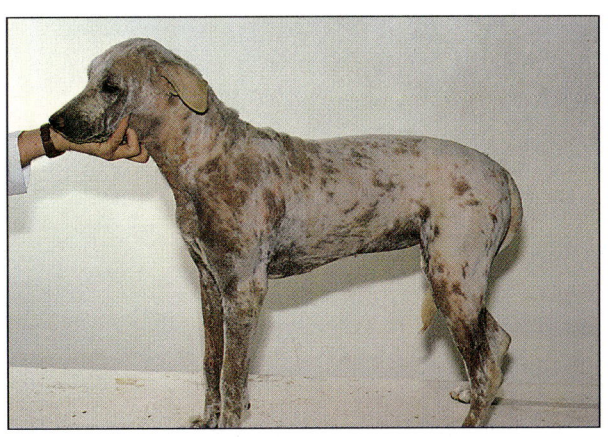

169   Demodicosis. Generalised demodicosis in a young Bull terrier. There are large patches of intense erythema and alopecia. The colloquial name is 'red mange'.

170   Demodicosis. Generalised demodicosis in a Labrador retriever bitch which has been clipped to illustrate the extent of the lesions.

171

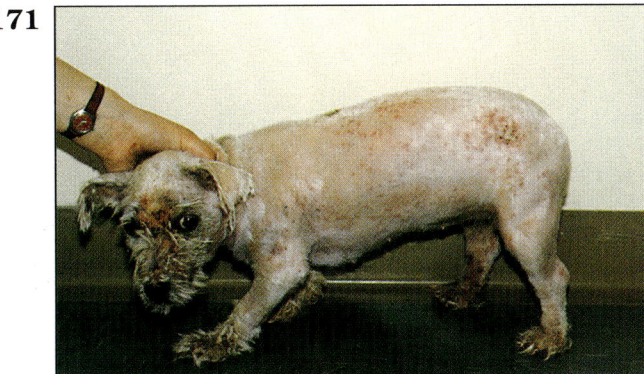

172

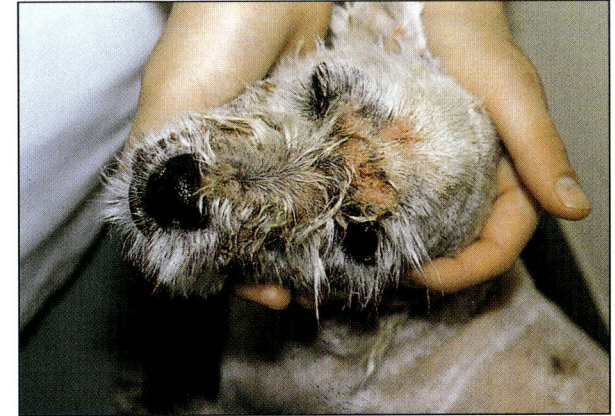

171 and 172   Demodicosis. Generalised demodicosis in a West Highland White terrier.

173

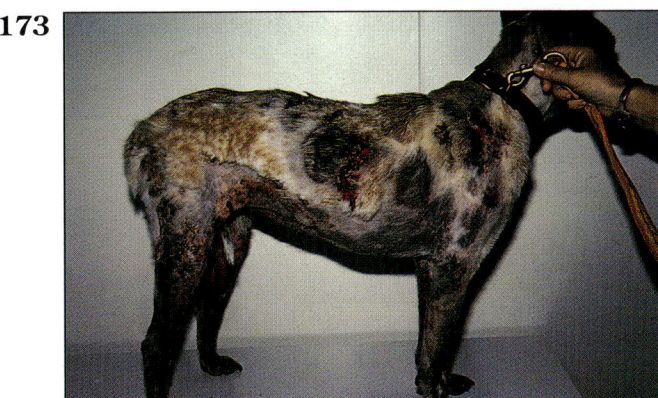

174

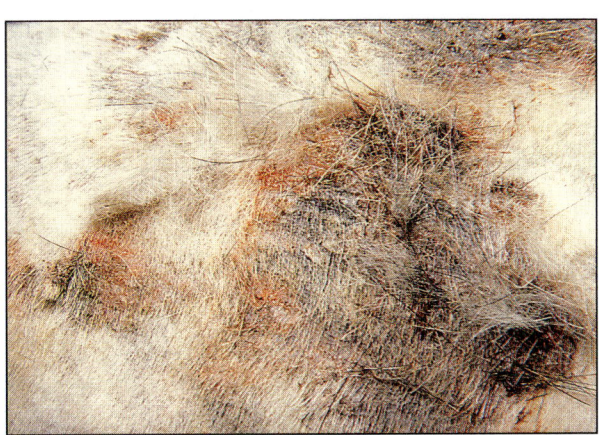

173   Demodicosis. Generalised demodicosis in an Australian kelpie which has been clipped.

174   Demodicosis. Typical plaque-like lesion showing hyperpigmentation, crusting, an erythematous margin and discharging fistulas.

175

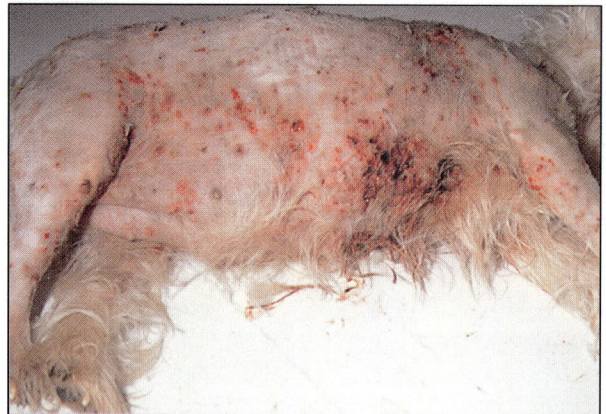

175   Demodicosis. Generalised demodicosis in a West Highland White terrier.

176

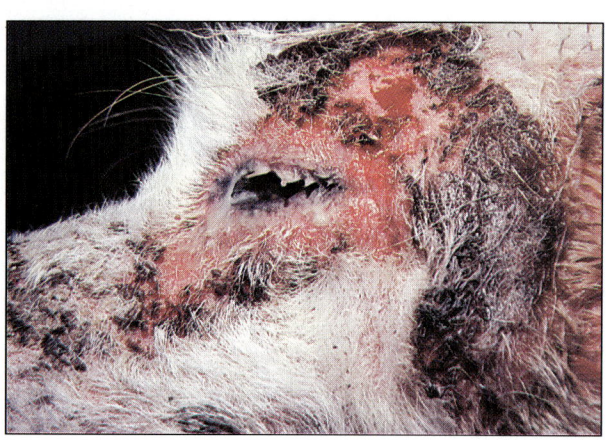

176   Demodicosis. Severe lesions on the face of a samoyed accompanying generalised demodicosis.

177

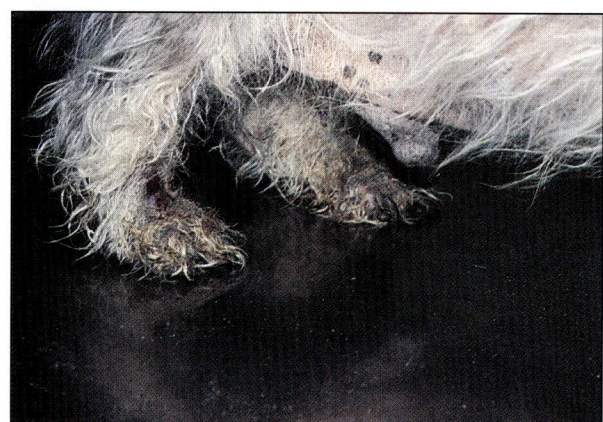

177   Pododemodicosis. Hyperpigmentation and crusting accompany this case of generalised demodicosis in which pedal lesions are very severe.

ed and remains as the squamous form of the condition. More commonly, infection, initially with *Staphylococcus intermedius,* and then later with Gram-negative organisms such as *Pseudomonas* spp., *Proteus* spp. and *Escherichia coli* occurs, producing either a pustular form or a deep pyoderma with draining tracts. The condition becomes chronic with crusted, pyogenic and haemorrhagic lesions over most of the body.[18,19] Animals are at risk from bacteraemia and polylymphadenopathy, pyrexia and weight loss are common findings.

Pedal lesions may be particularly severe and occasionally pododemodicosis in isolation may be encountered. Pododemodicosis, alone or as part of a more generalised condition (**177**) is particularly difficult to manage and many cases will remain in remission only with regular therapy and high doses of systemic antibacterial agents. Otodemodicosis has been described but appears to be rare.

Demodicosis is characterised by:
- Occurrence in young dogs.
- Focal non-pruritic patches of alopecia with scaling.
- Wide-spread plaque-like areas of pustules, furunculosis and deep pyoderma in the generalised form.

Differential diagnoses include
- Superficial pyoderma.
- Dermatophytosis.
- Deep pyoderma.
- Deep mycotic infections and atypical mycobacterial infections.

Diagnosis is made by
- Identification of the characteristic mite in skin scrapings or biopsy specimens.

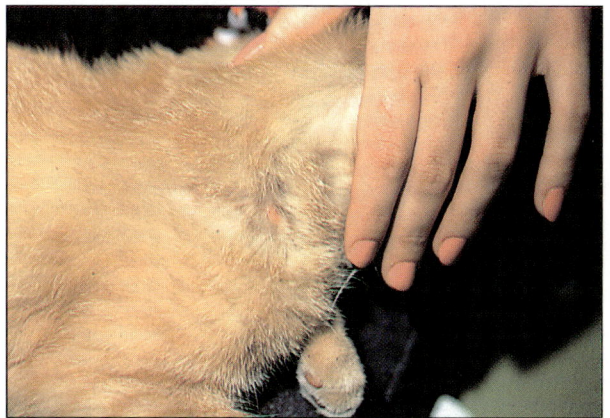

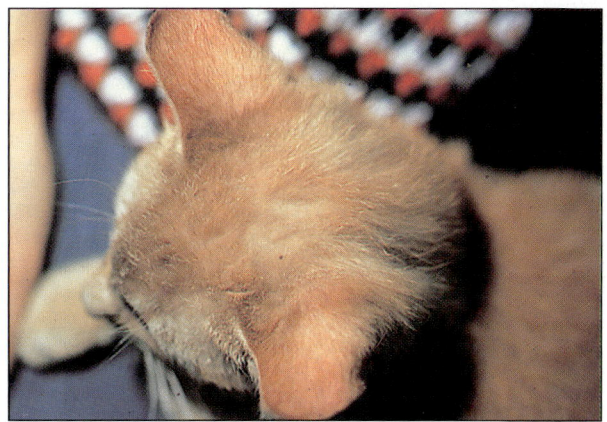

178 and 179   Feline demodicosis. Lesions on the head and neck due to *Demodex cati.*

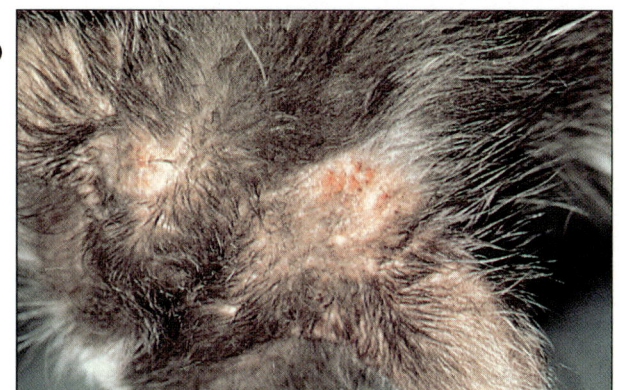

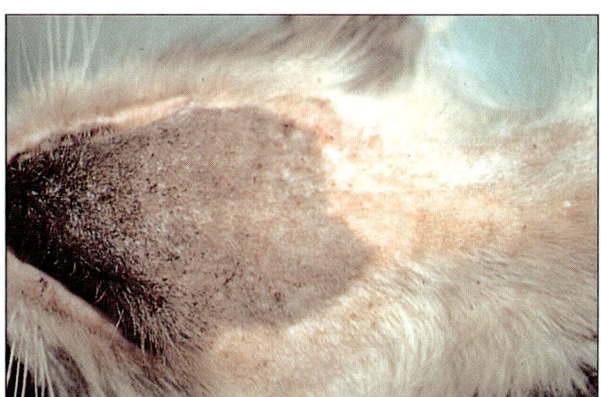

180 and 181   Feline demodicosis. More severe lesions in a cat with diabetes mellitus.

Feline demodicosis

Feline demodicosis is due to infestation with the mite *Demodex cati* or an as yet unnamed short species.[7,23] Disease due to the former species is an uncommon condition, but usually presents as a non-pruritic, hairless and slightly scaly lesion that is confined to the head, particularly around the eyes (**178** and **179**). Very rarely a generalised form occurs, especially in immunocompromised cats (**180** and **181**), but the severe, systemic disease which may be seen in the dog does not occur in the cat. Histological studies show that the mites are present in the hair follicles as in canine demodicosis.

Occasionally *D. cati* has been found in a cheesy exudate in cases of external otitis in cats. *D. cati* is morphologically similar to *D. canis* (**182** and **183**) although more slender with an elongated shape. The unnamed demodecid mite has been reported in association with the feline disease (**184** and **185**). This mite differs from *D.cati* in that it has a very short, stubby abdomen (**186**) and is found in the epidermal crypts rather than the hair follicles. A consequence of this change of habitat is that the presence of the mite evokes severe pruritus with consequent self-inflicted trauma to the skin. Infestation is again confined to the skin of the head in most cases although widespread, even symmetrical, alopecia may be found.

182

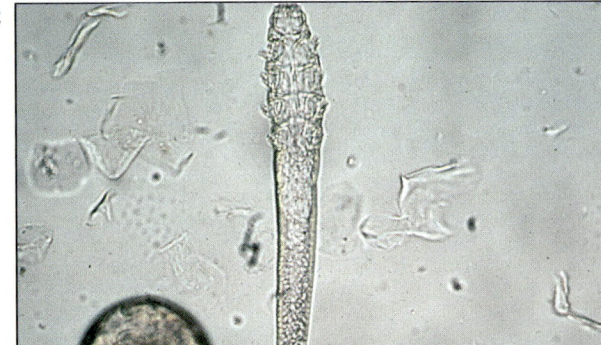

183

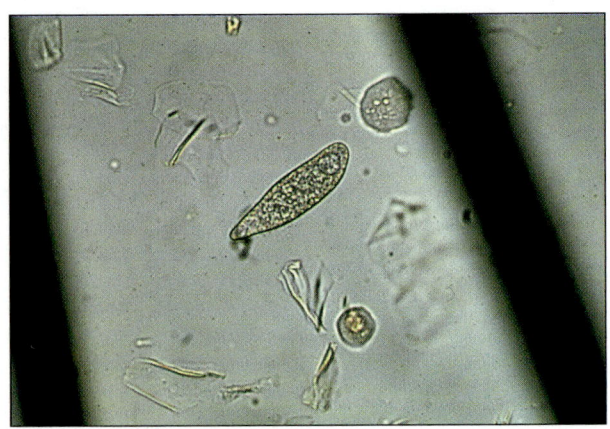

182 and 183   Feline demodicosis. Photomicrographs illustrating *Demodex cati* and its ovum. Note the long slender abdomen. (Illustrations from Scott, D. W. [1980]. Feline Dermatology 1900–1978: A monograph. *Journal of the American Animal Hospital Association*, **16**: 331–459.)

184

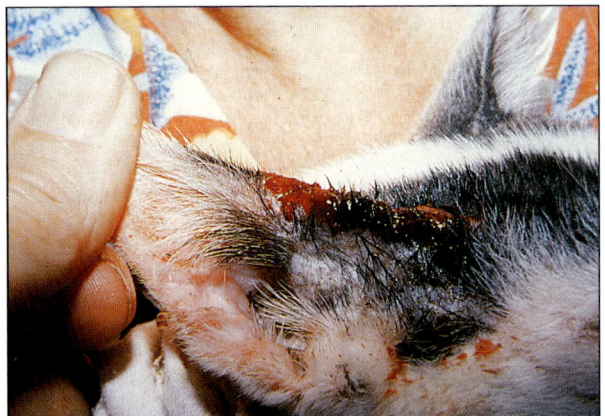

185

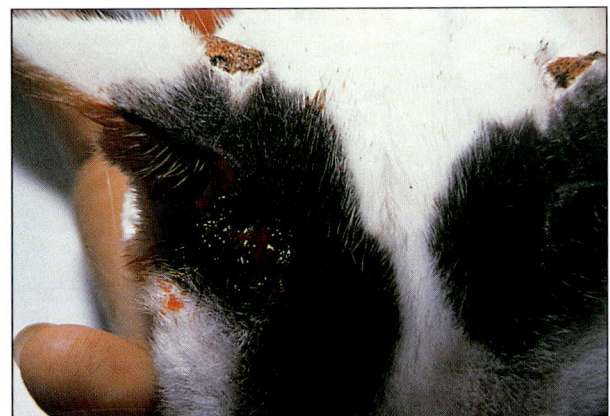

184 and 185   Feline demodicosis. Very pruritic bilateral lesions on the ears of a cat associated with the second, unnamed feline demodecid mite.

186

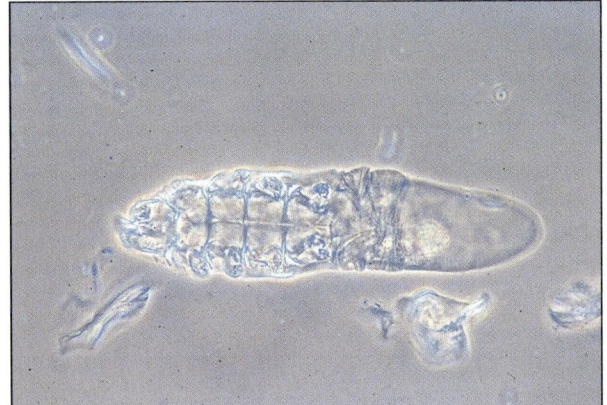

186   Feline demodicosis. Photomicrograph of the shorter feline demodicid mite. Note the short, broad, abdomen of this species and compare it with *D. cati* in **182**. This mite inhabits the epidermal crypts whereas *D. cati* inhabits the hair follicle. (Illustration courtesy of C. J. Chesney.)

Feline demodicosis is characterised by:
- Uncommon occurrence.
- Non-pruritic alopecic lesions mainly on head.
- Widespread multifocal or symmetrical alopecia.

Differential diagnoses include:
- Dermatophytosis.
- Food allergy.

Diagnosis can be made by:
- Demonstration of the mite in skin scrapings.

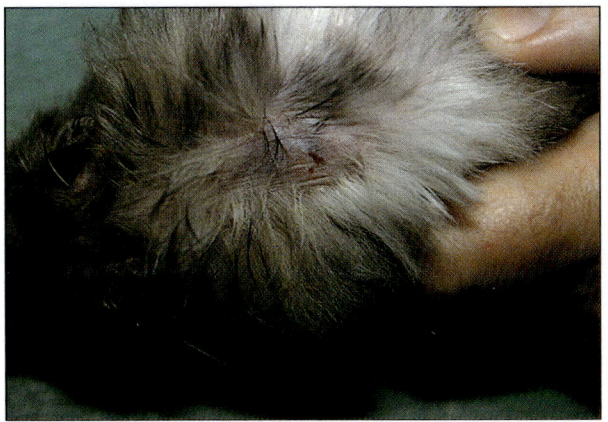

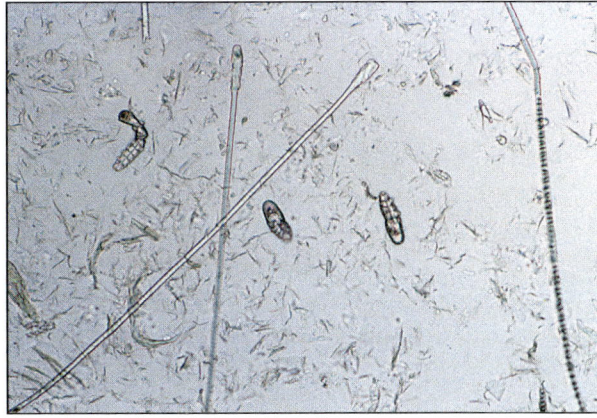

187 and 188   Patchy alopecia in hamsters due to demodicosis is usually non-pruritic. Two species are associated with the demodicosis in hamsters (**188**): *D. criceti* (a short form of the mite) and *D. aurati* (the elongated, typical demodecid mite).

Demodicosis in other species

Demodecid mites are commonly found on hamsters and gerbils and occasionally on rabbits. The hamster is host to two species; an elongated follicular inhabitant *D. aurati* and a short, broad mite *D. criceti*. Mixed infections are common (**187** to **188**). The disease is usually non-pruritic and is associated with a scaly alopecia.[10] Most cases arise as a result of intercurrent diseases or external stressors such as malocclusion or poor management. *D. meriones* of the Mongolian gerbil may be associated with a mildly pruritic alopecia. *D. cuniculi* is usually an incidental finding on rabbits.[17]

Demodicosis in small mammals is characterised by:
- Non-pruritic alopecia and scale formation.

Differential diagnoses
- Mycosis fungoides in elderly hamsters has a similar appearance but animals are pruritic.

Diagnosis of demodicosis in these species is the same as in the dog or cat
- Demonstration of the mite in skin scrapings.

Miscellaneous mite infestations

Infection with the red poultry mite *Dermanyssus gallinae* has been reported but is a very rare occurrence. Infection occurs when domestic pets enter infected chicken houses. Signs of pruritus and mild self trauma are to be expected. *Ophionyssus natricis,* the snake mite, is related to *D. gallinae*. It is a voracious blood sucker and may be a vector of *Aeromonas hydrophilia*. It is relatively common on captive reptiles, particularly snakes. It is usually found between the scales[8], often within the orbit.

Facial dermatitis due to *Pneumonyssoides caninum* has been reported.[24] The mite is a normal inhabitant of the nasal passages and sinuses.

Recurrent infestation of a cat with a free-living prostigmatic mite *Cheyletus eruditus* was noted. The presence of very large numbers of extremely mobile mites was not associated with clinical signs of discomfort.[21]

Forage mite infestation with *Acarus siro, Glycophagus domesticus*, and *Tyrophagus putrescentiae* has been recorded as a rare cause of diarrhoea in dogs which have eaten heavily infested foodstuffs.[12] However, these mites, and house dust mites such as *Dermatophagoides farinae,* are much more significant as sources of allergenic challenge to atopic dogs than as potential causes of papular dermatitis due to direct contact with the skin.

189

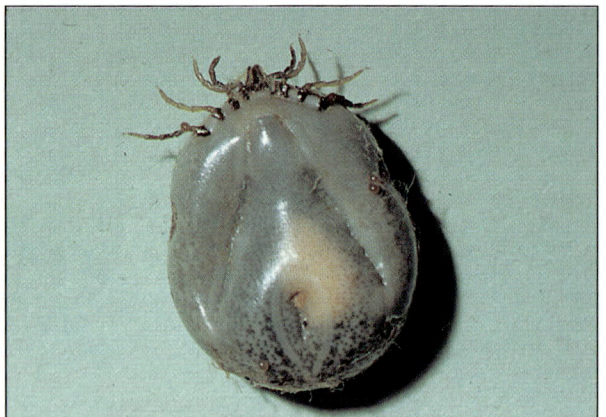

189   Tick infection. An adult *Ixodes holocyclus*.

190

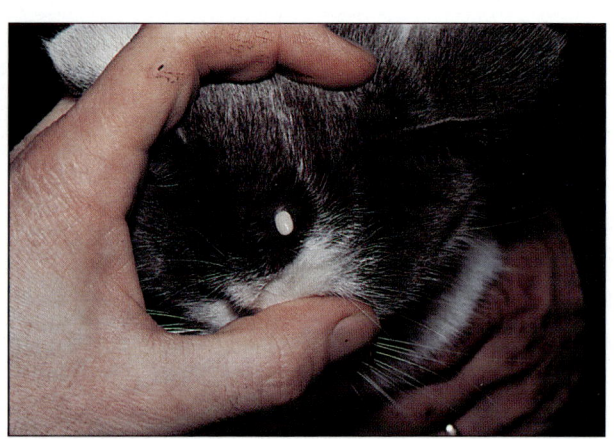

190   Tick infection. An ixodic tick on the head of a cat. This is the typical presentation with no apparent pruritus and no associated clinical signs.

191

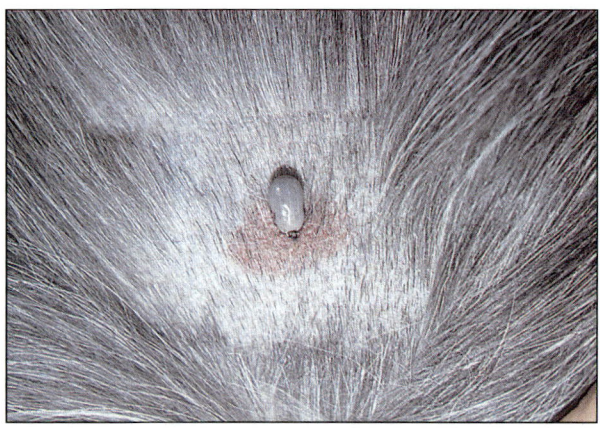

191   Tick infestation. Although non-pruritic, there is an erythematous halo around the ixodic tick on this cat.

192

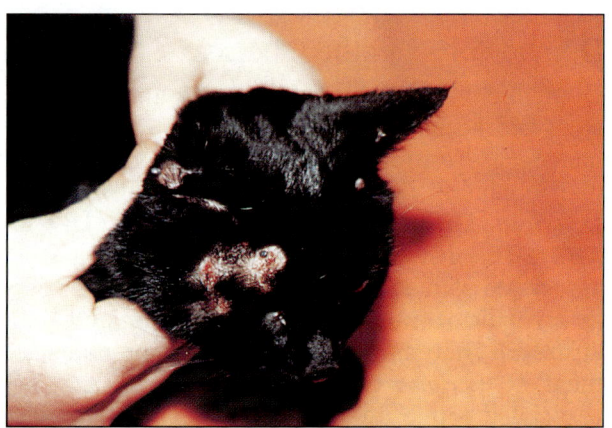

192   Tick infestation. Facial trauma secondary to presence of ticks on a cat's head. (Illustration courtesy D. C. Mactaggart.)

Tick infestation

Many different species of ticks may infest dogs and cats as the parasites are not host specific. The presence of a tick causes no clinical signs in the majority of animals (**189** and **190**) but the prolonged intimate contact with the host may induce signs in some cases. These vary from discrete patches of erythema around the tick to more severe reactions such as pruritus and self trauma (**191** and **192**). Foreign body reactions may occur when the tick is removed inexpertly leaving the head or mouth parts embedded in the skin and, occasionally, very florid, proliferative, granulomatous lesions may result. The prolonged contact with the host allows for infections to be passed and a number of disease may be associated with the tick, for example tick paralysis. Other diseases may be vectored by ticks and these include Borreliosis (*Borrelia bugdorferi*), Rocky Mountain spotted fever (*Rickettsia rickettsii*) and canine ehrlichiosis (*Ehrlichia canis*).[11,31] Heavy infection with ticks may produce anaemia.

Tick infestation is characterised by:
- The obvious presence of quite large parasites.

Differential diagnoses include:
- Tumours, i.e. basal cell carcinomas and cysts.

Diagnosis is made by:
- Observation, removal and identification of the tick.

193

194

195

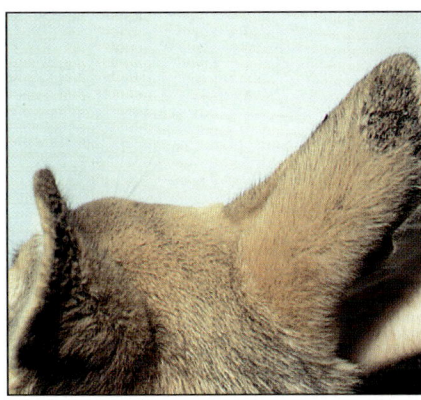

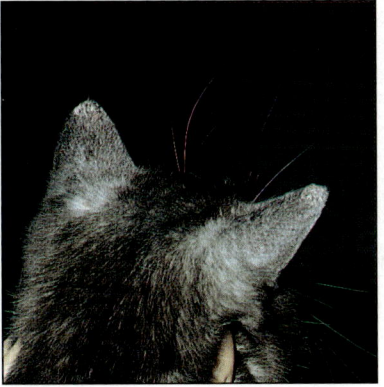

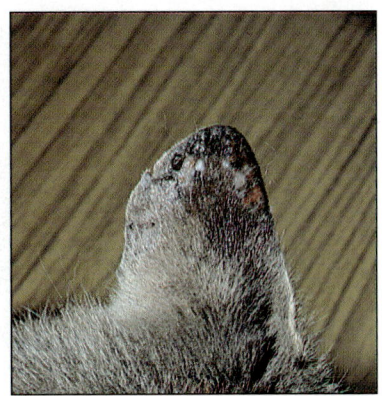

193 Fly bite dermatitis. Crusted haemorrhagic lesions on the ear tips of a German shepherd dog.

194 and 195 Fly bite dermatitis. An affected cat showing bilateral lesions on the pinnae and a close-up (**195**) of the ear lesion in a cat showing similar changes to those in the dog.

196

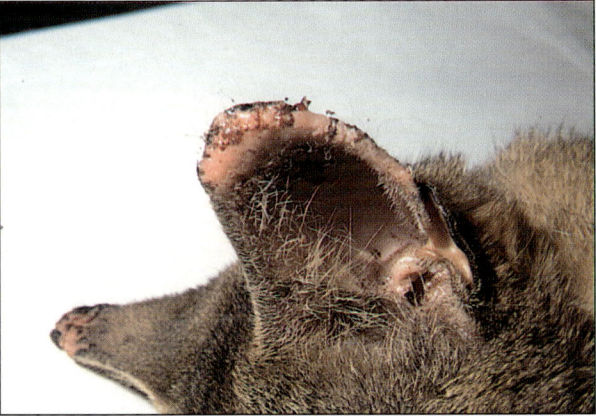

197

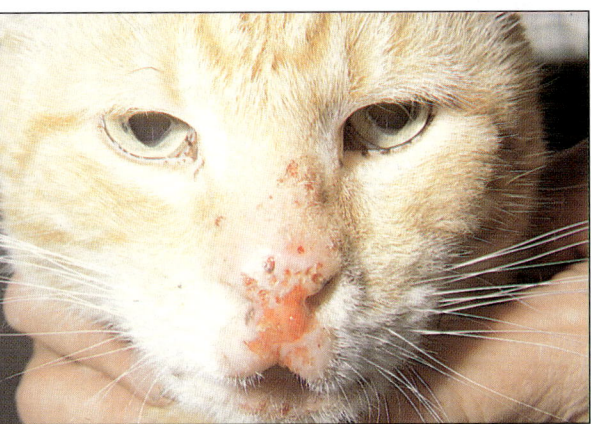

196 Fly bite dermatitis. Severe lesions on the pinna of an Abyssinian cat.

197 Fly bite dermatitis. Unusual severe fly bite damage to the planum nasale in a cat.

Biting insect dermatoses

Fly bite dermatitis

A condition caused by the stable fly *Stomoxys calcitrans* which bites the ear tips of dogs with erect ears during the summer months (**193**). In collies, Shetland sheepdogs and other breeds in which the tips of the pinnae bend over, the bites occur on the folded edge of the skin rather than the tip. There appears to be a higher incidence in the German shepherd dog. Lesions consist of erythema, hair loss and haemorrhagic crusting resulting from oozing of blood and serum. The condition is usually bilateral and is very irritant to the dog which reacts by shaking the head and rubbing and scratching at the ears, thus compounding the inflammation. A similar condition is seen in cats but the offending insect has not been positively identified (**194** to **196**). Occasionally, flies will attack the unpigmented planum nasale in cats (**197**).

Fly bite Dermatitis is characterised by:
- Dermatitis affecting tips and folds of pinnae.

Differential diagnoses include:
- Actinic dermatitis in white-eared cats.
- *Spilopsyllus cuniculi* infestation in cats.

Diagnosis can be made by:
- History of fly worry and compatible clinical signs.

198

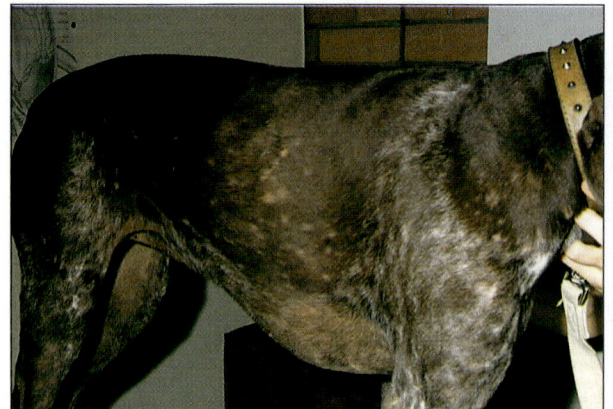

199

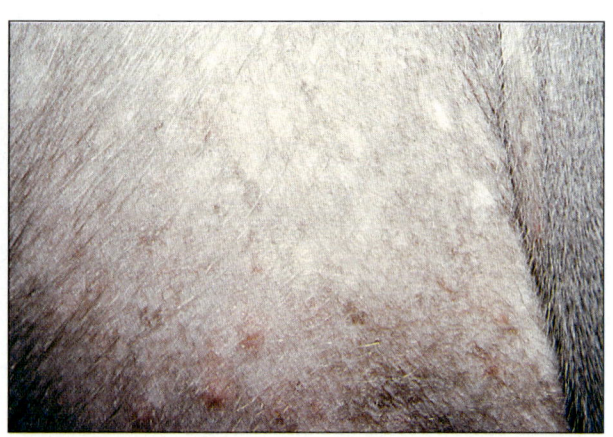

198   Insect bite dermatitis. Characteristic distribution on lateral trunk and upper limbs in a German short-haired pointer.

199   Insect bite dermatitis. Close-up of lesions in a Weimaraner dog showing papules, vesicles and alopecic, depigmented and hyperpigmented macules.

200

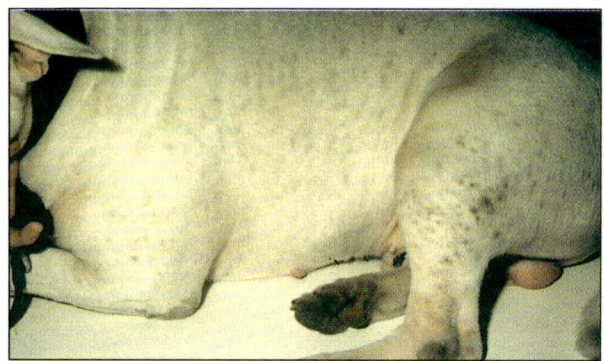

200   Insect bite dermatitis. A white Bull terrier dog showing the end result, with disfiguring hyperpigmented alopecic macules in characteristic distribution.

Insect bite dermatitis

A condition occurring in short-coated dogs, such as Weimaraners, Doberman pinschers, German short-haired pointers and Bull terriers, which are kept outdoors, especially in warm climates. The species of biting insect is not known, but is thought to be a mosquito, bush fly, sand fly or buffalo fly. The lesions have a characteristic distribution and are most obvious in Weimaraners and white bull terriers where they appear on the dorsum and lateral surfaces of the trunk and upper limbs. The head and the ventral surface of the trunk are spared.

The initial lesion is a vesicle or a papule which soon extends to form a circular, erythematous lesion, which later crusts over and finally heals, often with a focus of hyperpigmentation (**198** to **200**). The hair over the lesion is lost and regrowth is delayed, so that the dog appears 'moth eaten' or 'pock marked' with consequent deterioration in the cosmetic appearance of show dogs. There does not appear to be any marked irritation evoked by the bites in most cases. Often there is a history that flies are constantly worrying the dog.

Insect bite dermatitis is characterised by:
- Small foci of hair loss and hyperpigmentation and a characteristic distribution.

The differential diagnoses include:
- Superficial folliculitis.
- Demodicosis.
- Dermatophytosis.

Diagnosis can be made by:
- History of fly worry in dogs kept outdoors in warm climates.
- Characteristic pattern of distribution of lesions.
- Lack of response to appropriate antibacterial therapy.
- Skin biopsy shows eosinophilic infiltrate.

201

202

203

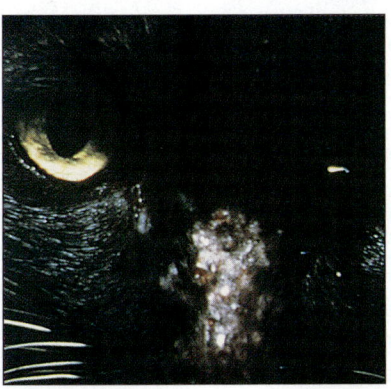

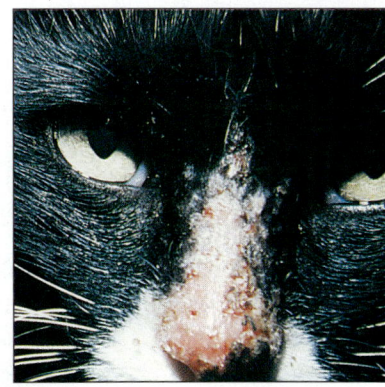

204

205

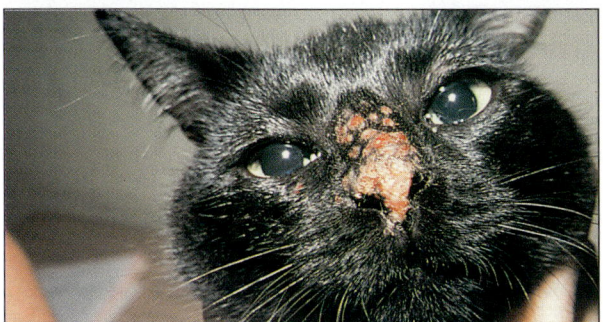
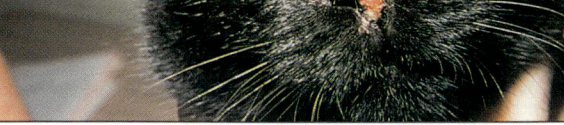

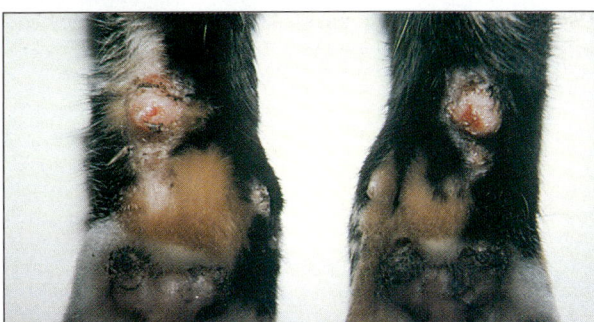

Feline mosquito bite allergy

A distinct clinical entity, occurring during the summer months in warm climates and resolving spontaneously in the winter or when the cat is housed in fly-screened accommodation. Cats of any age, either sex, and with pigmented or unpigmented coats may be affected. Typically the syndrome presents with a quintet of clinical signs (**201–205**):

1 A papular eruption on the outer and inner aspects of the pinnae.
2 A similar eruption on the bridge of the nose, but this soon worsens with the development of erosions, crusting, scaling and sometimes depigmentation. Occasionally the erosions extend on to the planum nasale.
3 Bilaterally symmetrical hyperkeratosis of all the pads of all four feet, preceded by swelling, tenderness, erythema and sometimes fissuring of the pads. The hyperkeratosis usually forms around the circumference of the pads and, unusually for the cat, is often hyperpigmented.
4 A peripheral lymphadenopathy.
5 A mild pyrexia.

Rarely the condition will be accompanied by a corneal eosinophilic granuloma.

201–205 Feline mosquito bite allergy. A variety of lesions may be seen in this condition such as papular eruptions on the pinna of a black cat (**201**), hair loss and papular eruption on the nose (**202**), more severe nasal lesion showing hair loss, depigmentation, erosions and crusting in a black cat (**203**) and extensive erosion of planum nasale due to coalescence of papular lesions (**204**). Figure **205** shows the characteristic, bilaterally symmetrical hyperpigmented hyperkeratosis mainly distributed on the margins of the foot pads. (Illustrations from Wilkinson, G. T. and Bate, M. J. (1984). A possible further clinical manifestation of the feline eosinophilic granuloma complex. *Journal of the American Animal Hospital Association*, **20**: 325–331.)

Feline mosquito bite allergy is characterised by:
- A clinical entity composed of a quintet of clinical signs occurring in cats in mosquito-infested areas.

Differential diagnoses include:
- Feline eosinophilic granuloma complex.
- Actinic dermatitis.
- Notoedric mange.
- Pemphigus erythematosus.
- Systemic lupus erythematosus.

Diagnosis can be made by:
- History and clinical signs.
- Rapid resolution of condition when patient is housed in insect screened accommodation.

206

207

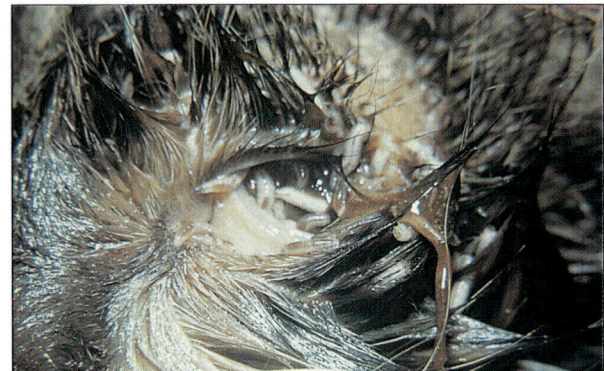

206 **Myiasis.** Maggot infestation of conjunctival sac following a purulent conjunctivitis.

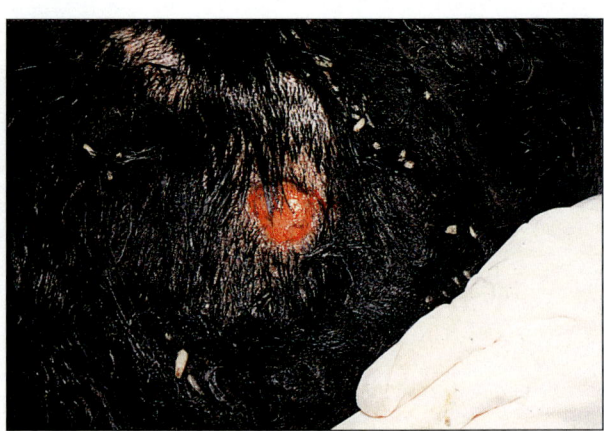

207 **Myiasis.** Punctate ulcers on the dorsal lumbo-sacral region of a dog are revealed after matted hair has been clipped.

Fly myiasis

Fly myiasis or fly strike occurs particularly in long-haired cats, elderly dogs and rabbits. Animals are often either unable to groom themselves or are elderly or ill. Owner neglect is often a cause. Animals with enteritis and perineal contamination with faeces are also victims. Flies belonging to the genera *Cuterebra* spp.*, Calliphora* spp. and *Sarcophaga* spp. lay their eggs which hatch rapidly

> **Diagnosis is obvious on examination of the affected region.**

(**206**). The maggots may invade the skin and, if so, they cause characteristic punched out ulcers (**207**). Secondary infection is surprisingly rare. There is often a foul odour.

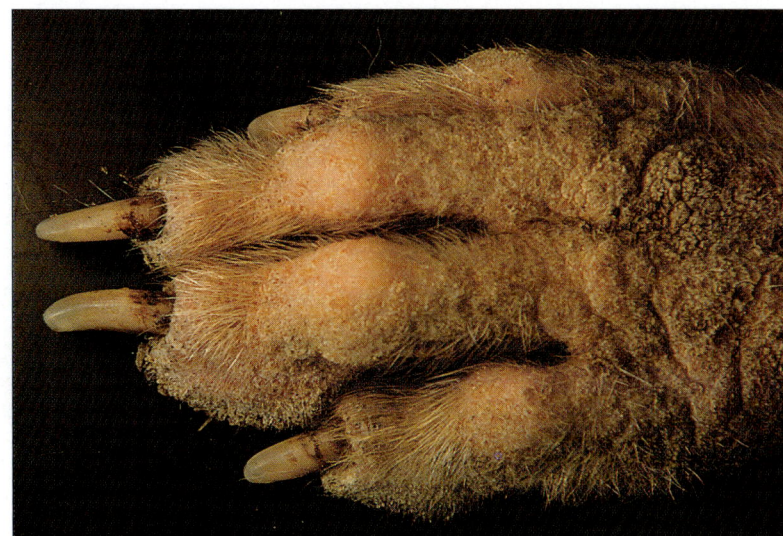

208

208 Hookworm larval dermatitis. Chronic hair loss, lichenification and crusting on the foot and lower leg.

Hookworm larval dermatitis

Hookworm dermatitis may be caused by the percutaneous passage of the larvae of *Uncinaria stenocephala* or *Ancylostoma* spp. although clinical signs are most commonly due to the former parasite.[6]

The larvae will penetrate the skin wherever it contacts the ground and signs are most frequently seen on the feet, particularly in the interdigital skin folds of dogs. The disease is seen most commonly in dogs that are housed in kennels with earth or grassed runs e.g. greyhound kennels. Faecal examination will reveal the presence of hookworm ova. The continuous exposure to the migrating larvae results in a chronic pruritic pododermatitis.

There is erythema of the interdigital web accompanied by loss of hair on the foot which may become encrusted (**208**). The margins of the pads may become thickened and hardened and the claws may appear necrotic at the base. Abnormalities of nail growth are common. There is local lymphadenopathy and there may be a peripheral eosinophilia. Pruritus is usually not marked and is manifested by persistent gentle chewing of the feet. Lesions on the feet may extend up the leg in severe cases; they are often persistent, resistant to treatment and may cause lameness. The migrating larvae are not found on microscopic examination of skin scrapings.

Hookworm dermatitis is characterised by:
- Chronic dermatitis affecting the lower limbs and feet.
- Hyperkeratosis of pads.
- Occurring in dogs allowed access to grassed runs.

Differential diagnoses include:
- Pododemodicosis.
- Trombiculidiasis.
- Atopy.
- Pelodera dermatitis.
- Autoimmune disease.
- Zinc responsive dermatosis.

Diagnosis can be made by:
- Consideration of the history and clinical signs.
- Faecal examination for hookworm ova is positive.
- Histopathological examination of biopsy specimens.

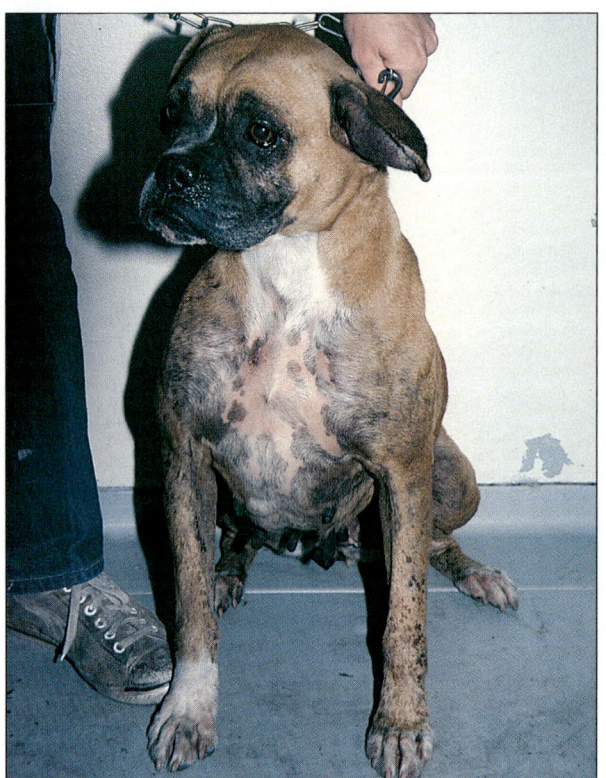

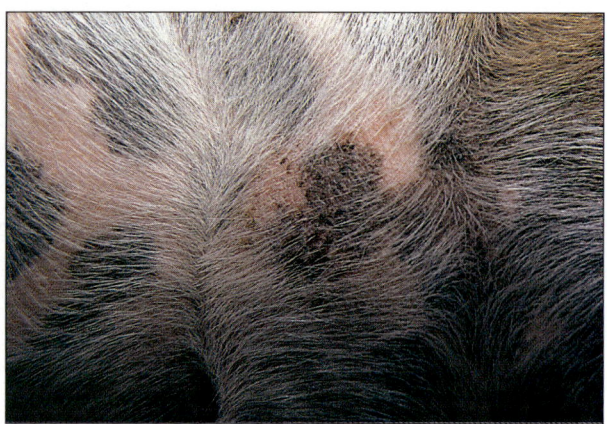

209 and 210   Heartworm dermatitis. Marked erythema, thickening and crusting of the presternal skin of a Boxer bitch associated with the presence of microfilaria of *Dirofilaria immitis* in the dermal capillaries and tissues.

Pelodera dermatitis

This is a rare condition caused by the infection of skin by the larvae of the free-living nematode *Pelodera strongyloides*. Infection results when the larvae pass from organic material into apposed skin and thus it occurs in situations where animals are poorly accommodated and lie directly on soil or vegetation. In contrast to hookworm dermatitis there is intense pruritus in infected areas. Microscopic examination of skin scrapings reveals the larvae.

Heartworm dermatitis

Microfilariae of the heartworm *Dirofilaria immitis*, which are usually present in the peripheral circulation, have been incriminated as a cause of a hypersensitivity reaction when they find their way into the dermis. Reported lesions have included chronic, ulcerated, multifocal nodules and pustular eruptions (**209** and **210**). Diagnosis can be made by demonstration of microfilaria in skin scrapings and within the dermis in skin biopsies, and resolution of the condition following microfilaricidal therapy.

References

1. Alexander, M. M. and Ihrke, P. J. (1982). Cheyletiella dermatitis in small animal practice: a review. *California Veterinarian*, **36**: 9–12.

2. Baker, B. B. and Stannard, A. A. (1974). A look at canine scabies. *Journal of the American Animal Hospital Association*, **10**: 513–515.

3. Baker, K. P. and Mulcahy, R. (1986). Fleas on hedgehogs and dogs in the Dublin area. *Veterinary Record*, **119**: 16–17.

4. Beresford-Jones, W. P. (1981). Prevalence of fleas on dogs and cats in an area of central London. *Journal of Small Animal Practice*, **22**: 27–29 5.

5. Bornstein, S. (1991). Experimental infection of dogs with *Sarcoptes scabiei* derived from naturally infected wild red foxes (*Vulpes vulpes*): clinical observations. *Veterinary Dermatology*, **2**: 151–159.

6. Bowman, D. W. (1992). Hookworm parasites of dogs and cats. *Compendium on Continuing Education*, **14**: 585–593.

7. Chesney, C. J. (1989). Demodicosis in the cat. *Journal of Small Animal Practice*, **30**: 689–695.

8. Cooper, J. E. (1992). Integument. In: Beynon, P. H., Lawton, M. P. C. and Cooper, J. C. (Eds.) *Manual of Reptiles*, pp. 73–79. British Small Animal Veterinary Association, Cheltenham.

9. Dryden, M. W. (1989). Biology of the cat flea, *Ctenocephalides felis felis*. *Companion Animal Practice*, **19**: 23–27.

10. Estes, P. C., Richter, C. B. and Franklin, J. A. (1971). Demodectic mange in the golden hamster. *Laboratory Animal Science*, **21**: 825–828.

11. Font, A., Closa, J. M. and Mascort, J. (1992). Tick-transmitted diseases: a comparative study of Lyme disease, canine ehrlichiosis and rickettsiosis in the dog. *Veterinary International*, **4**: 3–13.

12. Fox, M. T., Sykes, T. J. and Jacobs, D. E (1986). Forage mite infestation in the dog. *Veterinary Record*, **118**: 459–460.

13. Greve, J. H. and Gaafar, S, M. (1966). Natural transmission of *Demodex canis* in dogs. *Journal of the American Veterinary Medical Association*, **148**: 1043–1045.

14. Halliwell, R. E. W. (1986). Flea bite hypersensitivity in dogs and cats—the current status. *Tijdschrift voor Diergeneeskunde*, **111**: 84S–87S.

15. Halliwell, R. E., Preston, J. F. and Nesbitt, J. G. (1987). Aspects of immunopathogenesis of flea allergy dermatitis in dogs. *Veterinary Immunology and Immunopathology*, **17**: 483–494.

16. Harvey, R. G. (1990). Dermatitis in a cat associated with *Spilopsyllus cuniculi*. *The Veterinary Record*, **126**: 89–90.

17. Harvey, R. G. (1990). *Demodex cuniculi* in dwarf rabbits, (*Oryctolagus cuniculi*). *Journal of Small Animal Practice*, **31**: 204–207.

18. Henfrey, J. I. (1990). Canine demodicosis. *In Practice*, **12**: 187–192.

19. Kwochka, K. W. (1986). Canine demodicosis. In: Kirk, R. W. (Ed.) *Current Veterinary Therapy IX*, pp. 531–537.

20. Lumej, J. T. and Cremers, H. J. W. M. (1986). Anorexia and *Chirodiscoides caviae* infection in a guinea pig (*Cavia porcellus*). *Veterinary Record*, **119**: 432.

21. McGarry, J. W. (1989). Recurrent infestation of a cat by *Cheyletus eruditus* (Shrank 1791). *Veterinary Record*, **125**: 18.

22. McKeever, P. J. (1979). Dermatitis associated with *Cheyletiella* infestation in cats. *Journal of the American Veterinary Medical Association*, **174**: 718–720.

23. Medleau, L., Brown, C. A., Brown, S. A. and Jones, C. S. (1986). Demodicosis in cats. *Journal of the American Animal Hospital Association*, **24**: 85–91.

24. Mundell, A. C. and Ihrke, P. J. (1990). Ivermectin in the treatment of *Pneumonyssoides caninum*: a case report. *Journal of the American Animal Hospital Association*, **26**: 393–396.

25. Nesbitt, G. H and Schmitz, J. A. (1978). Fleabite allergic dermatitis: a review and survey of 330 cases. *Journal of the American Veterinary Medical Association*, **173**: 282–288.

26. Ossbrink, W. L. A. and Rust, M. K. (1984). Fecundity and longevity of the adult cat flea, *Ctenocephalides felis felis* (Siphonoptera: Pulicidae). *Journal of Medical Entomology*, **21**: 727–731.

27. Ottenschot, T. R. F. and Gil, D. (1978). Cheyletiellosis in long-haired cats. *Tijdschrift voor Diergeneeskunde*, **103**: 224–228.

28. Powell, M. B., Weisbroth, S. H., Roth, L. and Wilhelmsen, C. (1980). Reaginic hypersensitivity in *Otodectes cynotis* infestation of cats and mode of mite feeding. *American Journal of Veterinary Research*, **6**: 877–881.

29. Thoday, K. L and Beresford-Jones, W. P. (1977). The diagnosis and treatment of mange in the guinea-pig caused by *Trixacarus (Cavioptes) caviae* (Fain, Hovell & Hyatt, 1972). *Journal of Small Animal Practice*, **18**: 591–595.

30. Weisbroth, S. H., Friedman, S. and Scher, S. (1976). The parasitic ecology of the rodent mite, *Myobia musculi*. III. Lesions in certain host strains. *Laboratory Animal Science*, **26**: 725–735.

31. Weiser, I. B. and Green, C. E. (1989). Dermal necrosis associated with Rocky Mountain spotted fever in four dogs. *Journal of the American Veterinary Medical Association*, **195**: 1756–1758.

Chapter 5:

Bacterial skin diseases

Introduction

It is now generally accepted that almost all bacterial skin disease is secondary to some change in the local cutaneous environment or to a circumvention of host defences.[7] In some instances micro-organisms are inoculated directly into the skin, as in the case of cat bite abscessation or the infections due to atypical mycobacteria. Most commonly, however, there is a change in the local cutaneous environment which favours colonisation by potentially pathogenic bacteria. Changes may be local and transient, such as those which may follow exposure to a caustic irritant or an ectoparasite, whilst in other instances there may be a more generalised change in the micro-environment as a consequence of an underlying disease.

Thus in hypothyroidism there are a number of cutaneous changes such as an alteration in the rate of keratinisation, reduced follicular activity, reduced cutaneous metabolism and a reduced ability to resist infection, all of which may result in an increased incidence of pyoderma. In atopy the cutaneous erythema and increased humidity, particularly in the intertriginous regions, contribute to the increased carriage of micro-organisms and an increased incidence of pyoderma in these animals. Furthermore, the presence of coagulase-positive staphylococci on the surface of inflamed skin may result in pro-inflammatory, and potentially sensitising, metabolites diffusing through the defective epidermal barrier and provoking further inflammation.[11]

> **The diagnosis and management of bacterial skin disease rests on three principles:**
> - A recognition of the depth of the infection and a knowledge of the likely micro-organism involved.
> - The identification of any underlying disease that may be present.
> - An understanding of cutaneous ecology and the epidermal defence mechanisms and of the steps necessary in order to return the skin surface to normality.

The depth of the infection and the organism involved [3,7,19]

Bacterial skin disease is classified into three groups based on the depth of the infection in the skin (**Table 4**). A knowledge of the depth of the infection is important for two reasons.

Firstly, because a poorer prognosis accompanies the deeper bacterial infections since they may be associated with severe defects in the host's defences and may thus be life-threatening. In contrast, an acute episode of pyotraumatic dermatitis (a surface infection) that arises as a result of the animal attempting to ease the discomfort of impacted anal sacs will not be life-threatening and has a good prognosis.

The second advantage that stems from recognising the signs associated with the various depths of infection is that the approach to the therapy of each is well-documented.[7]

The pathogen most commonly isolated from canine bacterial skin disease is a coagulase-positive, Gram-positive coccus, *Staphylococcus intermedius*.[1,7,15] In an uncomplicated case of superficial pyoderma a narrow-spectrum antibacterial agent

> **Table 4:** *The classification of bacterial skin disease according to the depth of the infection.*
> *(after Ihrke, 1990)*
>
> 1. **Surface infections**
>   i. pyotraumatic dermatitis
>   ii. body fold pyoderma such as lip-fold and facial-fold pyoderma
> 2. **Superficial infections**
>   i. impetigo
>   ii. superficial folliculitis
> 3. **Deep infections**
>   i. localised deep folliculitis and furunculosis such as canine acne and nasal pyoderma
>   ii. generalised deep pyoderma
>   iii. cellulitis
>   iv. mycobacterial infections
> 4. **Subcutaneous abscesses**
>   i. cat bite abscess
>   ii. botriomycosis, actinomycosis and nocardiosis

that is active against Gram-positive cocci (in particular the staphylococci) is a good empirical choice of treatment. Even in mixed infections it is often only necessary to kill the staphylococci in order for the host defences to then remove the other, typically Gram-negative, organisms.

Cutaneous infections associated with staphylococci are unusual in the cat.[7,12,18] The primary pathogens associated with feline skin disease are *Pasteurella multocida* and *Bacteroides* spp. These organisms are resident of the feline oral cavity and are inoculated into the skin by cat bite.

There are a number of cutaneous infections in the dog and cat, some with very characteristic clinical signs, which are recognised to be due to specific bacteria such as *Mycobacterium* spp., *Actinobacillus* spp. or *Nocardia* spp.[7] These are ubiquitous organisms which occasionally may be found as transients or contaminants on normal skin.[10,14] They are associated with deep infections, often chronic in nature, and usually associated with a discharging fistula. Most cases are due to contamination of penetrating wounds.

Recognising the underlying disorder

The underlying disorder may be readily apparent to the clinician in the case of the surface bacterial infections: a humid environment and maceration of tissues deep within body folds is accompanied by a low-grade, chronic, increased carriage of bacteria. They are not considered to be true bacterial infections. While gentle cleansing, perhaps with benzoyl peroxide gel, may provide temporary improvement, only surgical ablation of the fold will be curative. Determining the underlying cause in the case of a superficial bacterial infection is more difficult. In some cases the cause will be transient and the infection responds to a single course of treatment. In others a generalised change in the cutaneous environment, such as that accompanying the hypersensitivities, endocrinopathies and keratinisation defects, will need to be considered.

A failure to address these underlying disorders will result in continued aberrations in the micro- climate and recurrent infections. Similarly, in the case of the deep bacterial infections it is imperative to identify any associated immunosuppressive conditions such as demodicosis or an endocrinopathy at an early stage if management is to be successful.

The epidermal defences and cutaneous ecosystem

The epidermal defence against micro-organisms is dependent on physical barriers, chemical defences and the presence of a normal resident flora. Physical defences such as the hair coat, surface lipid and the stratum corneum act as barriers to the inward movement of micro-organisms. Surface chemicals such as immunoglobulins, fatty acids and inorganic ions hinder the ability of transient micro-organisms to establish on the surface.

The protective effect of a resident population of micro-organisms, itself dependent on local humidity, pH, fatty acids and inorganic ions, is a result of a number of factors: The normal flora in the dog consists of coagulase-negative staphylococci, β−haemolytic streptococci and anaerobic bacteria and these organisms are adapted to the local conditions, occupy available ecological niches, utilise available nutrients and may produce antibacterial substances, all of which reduce the likelihood that transient and contaminant organisms will establish.

The restoration of a normal cutaneous environment is a major target in the management of pyoderma and principally is achieved by attending to any underlying disease that may be present and by killing the pathogenic organisms, usually with systemic antibacterial therapy. However, appropriate use of topical therapeutics can hasten the restoration to normality by removing dirt and exudate, killing pathogenic bacteria and fungi, reducing epidermal proliferation, reducing percutaneous water loss, increasing epidermal hydration and by reducing pruritus.

Surface infections

Pyotraumatic dermatitis (hot spot, wet eczema, acute moist pyoderma).

Pyotraumatic dermatitis is an acute, highly pruritic dermatitis which rapidly spreads peripherally. No primary lesions are present. The affected area is moist, shiny, erythematous and often has an adherent crust (**211–213**). The self trauma may be intense. There is a well-defined boundary, although clipping of surrounding hair may be necessary to reveal this. There is an increased incidence in dogs with thick, dense, coats[19] such as Labrador retrievers, Golden retrievers, Chow-Chows, German shepherd dogs and Newfoundlands.

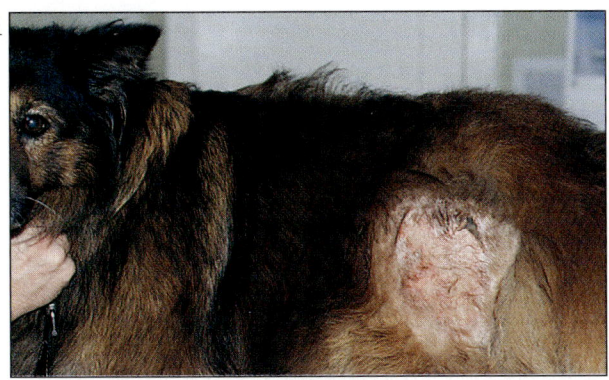

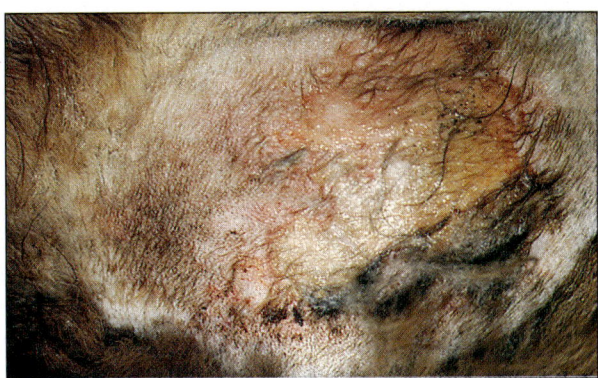

211 and 212   Pyotraumatic dermatitis. Note the erythema, the shiny, moist appearance and the adherent hairs. Close-up (**212**) of the lesion after clipping the surrounding hair. Note the well-demarcated area of erythema, moist appearance and adherent crust.

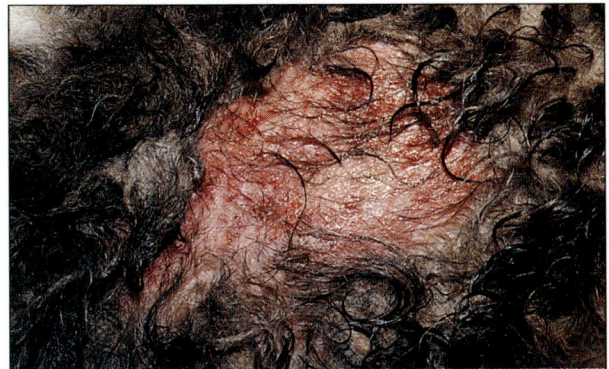

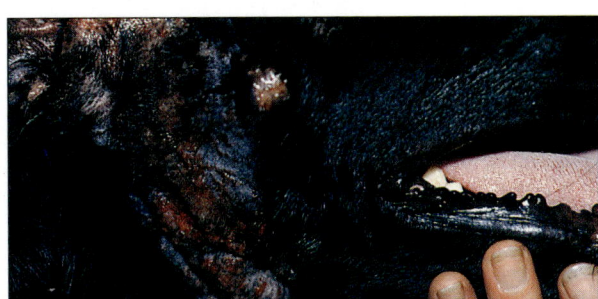

214   Pyotraumatic dermatitis and accompanying deep folliculitis in a Labrador retriever. Note the satellite lesion rostral to the main area of inflammation. This breed appears to be predisposed to be one in which there is a tendency for the lesion to be accompanied by deep folliculitis. It is not known if one is a consequence of the other.

213   Pyotraumatic dermatitis. A large lesion on the lateral thigh of a cross-bred dog with sarcoptic mange. Note that this dog has a thick, heavy coat. This type of coat appears to predispose the dog to this condition.

These heavy coats are thought to favour an increased humidity at the skin surface, and, perhaps, trap the dirt and foreign bodies, which may be involved in the pathogenesis of the lesion.

Although the cause of these lesions is not completely understood, it is known that any localised pain or discomfort such as otitis externa, impacted anal sacs or the presence of an ectoparasite may elicit the attention which results in localised trauma to the skin. Given the right conditions, a hot spot will develop.

In some animals, particularly Labrador retrievers and St. Bernards there may not be a rapid response to treatment. Histopathological examination of samples from these cases reveals deep folliculitis, furunculosis and panniculitis although whether these lesions result as an extension to the pyotraumatic dermatitis is not known.[17] Suspicion may be aroused by the breed and by the occurrence of satellite lesions which are uncommon in pyotraumatic dermatitis (**214**). Systemic antibacterial therapy is indicated in these cases.

Pyotraumatic dermatitis is characterised by:
- Acute onset.
- Severe pruritus.
- Rapid lateral progression.
- Occasional deep progression.

The major differential diagnoses are:
- Deep folliculitis and accompanying furunculosis in some breeds.
- Calcinosis cutis.

Diagnosis is made by:
- Typical history and clinical signs and identifying an underlying cause.

215

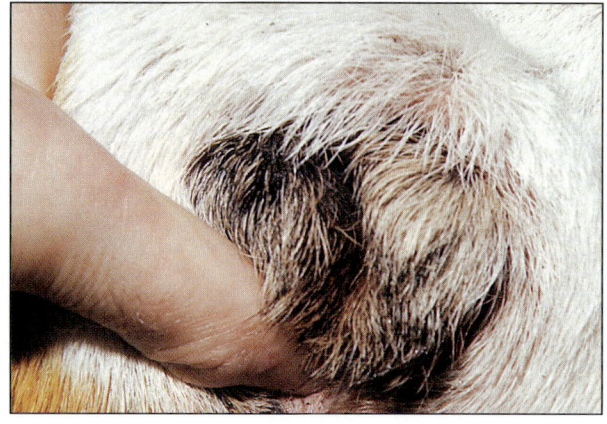

216

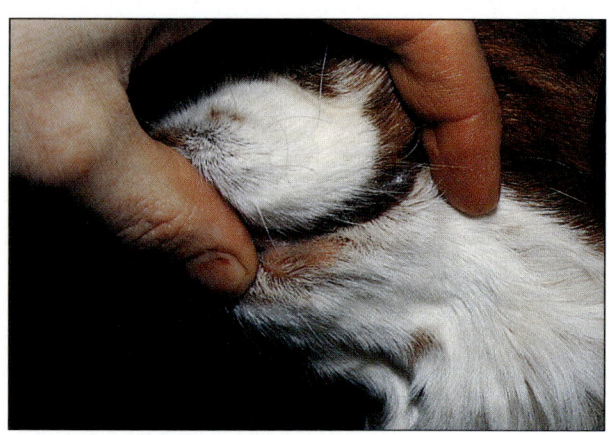

215   Fold pyoderma. Corkscrew tail in a bulldog is often associated with fold pyoderma.

216   Fold pyoderma. A small patch of erythema and surface maceration in the lip fold of a Springer spaniel.

217

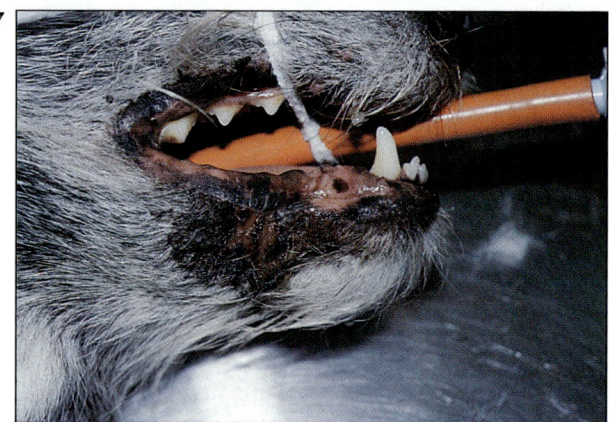

217   Fold pyoderma. Lip fold pyoderma in a Lurcher. The affected area is about to be prepared for surgical resection.

Fold pyoderma

In contrast to pyotraumatic dermatitis these surface infections are characterised by a chronic course and little pruritus. The inflammation results from maceration of epithelial tissues and surface infection as a consequence of increased humidity and friction between closely apposed folds of skin. Odour may be significant, particularly in lip fold pyoderma. The infected areas are erythematous, often with adherent, white, macerated skin visible as a greasy film on the surface. Although topical therapeutics may be useful surgical resection is curative. Body folds may be found in any area but typically are found around the vulva in obese bitches and between the tightly apposed folds of the tail in bulldogs (**215**).

The two most common sites of fold pyoderma are the lip fold and facial fold. Lip fold pyoderma occurs on the lower lip, adjacent to the canine tooth. Animals with excessive skin around the mandible may be predisposed, particularly Springer and Cocker spaniels (**216** and **217**). The inflamed fold may be hard to see until the skin is stretched open. Odour may be foul and owners will frequently need to be convinced that the odour

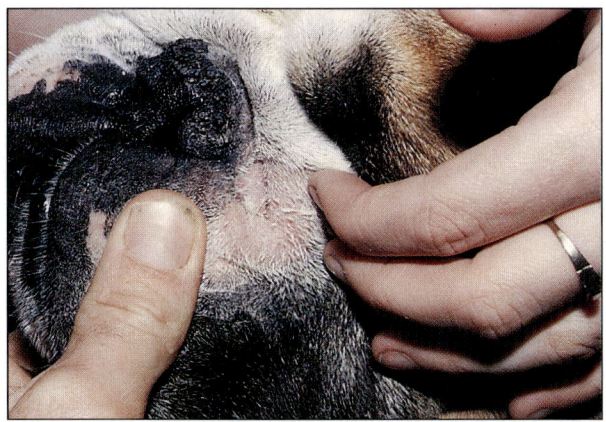

218   Fold pyoderma. Facial fold pyoderma immediately caudal to the planum nasale of a bulldog.

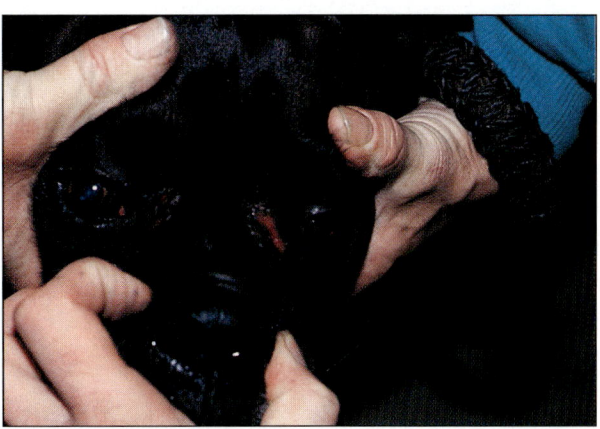

219   Fold pyoderma. Facial fold in a Boxer adjacent to the medial canthus of the left eye.

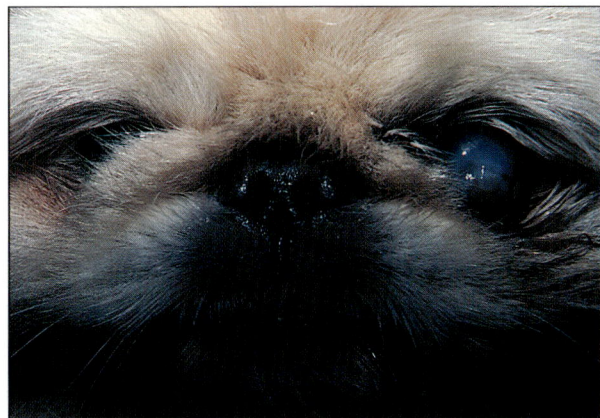

220   Fold pyoderma. Facial fold in a Pekinese resulting in prolonged contact between hairs and the cornea. A chronic keratitis has resulted.

originates from the lip fold and not the teeth.

Facial folds are particularly common in the brachycephalic breeds (**218** and **219**). Transverse folds are found caudal to the planum nasale and rostral to the eyes, whilst longitudinal folds may be present on the frontal region of the head. Facial fold pyoderma is less malodorous than those in lip folds. However, they may have a more serious clinical sequel if the folds result in hair lying in contact with the cornea, as a keratitis may result (**220**).

Surface infections are characterised by:
- Chronicity.
- Very slow lateral progression.
- Low grade pruritus.
- Foul odour, particularly in the case of lip fold pyoderma.

Major differential diagnoses are:
- Demodicosis.
- Mucocutanous candidiasis, particularly in the case of lip fold pyoderma.
- Mycosis fungoides, particularly in the case of lip fold pyoderma.

Diagnosis is made by:
- History and demonstration of an intertriginous area between apposing body surfaces.
- Impression smears to rule out candidiasis.

221

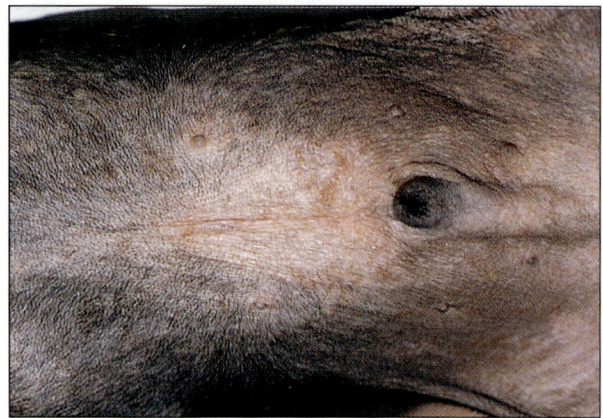

222

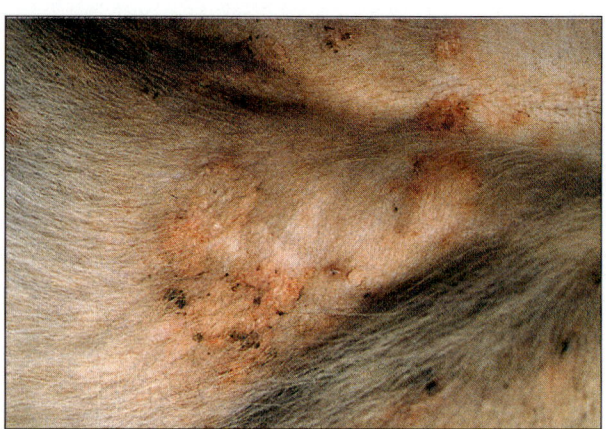

221 Impetigo. A Staffordshire Bull terrier pup with impetigo. The lesions are barely visible at this distance.

222 Superficial folliculitis. Pyoderma in the groin of a German shepherd bitch. Note the lack of erythema and the well-defined lesions, principally inflammatory papules.

Superficial bacterial infections

A superficial pyoderma is defined as a bacterial skin infection situated within the stratum corneum or the intact hair follicle. Superficial pyoderma is often pruritic. In contrast to both surface and deep infections they can be difficult to recognise, principally because of the all-too-common absence of primary lesions. It is important to remember that erythematous macules and papules precede pustules and that crusted papules, epidermal collarettes, post-inflammatory hyperpigmented patches and focal alopecia may follow pustules. The presence of any of these lesions alone, or in combination, may indicate a superficial pyoderma.

Treatment is usually straightforward provided that the temptation to use glucocorticoids is resisted. Systemic glucocorticoids will confuse evaluation of any response to antibacterial therapy, will compromise immunity and decrease keratinisation and sebum production. These effects tend to result in a partial improvement followed by a severe deterioration.

Recurrence of superficial pyoderma after adequate treatment should prompt a search for the underlying disease, which is often present.

Impetigo

This is a condition of young animals and is typically confined to the glabrous skin of the abdomen and groin. Papules and small pustules may be found but the commonest lesions are tiny yellowish-brown epidermal collarettes and scale (**221**). Pruritus is minimal. Lesions may be very difficult to see from a distance. The condition is traditionally associated with young animals kept in insanitary conditions.

Impetigo is characterised by:
- Crusts and scale.
- Minimal pruritus.

The differential diagnoses are:
- Demodicosis.
- Dermatophytosis.

The diagnosis is made by:
- Consideration of the age and the typical signs.
- (Skin scrapings should be made to rule out the differential diagnoses.)

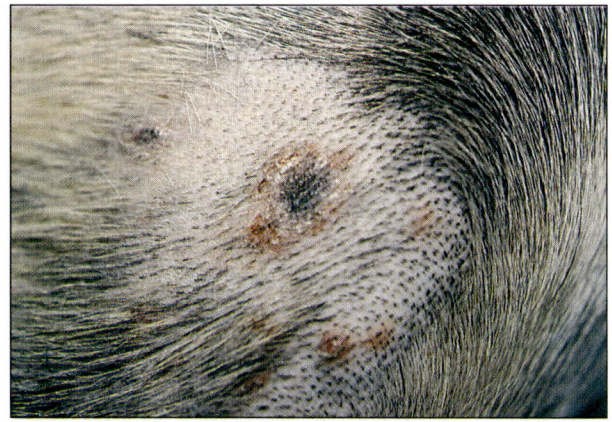

223   Superficial folliculitis. A central area of post-inflammatory hyperpigmentation surrounded by an erythematous zone. Note that the majority of the lesions precede or follow the pustular phase: erythematous macules and papules and post-pustular lesions outnumber the solitary pustule.

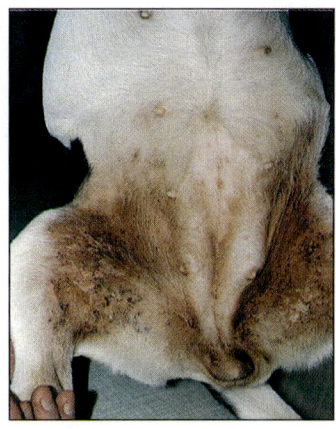

224   Superficial folliculitis. Pyoderma in the groin of a Labrador retriever with atopy. Note the similar distribution of the lesions but that in this case there is extensive saliva staining.

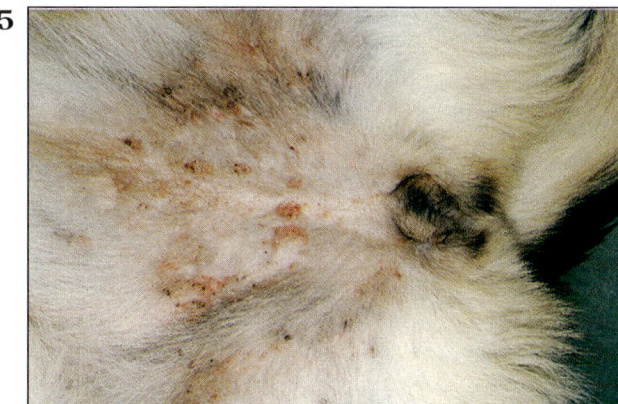

225   Superficial folliculitis. Close up demonstrating the range of lesions in a typical case. Note the erythematous macules, papules, pustules. A few epidermal collarettes are visible.

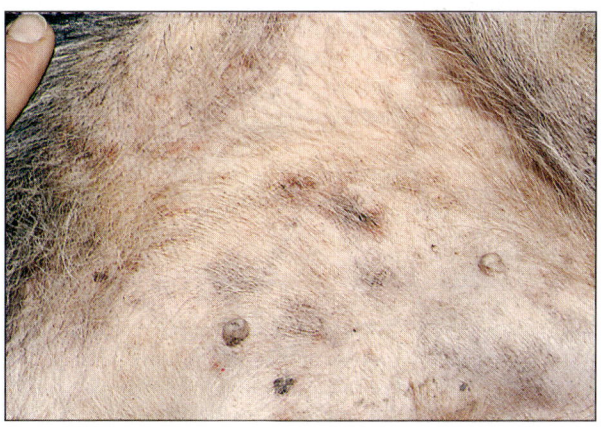

226   Superficial folliculitis. Close up demonstrating another case in which the predominant lesion is a small post-inflammatory hyperpigmented patch.

Superficial pyoderma

The primary lesions of superficial pyoderma are inflammatory macules progressing to papules and pustules (**222–226**). There may also be crusted papules, epidermal collarettes and post-inflammatory hyperpigmentation, scale and patchy alopecia. Pruritus is variable. All of these lesions may be present on the same animal at one time but their relative proportions will vary. Inflammatory papules will be the commonest finding and crusted papules and epidermal collarettes will also be more frequent than pustules in many cases (**227–230**).

227

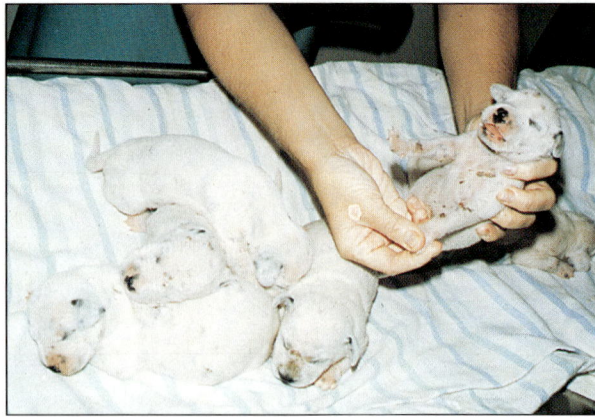

227   Superficial pyoderma. Extensive superficial pyoderma in a litter of young Dalmatian pups.

228

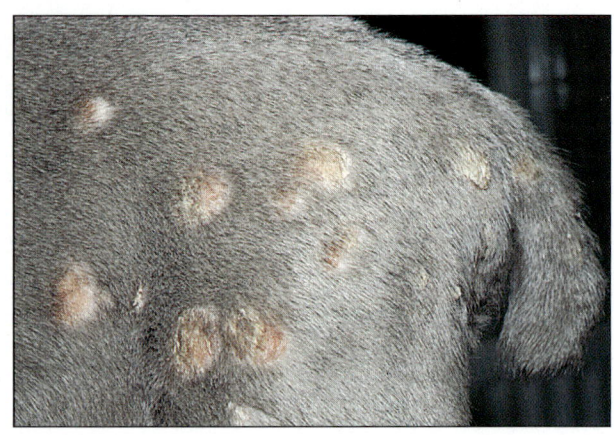

228   Superficial folliculitis in a Great Dane puppy. Note the coalescing, almost plaque-like epidermal collarettes.

229

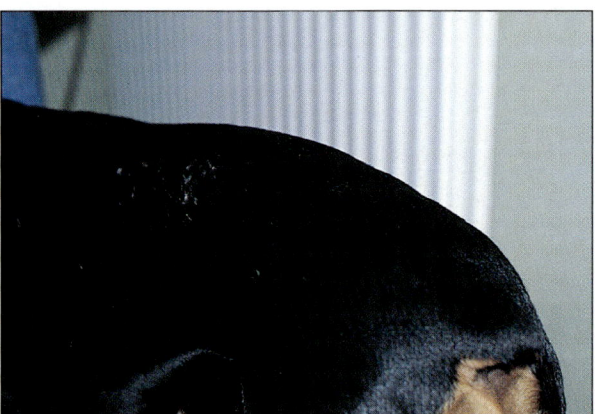

230

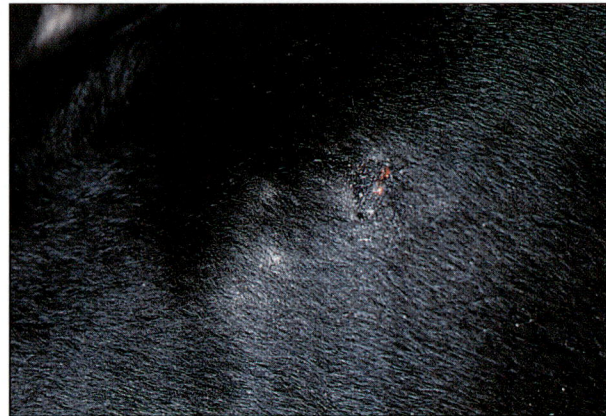

229 and 230   Superficial folliculitis in a Doberman pinscher. In this breed the initial signs are typically raised papules with elevated groups of hairs. Hives (oedematous papules) is a common diagnosis. Careful examination of the skin will reveal the primary lesion, an inflammatory papule centred over a hair follicle (**230**).

231

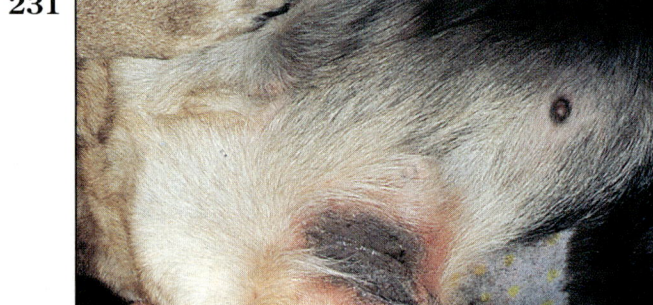

231   Superficial pyoderma in a German shepherd dog with atopy. Note large erythematous patch in the axilla with papules and post-inflammatory hyperpigmentation clearly visible.

Florid lesions may be found in the intertriginae, particularly the axillae (**231**). Rarely, florid pustules of varying colour, often surrounded by an erythematous ring, may be found. Large pustules with no evidence of accompanying inflammation should prompt suspicion of immunosuppression such as hyperadrenocorticism. Erosions and ulcers may also be seen in cases of folliculitis and superficial pyoderma (**232**). Healing occurs without scar formation.

The commonest underlying cause of superficial pyoderma is a change in the cutaneous environment.[7,19] Flea bite hypersensitivity and atopy (**233**) are the main causes of such aberrations in cutaneous homeostasis but immaturity, physiological endocrine changes at puberty and oestrus (**234**), endocrinopathies, ectoparasites and

232

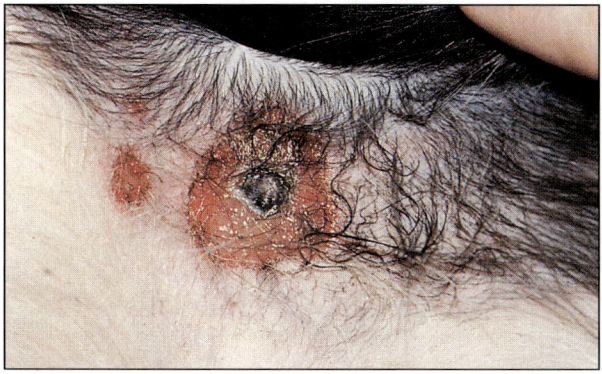

232 Superficial pyoderma in the pre-crural fold of a Border collie. Note deeper, erosive lesions, one of which has a clearing central area of post-inflammatory hyperpigmentation.

233

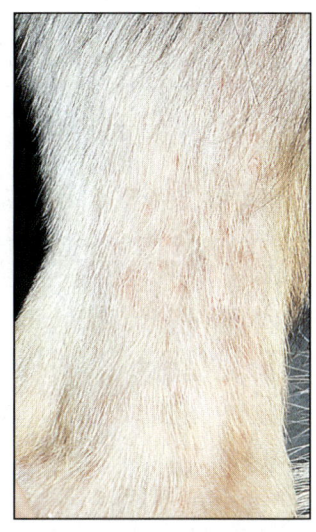

233 Superficial pyoderma over the hock of a German shepherd dog with atopy. Inflammatory papules are the predominant lesion.

234

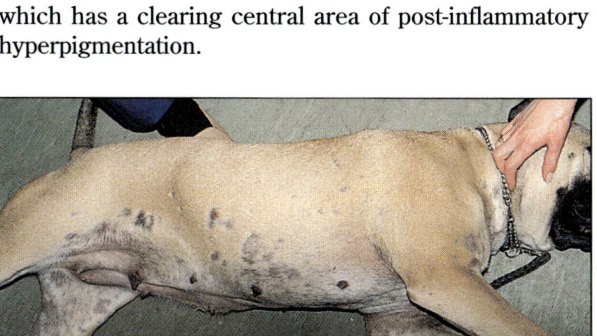

234 Superficial folliculitis. In this Bull mastiff bitch there are well circumscribed patches of post-inflammatory hyperpigmentation and alopecia on the flanks. These were a regular problem, occurring in the period immediately preceding oestrus. Topical antibacterial shampoo prevented the problem in succeeding years.

235

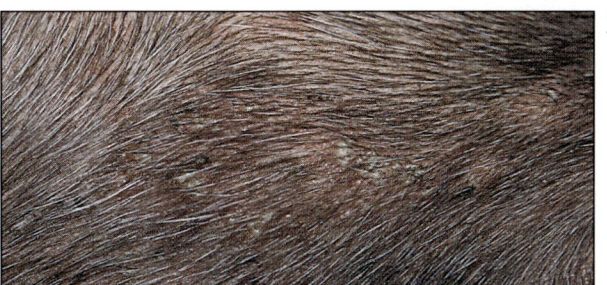

235 Superficial pyoderma in a German short-haired pointer. Note the discrete pustules on the flank, a consequence of micro-trauma caused by working in rough vegetation. This type of superficial pyoderma is also known as 'hunting dog pyoderma'. Lesions are predominantly found on the rostral and lateral body surfaces and appear 24 to 48 hours after work. They usually resolve without systemic treatment.

Superficial pyodermas are characterised by:
- Papules, pustules, epidermal collarettes and post-inflammatory hyperpigmentation.
- Scale and crust in many cases.
- Variable, often severe pruritus.

The major differential diagnoses are:
- Demodicosis.
- Dermatophytosis.
- Pemphigus foliaceus.

The diagnosis is made by:
- Skin scrapings to rule out demodicosis.
- Identification of characteristic spectrum of lesions.
- Aspiration and microscopic examination of pustule contents.
- Culture of pustule contents should yield *Staphylococcus intermedius*.

defects in keratinisation should all be considered in recurrent cases.

'Hunting dog pyoderma' is a superficial pyoderma which typically presents on Tuesdays after a weekend working to the gun. The dogs are presented with florid pustules on the anterior aspects of the limbs and the ventrum (**235**). The lesions result from inoculation of bacteria into the skin by vegetation. Short-haired dogs such as pointers are predisposed.

236

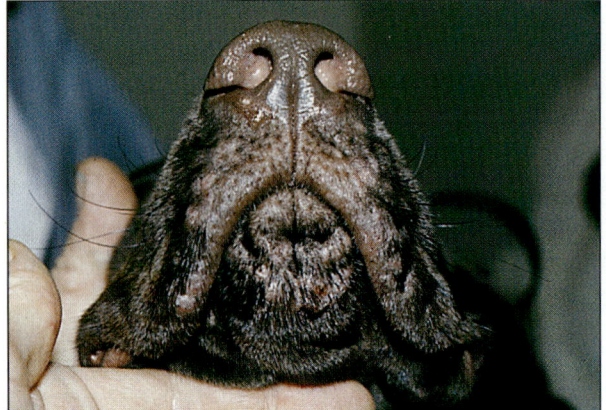

236 **Acne** in the dog is regarded as a localised form of deep pyoderma. Mild cases such as in this Labrador retriever may only require local treatment with benzoyl peroxide gel for example.

237

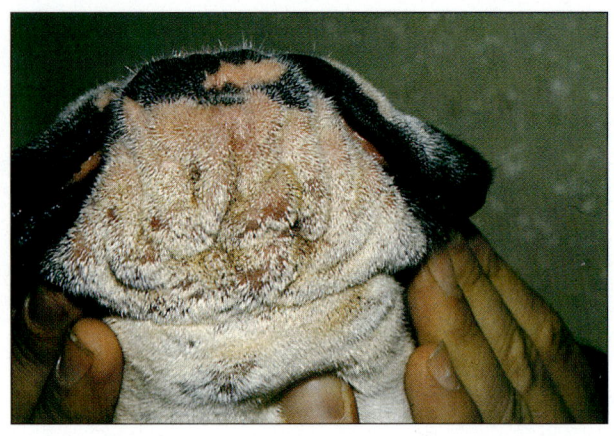

237 **Acne in a bulldog.** More severe with a few large pustules visible. Fibrosed papules and nodules are apparent.

Deep bacterial infections

Bacterial infection that lies below the level of the basement membrane is regarded as deep. The micro-organisms are potentially in direct contact with the vascular system and bacteraemia is a real risk. The local cutaneous defences are of little value and the animal must rely on systemic immune systems. Many cases are, however, immunosuppressed and thus the prognosis for this disease group is always guarded and may be poor.

Deep infections may occur as extensions of both surface or superficial infections through the follicle (furunculosis) or via the interfollicular epidermis. Direct inoculation from contaminated bite wounds or penetrating foreign bodies is a common aetiology. As with the other classifications of pyoderma the principal organism is *Staphylococcus intermedius* but other micro-organisms may be found. Culture and sensitivity is mandatory when investigating deep pyoderma.

In contrast to superficial pyoderma the deep infections are easily recognised. Treatment is often difficult and prolonged and management is helped by classification into a number of subgroups. In addition to treating the infection a determined search for underlying disease should be made. Demodicosis[19] should be always be considered until ruled out by skin scrapings. Other causes such as hypothyroidism and hyperadrenocorticism should also be considered. Misuse of glucocorticoids for the symptomatic control of pruritic dermatoses such as atopy or internal disease such as musculoskeletal problems may also be contributory.

238

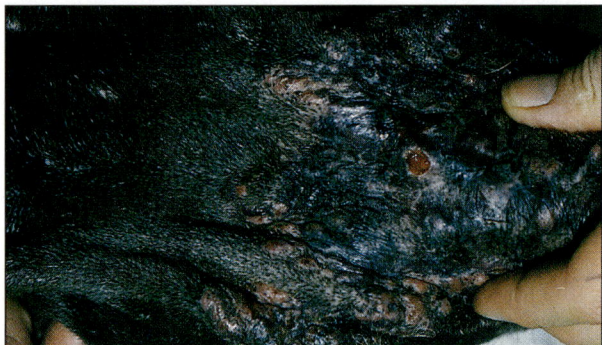

238 **Severe acne in a Great Dane.** The heavy discharge of purulent fluid from the fistulae is aesthetically unpleasant and unhygienic and systemic antibacterial therapy would be warranted.

Localised deep folliculitis and furunculosis

These conditions may occur as localised extensions of any surface pyoderma or superficial folliculitis wherein the follicle ruptures (furunculosis) liberating keratin debris and micro-organisms into the surrounding dermis. A number of more or less well-defined variants are recognised such as canine acne (**236–238**), nasal pyoderma (**239–241**), callus pyoderma (**242**), pododermatitis (**243–247**) and anal furunculosis (**248** and **249**). These conditions show little tendency to generalise and whilst local lymphadenopathy is common, other systemic signs are not, with the obvious exception of dyschezia due to anal furunculosis and lameness with multiple pododermatitis.

239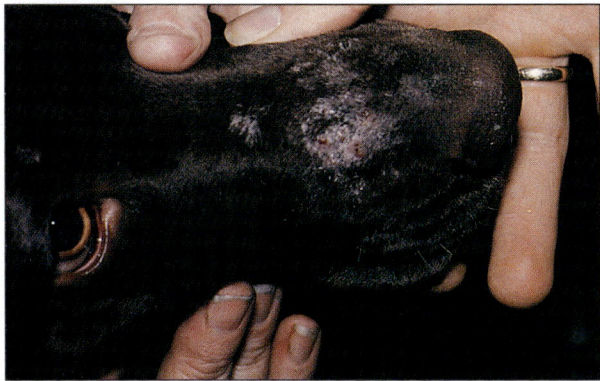

240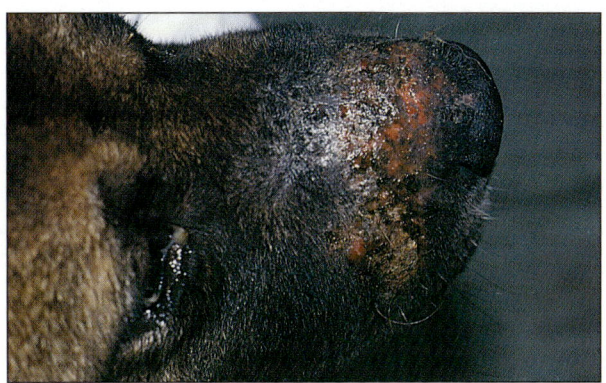

239   Nasal pyoderma may have a peracute onset and dogs exhibit severe discomfort. Although direct inoculation from penetrating wounds has been considered the principal cause of this condition a number of cases may result from insect bites and stings.

240   Nasal pyoderma in a Japanese Akita. Lesions in this case are more typical of deep infection with maceration of the surface tissue and fistula formation.

241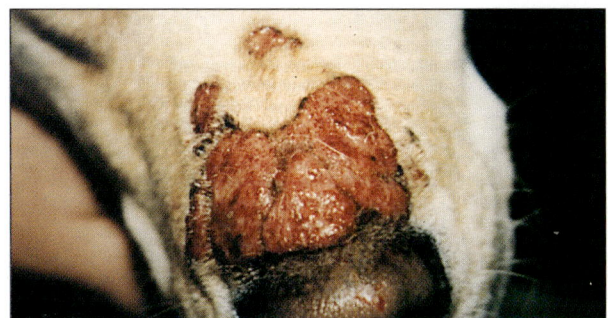

241   Nasal pyoderma will often result in scarring if the hair follicles are destroyed, as was the case in this Labrador retriever.

242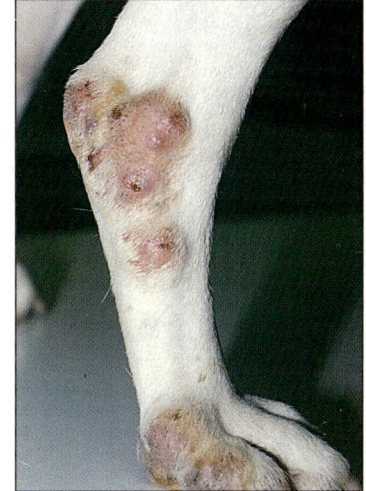

242   Callus pyoderma on the lateral surface of the hock joint. Note the discharging fistulae. Deep pododermatitis is visible on the lateral aspect of the foot.

Localised deep pyodermas are characterised by:
- Papules, pustules, discharging fistulae.
- Little tendency to progress laterally.
- Generally non-pruritic but may be very painful, particularly perianal and pedal lesions.

The general differential diagnoses for localised deep pyoderma are
- Demodicosis.
- Dermatophytosis.

For nasal pyoderma consider also scabies, actinic dermatitis, the autoimmune and immune-mediated dermatoses and zinc-responsive dermatoses.

For pododermatitis consider hookworm (*Ancylostoma* spp. and *Uncinaria* sp.), trombiculidiasis, autoimmune, immune mediated diseases, zinc responsive dermatoses and the hepatocutaneous syndrome.

The diagnosis is made by:
- Typical history and clinical signs.
- Skin scrapings to rule out demodicosis.

243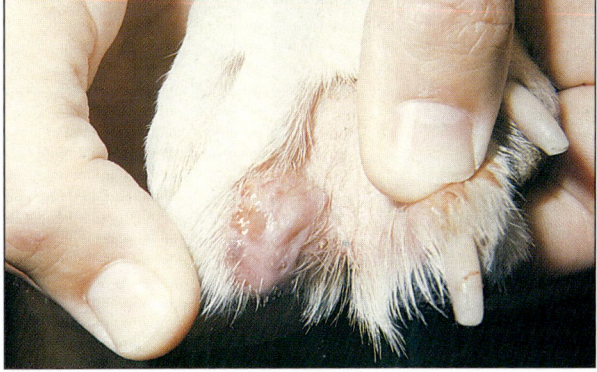

243   Pododermatitis is most frequently seen as an interdigital swelling which later fistulates, interdigital granuloma. Chronic cases may develop sinuses. Penetrating grass awns are a common cause.

244

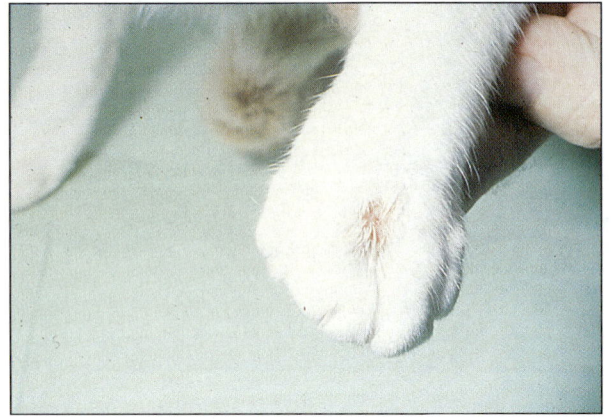

245

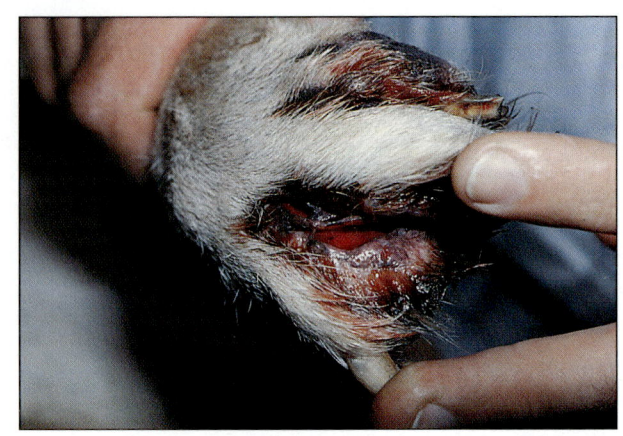

244 **Interdigital granuloma** is rare in the cat but occasional cases will be encountered.

245 **Severe interdigital pododermatitis** in a German shepherd dog.

246

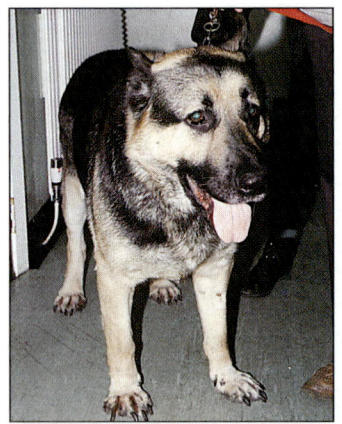

247

246 and 247 **Multiple pododermatitis** in a German shepherd dog. Note the very swollen feet. This dog was atopic and systemic glucocorticoids resulted in immunosuppression. The excessive weight of the dog was also attributable to the glucocorticoids. Close examination (**247**) of the clipped left fore foot reveals all the signs of deep pyoderma.

248

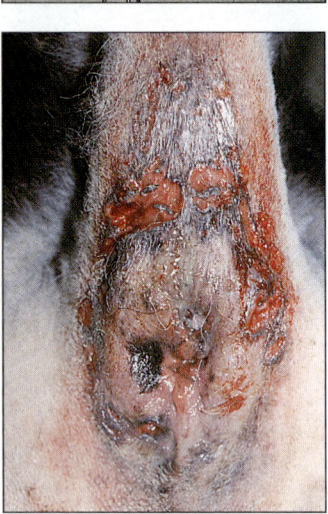

249

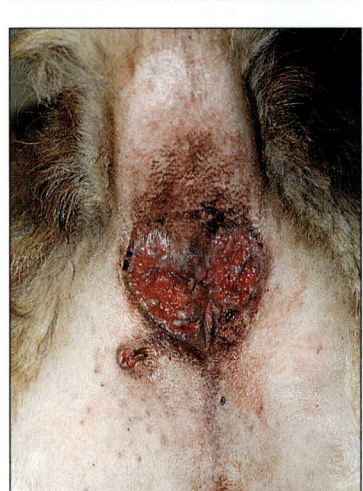

248 **Anal furunculosis** is seen almost exclusively in German shepherd dogs. Loss of cutaneous integrity with underunning and fistulation is common. The cause is not understood and cases may be very refractory to treatment.

249 **Anal furunculosis** involving the entire circumference of the anal ring. Severe lesions such as these may result in tenesmus and dyschezia.

250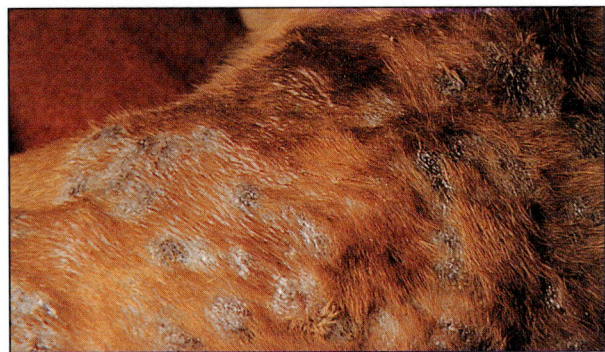

251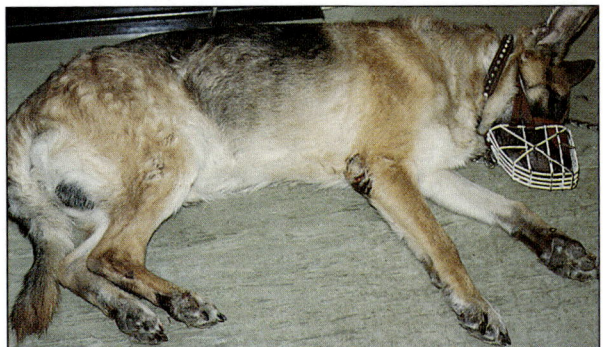

252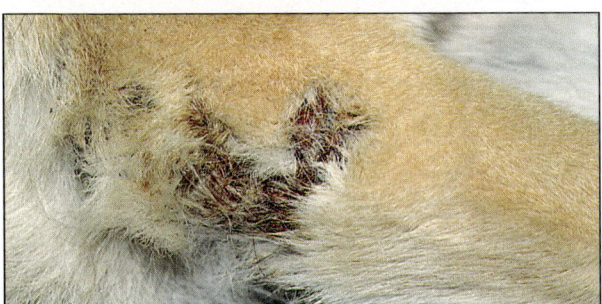

253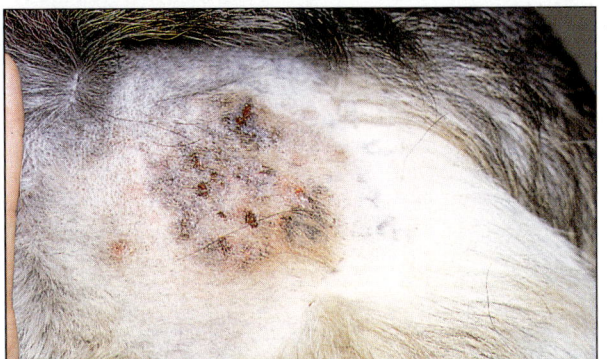

254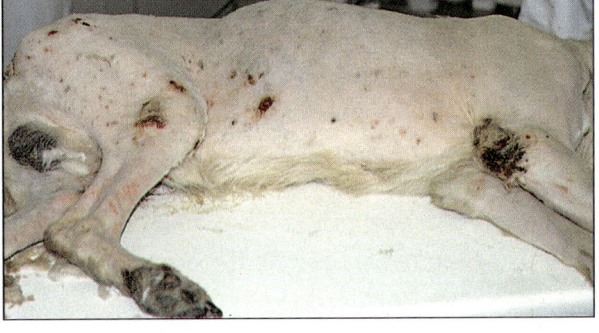

250   Generalised deep pyoderma may occur as an extension of a folliculitis and is often seen in cases of generalised demodectic mange. Numerous raised, hyperpigmented alopecic patches associated with fistulae on this foreleg of a Boxer are typical.

251–254   German shepherd dog pyoderma may be difficult to visualise in the unclipped dog. This German shepherd dog has been sedated for examination and only the right elbow was readily abnormal to the owner. Close examination of the elbow (**252**) revealed typical signs of deep pyoderma. Another area was found on the skin overlying the tuber coxae (**253**). The full extent of the infection was only apparent after a body clip had been performed (**254**). Multiple lesions of deep pyoderma are visible.

Generalised deep pyoderma

Generalised deep pyoderma may occur in any dog which is immunoincompetent and is most often seen in animals with demodicosis (**250**). A clinically well-defined but otherwise poorly understood condition known as German shepherd dog pyoderma is a variant of generalised deep pyoderma[13,20] (**251–254**). In contrast to the above group these conditions are frequently associated with systemic signs and septicaemia and bacteraemia are often encountered. Lesions may be hard to see under a thick coat and extensive clipping will allow assessment of the degree of infection and also simplify topical cleansing.

Generalised deep pyoderma is characterised by:
- Systemic signs such as pyrexia and lymphadenopathy.
- Discharging fistulae, sinus formation, bleeding and crust formation.
- Pruritus is variable but pain is often present.

The differential diagnoses are:
- Demodicosis.
- Dermatophytosis and subcutaneous mycoses.

The diagnosis is made by:
- Skin scrapings to rule out ectoparasites.
- Impression smears.
- Bacteriological culture.
- Histopathological examination of biopsy material.

255

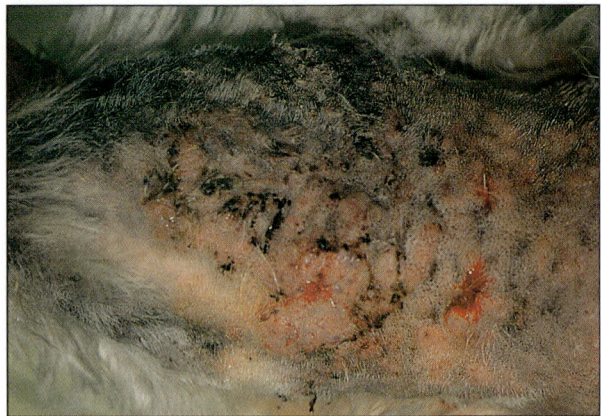

256

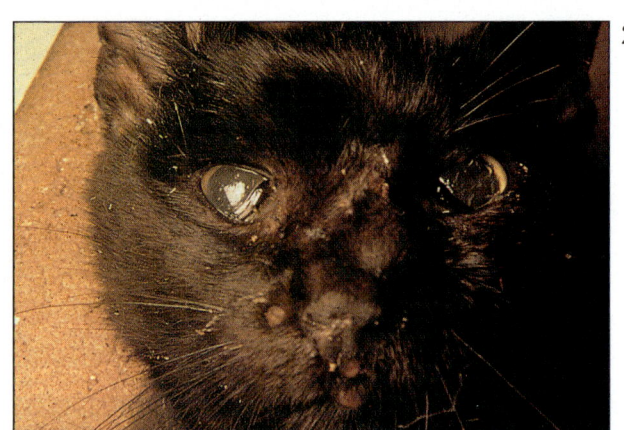

255   Cellulitis on the ventral neck of a West Highland White terrier with generalised demodicosis. There is multiple fistula formation; incipient lesions are apparent as greyish areas on the skin. The area of the infection is poorly defined.

Cellulitis

Cellulitis is seen occasionally following cat bites and in some cases of deep pyoderma. The infections are poorly localised and are not confined to tissue planes. Demodicosis is often associated with cellulitis (**255**).

257

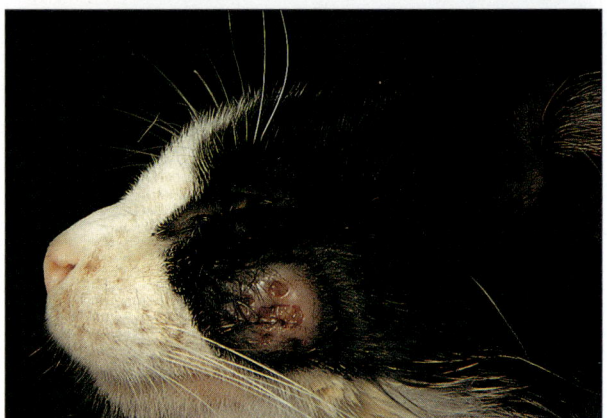

258

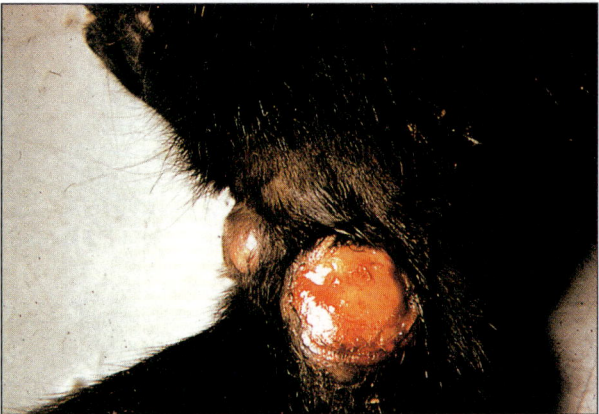

Cellulitis is characterised by:
- Systemic signs such as pyrexia and local lymphadenopathy.
- Poorly defined swelling and maceration of the skin.
- The presence of discharging fistulae and sinus formation.

The differential diagnoses are:
- Demodicosis.
- Subcutaneous mycoses.
- Atypical mycobacterial infections.
- Mycosis fungoides.

The diagnosis is made by:
- Skin scrapings.
- Bacteriological culture.
- Aspiration and impression smears.
- Histopathological examination of biopsy material.

256–258   Feline leprosy is caused by the rat leprosy bacillus *M. lepraemurium*. Rapidly growing, painless, mobile nodules which may ulcerate are typically found on the head (**256** and **257**) and limbs (**258**).

259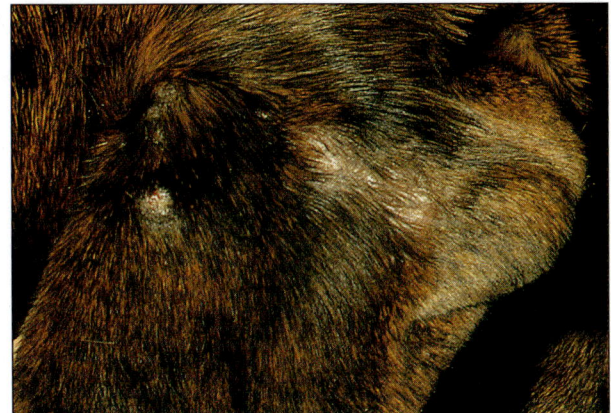

260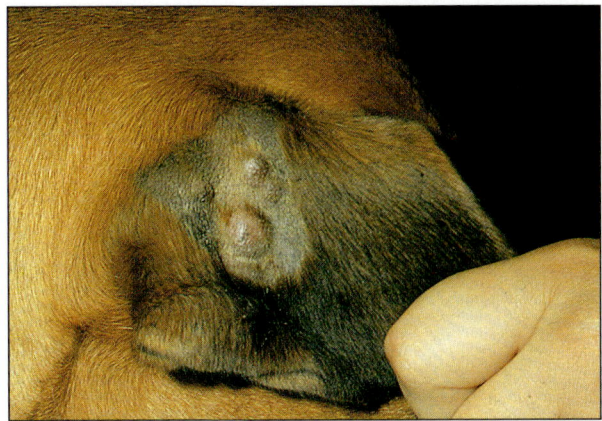

259 and 260   Canine leprosy. Multiple, painless nodules on the pinna of a Boxer and a Foxhound. (Illustrations courtesy S. E. Shaw.)

Mycobacterial infections

These are uncommon in small animals and may be classified into three groups.[10,14] On rare occasions cutaneous tuberculosis may be diagnosed and in these cases the classic species of mycobacteria (*M. tuberculosis*, *M. bovis* and *M. avium*) are isolated. These cases have a poor prognosis and a zoonotic potential and euthanasia is recommended. The second group comprises infections due to the obligate pathogen *M. lepraemurium* which have been reported in cats ('feline leprosy') and present as rapidly growing, mobile, painless, cutaneous nodules which often ulcerate (**256–258**). There may be a predilection for the head and limbs. Canine leprosy is associated with an unidentified mycobacterium and presents as nodules similar to those seen in feline leprosy. The nodules have been recorded on the pinnae of boxers and foxhounds (**259** and **260**). The final group of diseases are due to infection with members of Runyon's Group IV mycobacteria. These include *M. fortuitum*, *M. chelonei*, *M. phlei*, *M. smegmatis* and *M. vaccae* which are ubiquitous organisms causing lesions collectively known as the atypical mycobacterial granulomas. The organisms are introduced by bites or penetrating wounds and are most commonly found on the lateral and ventral trunk and the limbs. They typically present as single or multiple ulcers or as draining tracts (**261–264**).

Mycobacterial infections are rare and are characterised by:
- Chronic granulomatous lesions which may be accompanied by discharge and ulceration.
- Local lymphadenopathy.
- Little tendency to spread systemically although local infiltration is often seen.

The differential diagnoses are:
- Chronic abscessation in immunosuppressed individuals.
- Subcutaneous abscesses due to botriomycosis, actinomycosis or nocardiosis.
- Subcutaneous fungal infections.
- Ulcerative neoplasia.

The diagnosis is made by:
- Microscopic examination of smears.
- Histopathological examination of biopsy specimens.
- Culture and sensitivity.

261

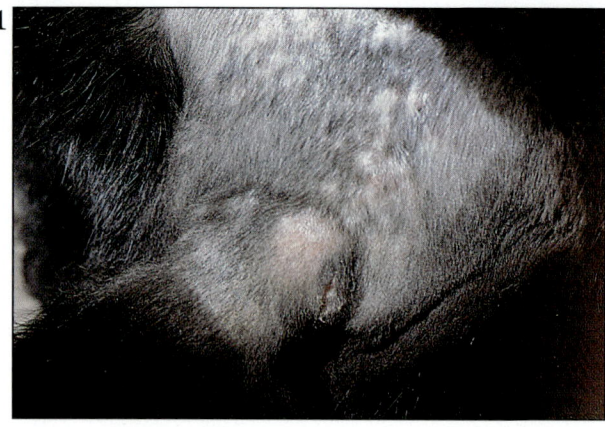

261   Atypical mycobacterial infection in a cat due to *M. fortuitum* usually presents as a chronic abscess which may discharge.

262

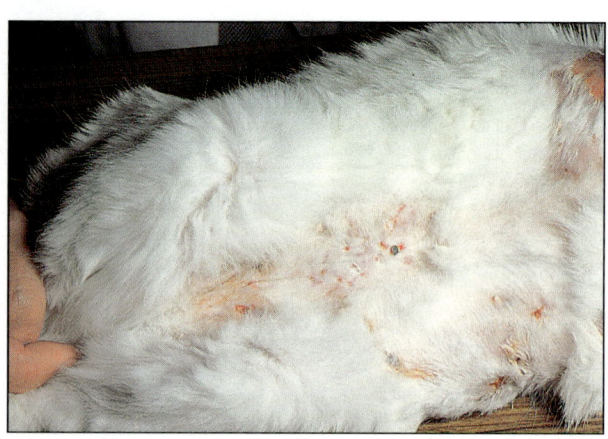

262   Atypical mycobacterial infection in a cat due to *M. smegmatis* produces a pyogranulomatous panniculitis seen here on the ventral abdomen.

263

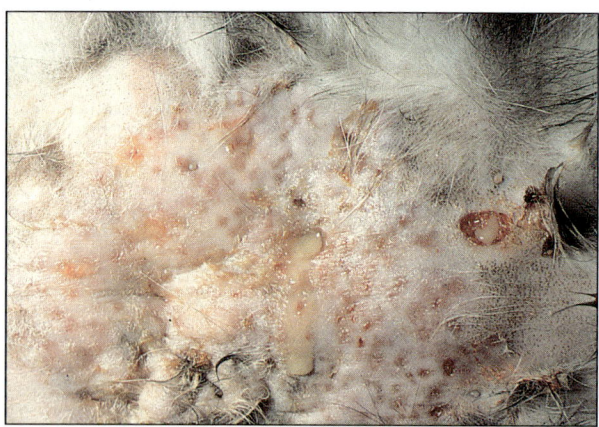

263   Atypical mycobacterial infection due to *M. smegmatis* with grossly thickened skin and discharging fistulae.

264

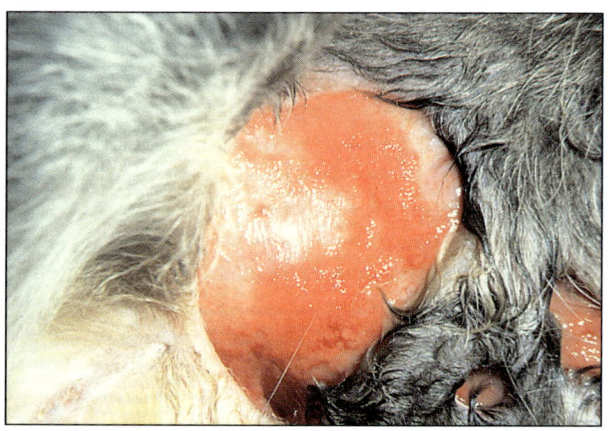

264   Infection with atypical mycobacteria may be refractory to treatment. Radical excision in this case was followed by recurrence of large non-healing ulcers one year after surgery.

Subcutaneous abscesses

Cat bite abscess is common and is typically treated by establishing drainage and administering systemic antibacterial agents for 3 to 5 days. The most commonly-isolated bacteria are *Pasteurella multocida*, *Bacteroides* spp. and β-haemolytic streptococci. Since β-lactamase producing staphylococci are not commonly involved depot ampicillin injections are frequently curative. Lesions are most common on the head, limbs and dorsal trunk (**265** and **266**). Occasionally recurrent or poorly responsive abscesses will be encountered. Infection with feline leukaemia virus or feline immunosuppressive virus should be considered in these cases. In addition there is a report of bacterial *L*-forms causing chronic abscesses unresponsive to all antibacterial treatment with the exception of tetracycline.[2]

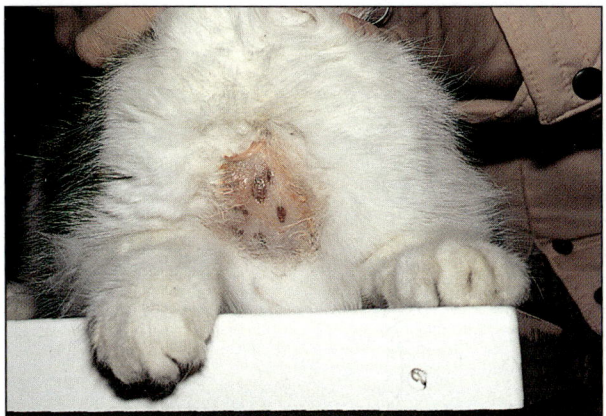

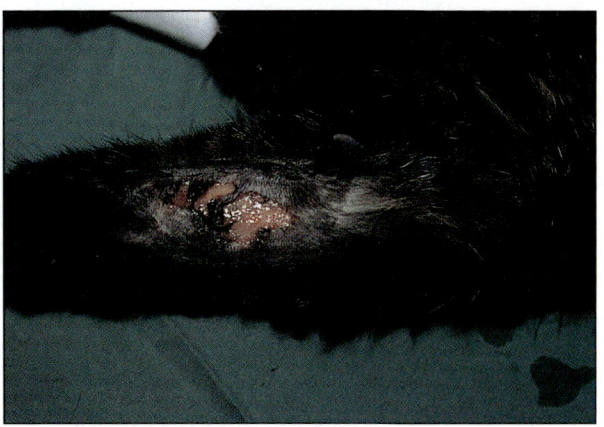

265 Cat bite abscess on the ventral neck of a cat. The puncture wounds are readily visible.

266 Cat bite abscess may not resolve rapidly. This abscess on the foreleg of a cat was still open three months after initial presentation. Culture and sensitivity revealed a mixed growth of *Pasteurella multocida* and coagulase-negative staphylococcus. Tests for feline leukaemia virus and feline immunosuppressive virus were negative.

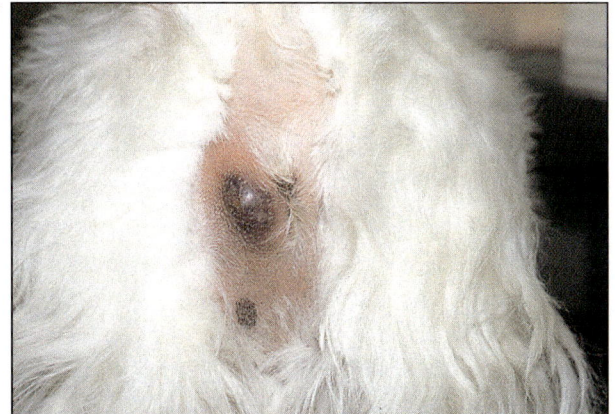

267 Anal sac abscessation. The anal sacs are a common site of spontaneous abscess formation in the dog. They rapidly come to a head and usually present having just burst.

Dog bite wounds, like cat bite wounds, principally occur on the head and extremities.[2,8] The anal sacs are common sites of spontaneous abscess formation in the dog (**267**). They are usually very painful. Botriomycosis, actinomycosis and nocardiosis are rare pyogranulomatous infections at the inoculation site of transient or contaminant bacteria into the skin. They follow bites and penetrating wounds and are characterised by subcutaneous abscessation and draining tracts. Discharges frequently contain tissue grains, white in botriomycosis and yellow in actinomycosis. Nocardiosis is often associated with a reddish brown discharge (**268–270**).

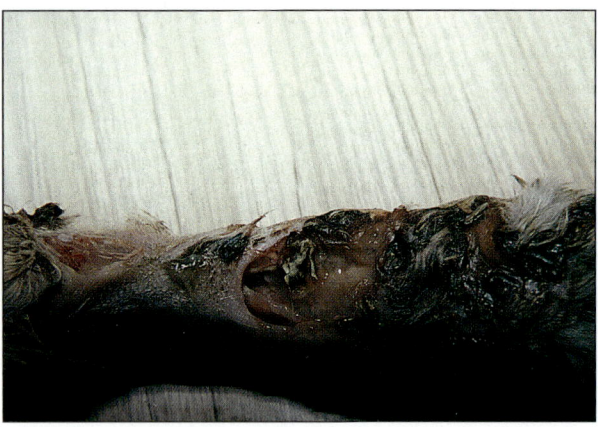

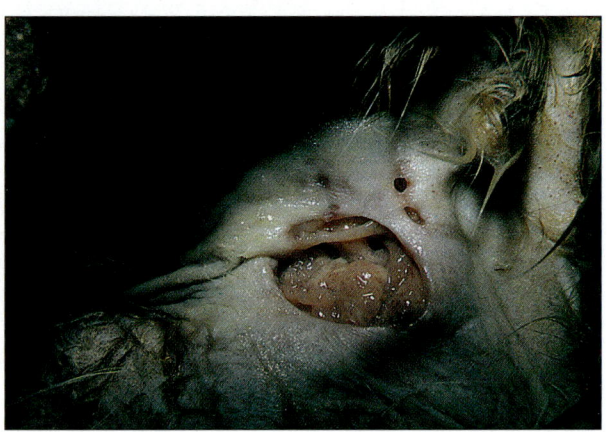

268 *Nocardia asteroides* is rare in the dog and cat and usually presents as non-healing discharging ulcers on the trunk and limbs. Area of chronic ulceration on the medial aspect of the hind limb of a cat.

269 Nocardiosis in a cat. Deep discharging ulcerative lesion on the medial aspect of the hind limb proximal to **268**.

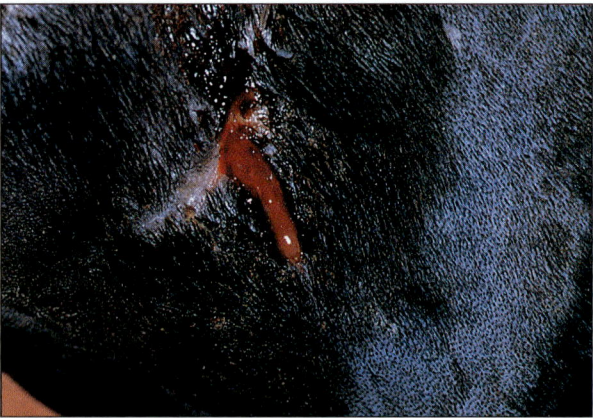

270 Reddish colour of discharge in a case of canine nocardiosis. (Illustration courtesy of R. Bond.)

Subcutaneous abscessation is characterised by:
- Usually a history of bite or penetrating wound.
- Varying degrees of abscessation, discharge and cellulitis.
- There may be a fluctuating course to the diseases with alternating healing and discharge.
- Pyrexia and pain may be apparent.

Differential diagnoses are:
- Atypical mycobacterial infections.
- Subcutaneous mycoses.

Diagnosis is made by:
- Consideration of the history and clinical signs.
- Microscopic examination of discharges.
- Histopathological examinations of biopsies.
- Culture and sensitivity.

Bacterial dermatoses of other animals

A number of micro-organisms, principally *Staphylococcus aureus*, have been isolated from lesions on small mammals although primary bacterial skin disease is rare. The vast majority of the diseases in which staphylococci are implicated are multifactorial, with hygiene and management playing a major part in the aetiology.[4,6] Common causes include bite wounds, puncture wounds, abrasions and urine scald. Some conditions are less easy to comprehend and 'wet nose' of gerbils, 'wet dewlap' in rabbits, ulcerative dermatitis in rats and chronic pododermatitis in rabbits and guinea-pigs are associated with, amongst other things, chronic trauma, poor housing, social stress and continual wetting. Chronic dental disease or conjunctivitis may result in moist lesions from which *Pseudomonas* spp. may be isolated in addition to *Staphylococcus aureus*.

Subcutaneous abscesses, septicaemia and internal abscessation (staphylococcosis) may be seen in individual pet rabbits or as a contagious disease in commercial rabbit colonies.[16] The disease carries a poor prognosis as staphylococcosis appears to be precipitated by stress in these cases.

In reptiles and lower vertebrates the major pathogens associated with dermatoses are *Aeromonas* spp. and *Pseudomonas* spp. which rapidly colonise abrasions, burns and wounds. Cellulitis ('red leg') is a common sequel to compromised barrier function and secondary infection. As with dermatoses associated with *Staphylococcus* spp. in mammals, it is important to search for the underlying cause as well as treating the infection.

References

1. Berg, J. N., Wendell, D. E., Vogelweid, C. and Fales, W. H. (1984). Identification of the major coagulase-positive Staphylococcus sp. of dogs as *Staphylococcus intermedius*. *American Journal of Veterinary Research*, **45**: 1307–1309.

2. Carro, T., Pederson, N. C., Beaman, B. L. and Munn, R. (1989). Subcutaneous abscesses and arthritis caused by a probable bacterial L-form in cats. *Journal of the American Veterinary Medical Association*, **194**: 1583–1588.

3. Codner, E. C. (1988). Classifying and diagnosing cases of canine pyoderma *Veterinary Medicine*, **83**: 984–994.

4. Collins, R. R. (1987). Dermatologic Disorders of Common Small Nondomestic Animals. In: Nesbitt, G. H. (Ed.) *Contemporary Issues in Small Animal Practice, Dermatology*, pp. 235–294. Churchill Livingstone, New York.

5. Cowell, A. K. and Penwick, R. C. (1989). Dog bite wounds: a study of 93 cases. *Compendium on Continuing Education*, **11**: 313–318.

6. Harkness, J. E. and Wagner, J. E. (1983). *The Biology and Medicine of Rabbits and Rodents*, pp. 169–171. Lea and Febiger, Philadelphia.

7. Ihrke, P. J. (1990). Integumentary Infections. In: Greene, G. E. (Ed.) *Infectious Diseases of the Dog and Cat*, pp. 72–78. W. B. Saunders, Philadelphia.

8. Kirpensteijn, J. and Fingland, R. B. (1992). Cutaneous actinomycosis and nocardiosis in dogs: 48 cases (1980–1990). *Journal of the American Veterinary Medical Association*, **201**: 917–920.

9. Kelly, P. J., Mason, P. R., Els, J. and Matthewman, L. A. (1992). Pathogens in dog bite wounds in dogs in Harare, Zimbabwe. *Veterinary Record*, **131**: 464–466.

10. Kunkle, G. A., Gulbas, N. K., Fadok, V., Halliwell, R. E. W. and Connelly, M. (1983). Rapidly growing mycobacteria as a cause of cutaneous granulomas: report of five cases. *Journal of the American Animal Hospital Association*, **19**: 513–521.

11. Mason, I. S. and Lloyd, D. H. (1989). The role of allergy in the development of canine pyoderma. *Journal of Small Animal Practice*, **30**: 216–218.

12. Medleau, L. and Blue, J. L. (1988). Frequency and antimicrobial susceptibility of *Staphylococcus* spp. isolated from feline skin lesions. *Journal of the American Veterinary Medical Association*, **193**: 1080–1081.

13. Miller, W. H. (1991). Deep pyoderma in two German shepherd dogs associated with a cell-mediated immunodeficiency. *Journal of the American Animal Hospital Association*, **27**: 513–517.

14. Monroe, W. E. and Chickering, W. R. (1988). Atypical mycobacterial infections in cats. *Compendium on Continuing Education*, **10**: 1044–1047.

15. Noble, W. C. (1989). Bacterial Skin Infections in Domestic Animals and Man. In: von Tscharner, C and Halliwell, R. E. W. (Eds.) *Advances in Veterinary Dermatology*, **1**: 312–326.

16. Okerman, L., Devriese, L. A., Maertens, L., Okerman, F. and Godard, C. (1984). Cutaneous staphylococcosis in rabbits. *Veterinary Record*, **114**: 313–315.

17. Reinke, S. I., Stannard, A. A., Ihrke, P. J. and Reinke, J. D. (1987). Histopathologic features of pyotraumatic dermatitis. *Journal of the American Veterinary Medical Association*, **190**: 57–60.

18. Rosser, E. J and Ihrke, P. J. (1983). Infectious Skin Diseases. In: Pratt, P. W. (Ed.) *Feline Medicine*, pp. 562–567. American Veterinary Publications Inc, California.

19. White, S. D. and Ihrke, P. J. (1987). Pyoderma. In: Nesbitt, G. H. (Ed.) *Contemporary Issues in Small Animal Practice, Dermatology*, pp. 95–121. Churchill Livingstone, New York.

20. Wisselink, M. A., Willemse, A. and Koeman, J. P. (1985). Deep pyoderma in the German shepherd dog. *Journal of the American Animal Hospital Association*, **21**: 773–776.

Chapter 6:

Viral, protozoal and rickettsial skin diseases

Viral skin diseases

There are a number of viruses associated with dermatoses in dogs and cats. Some, such as Aujeszky's disease and contagious ecthyma, are extremely rare. Others such as Feline Leukaemia Virus and Feline Immunosuppressive Virus are more common, but are not associated with cutaneous lesions in their own right: they cause immunosuppression and infected cats may suffer from recurrent abscesses, chronic paronychia and non-healing wounds. Feline Sarcoma Virus is associated with multicentric fibrosarcoma in young animals but is not associated with fibrosarcoma in adult cats. Both feline herpes virus and feline calicivirus infections have been associated with ulcerated skin lesions and with swollen footpads. In most cases there has been concurrent viral upper respiratory tract infection.

In dogs and cats there are three viruses that are associated with more specific skin lesions; poxvirus infection in cats, canine distemper virus and canine papovavirus. It is unlikely that viral diseases will be encountered in the smaller mammals and reptiles which are kept as pets, although there are conditions, such as myxomatosis, which are associated with cutaneous lesions.[2,5]

Poxvirus

Feline poxvirus is presumed to originate from a rodent reservoir and to be inoculated by bite wounds.[1] The initial lesion is usually found on the anterior part of the body and is typically a small plaque-like granuloma or ulceration (**271–274**). Most cases exhibit generalised secondary lesions within 14 days. These are small papules which ulcerate and then crust. A few cases exhibit systemic disease, in particular respiratory disorders. Concurrent immunosuppression, viral or iatrogenic, is more likely to be associated with severe systemic disease and even death. The disease is confined to Europe and exhibits a regional distribution. There is also a seasonal bias, with peak inci-

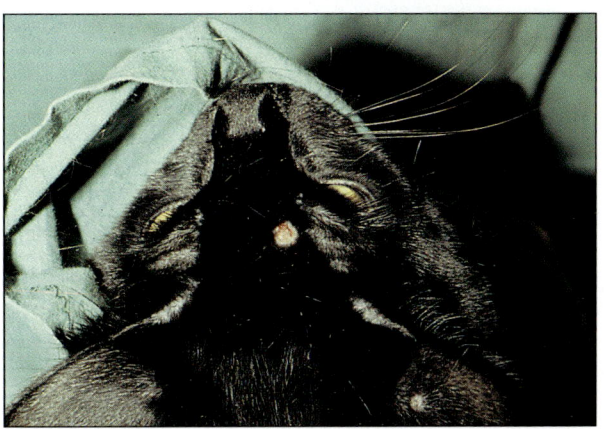

271

271 Feline poxvirus infection. Multiple, ulcerated nodules on the head of a cat.

272

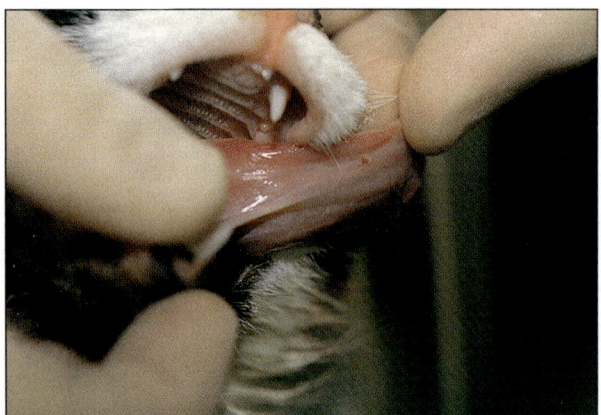

273

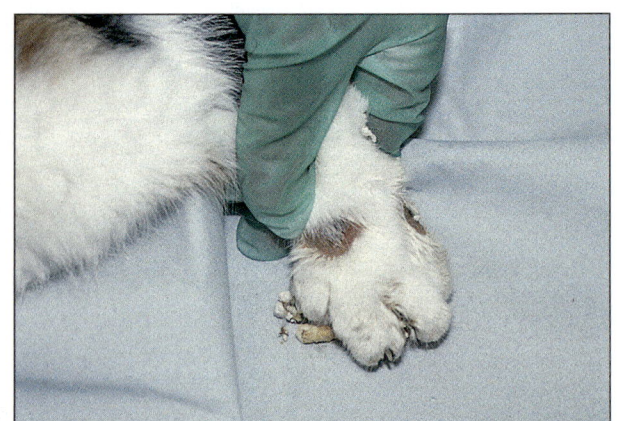

274

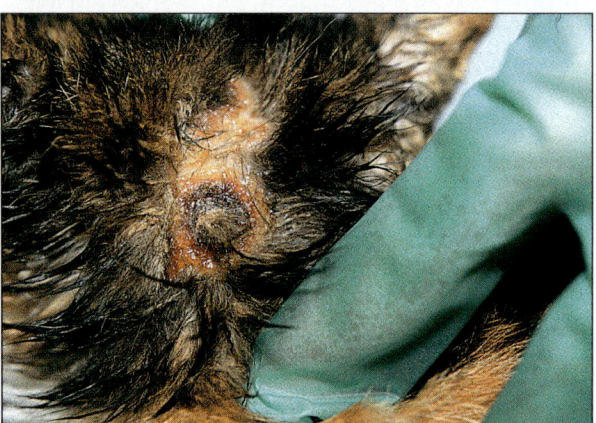

275

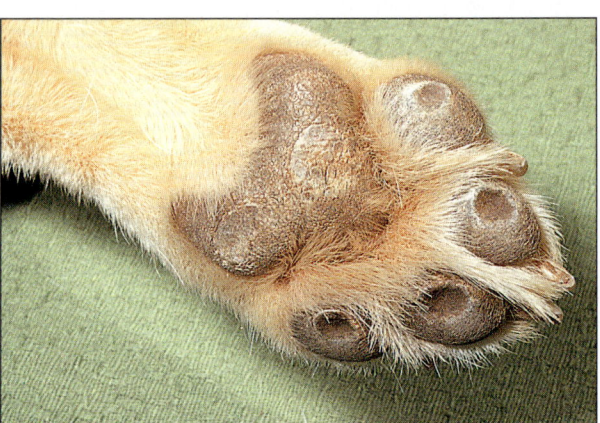

272–274   Feline poxvirus infection. A primary lesion (a small vesicle) on the ventral aspect of the tongue (**272**). More commonly secondary lesions such as haemorrhagic erosions (**273**) and crusted papules (**274**) are seen.

275   Canine distemper virus infection. Circular areas of hyperkeratosis on the footpads of a dog with 'hardpad'.

dence in the late summer and autumn. Diagnosis is based on local knowledge, clinical signs, serological measurement of rising titres, demonstration of the viral particles in infected material by electron microscopy and by virus isolation. The disease has a zoonotic potential and care should be taken when handling infected material.

Canine distemper virus

Canine distemper virus infection may be accompanied by hyperkeratosis of the planum nasale and, often, the footpads, hence the synonym of 'hardpad' for canine distemper virus infection. Normally the surface of the footpad is rounded and the individual papillae are prominent. With hardpad the central area of the footpad becomes flat and smooth, the papillae disappear and hyperkeratotic plaque forms (**275**). The pads become so hard that an affected dog produces a distinct tapping sound when walking over bare floors. If recovery from distemper virus infection occurs the footpads may return to normal but the nasal changes are usually permanent.

Diagnosis is readily apparent if canine distemper virus infection is recognised. Major differential diagnoses that should be borne in mind are zinc-responsive dermatosis, idiopathic nasodigital hyperkeratosis and pemphigus foliaceus.

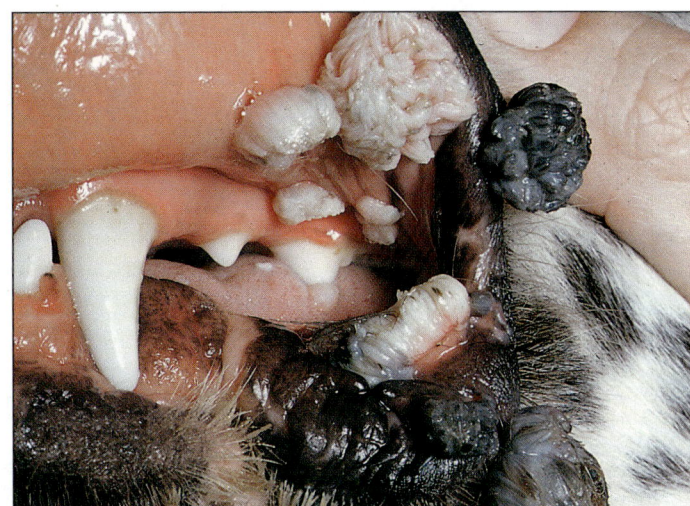

276   Canine viral papillomatosis. White proliferative growths on the oral mucosa and gingival margins.

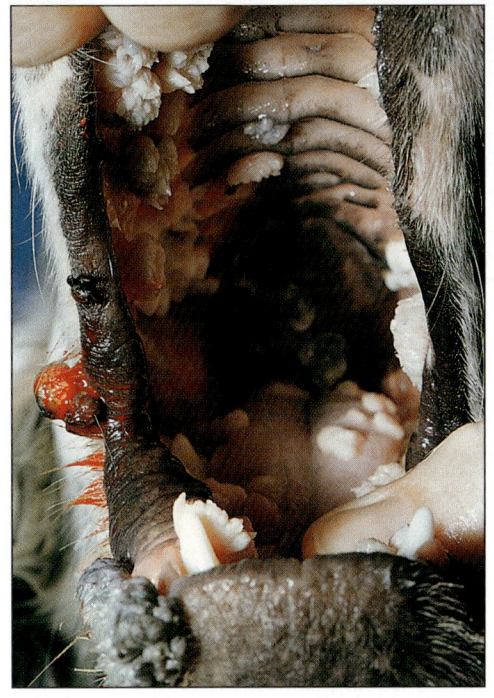

277

277   Canine viral papillomatosis. Lesions on the tongue, gums, hard palate and the oropharynx. Notice the haemorrhagic appearance of the lesions at the right oral commissure. Papillomas are friable and bleed easily.

Canine viral papillomatosis

This is a common disease in young dogs and is caused by a DNA papovavirus. Infection is transmitted by direct contact and the incubation period is at least 30 days. Lesions have a characteristic appearance and are most frequently found on the oral mucosae, the lips, the conjunctivae and the eyelids (**276** and **277**). Very large lesions, or close apposition of many smaller ones, may impair prehension and mastication of food. Larger lesions in particular may be very friable and are prone to haemorrhag. Spontaneous regression usually occurs but may take manymonths. Animals which recover have lifelong immunity. Note that the smaller, usually discrete, but often multiple, papillomas in old dogs are not of viral aetiology.

278 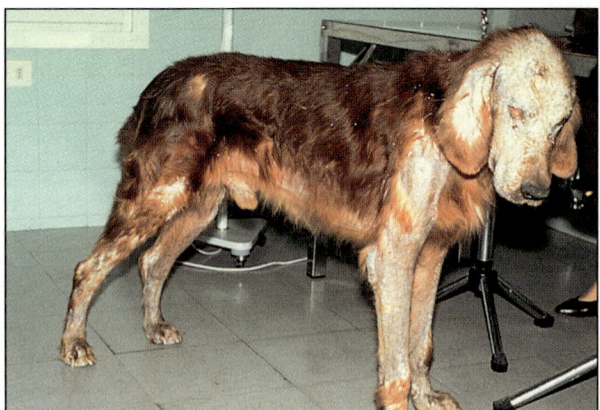 **279**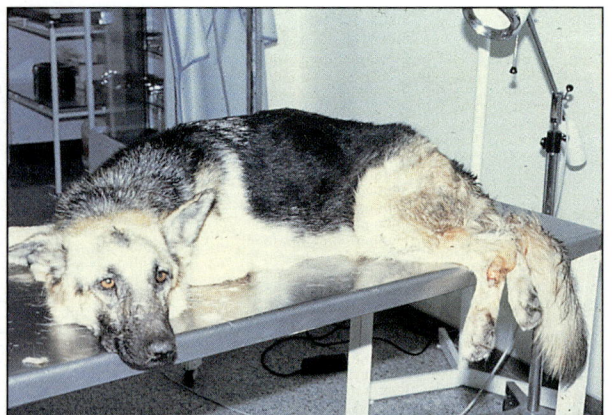

280 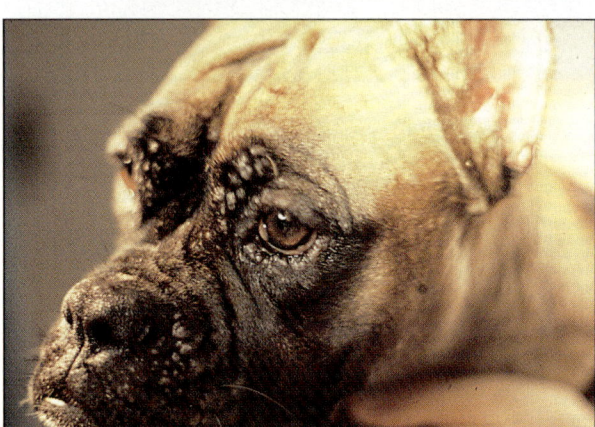 **281**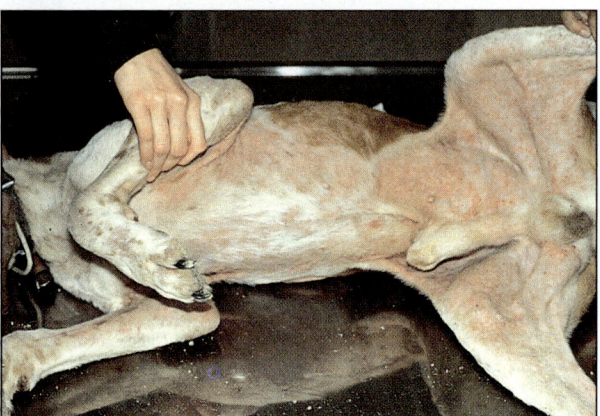

278–281 **Leishmaniasis.** Bilaterally symmetrical alopecia, hyperkeratosis and desquamation in an Irish setter (**278**), ulcerative dermatosis form in a German shepherd dog (**279**), generalised nodular form in a Boxer bitch (**280**) and generalised pustular form in a mongrel (**281**). (Illustrations from Ferrer, L., Rabanal, R., Fondevila, D., Ramos, J. A. and Domingo, M. [1988]. Skin lesions in canine leishmaniasis. *Journal of Small Animal Practice*, **29**: 381–388.)

Protozoal diseases

Canine leishmaniasis

Leishmaniasis is a severe and often fatal disease of dogs, and occasionally cats, which occurs in countries of the Mediterranean basin, the Middle and Far East, South America and in some States of the USA. The disease is caused by infection with the protozoal parasites *Leishmania donovani* and *L. chagasi*. The disease is transmitted by bloodsucking sandflies of the genus *Phlebotomus* in the Old World and *Lutzomia* in the New.

Leishmaniasis is a systemic disease although clinical signs may be confined to the skin and mucous membranes only in some cases. The organism multiplies within macrophages and other cells of the mononuclear-phagocyte system causing granulomatous lesions. Systemic signs include pyrexia, weight loss, occasional epistaxis and lymphadenopathy. The disease has a zoonotic potential.

Skin lesions may be of four main types[3]:

- Alopecia and an exfoliative dermatitis which is often symmetrical in distribution. The classic sign is of periorbital alopecia (**278**).
- Ulcerative dermatoses, particularly over the limb joints, occasionally with facial alopecia (**279**).
- Generalised non-ulcerated nodules (**280**).
- Bacteriologically sterile pustules, predominantly over the trunk (**281**).

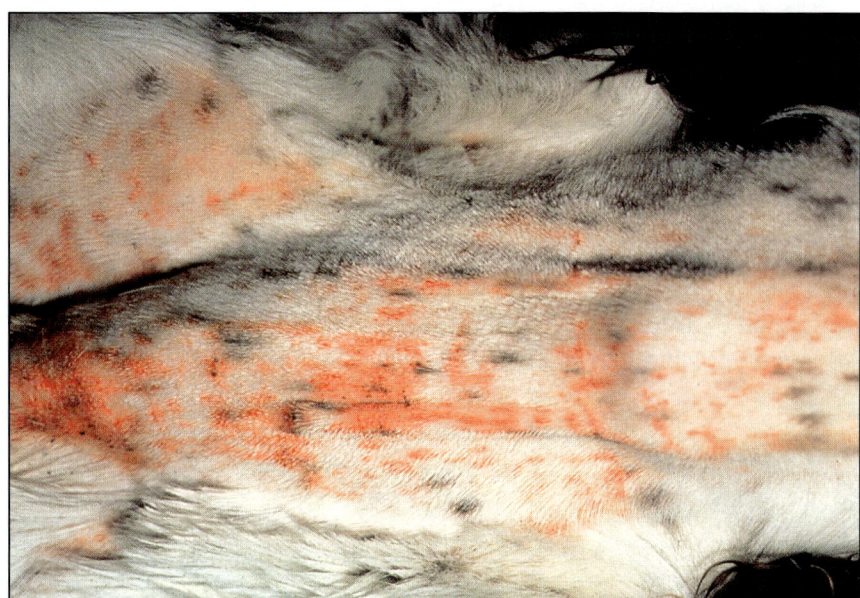

282 Ehrlichiosis.
Cutaneous lesions are due to a loss of vascular integrity resulting in petechiae and ecchymoses. (Illustration courtesy E. B. Breitschwerdt.)

Leishmaniasis is characterised by:
- Chronic dermatoses in association with wasting and lymphadenopathy.

Major differential diagnoses are:
- Demodicosis.
- Sarcoptic mange.
- Systemic lupus erythematosus.
- Mycosis fungoides.

The diagnosis is made by:
- Consideration of the history and clinical signs.
- Demonstration of the causal organism in aspirates and in sections.
- Serology.

Rickettsial diseases

Rickettsiae are tick-borne, obligate intracellular parasites of canine mononuclear cells. Two members of the group, *Ehrlichia canis* and *Rickettsia rickettsii,* have been associated with cutaneous lesions in addition to systemic disease in dogs, ehrlichiosis and Rocky Mountain spotted fever (RMSF) respectively.[4,6] The diseases are acute and cause rather non-specific signs such as pyrexia, anorexia and lymphadenopathy. Some 20% of cases exhibit petechiae and ecchymoses (**282**). It has been suggested that the cutaneous lesions in RMSF are a manifestation of vasculitis whereas those seen in ehrlichiosis are due to thrombocytopaenia. Diagnosis is suggested by clinical signs and laboratory findings. The organisms may be demonstrated in peripheral blood smears and there are also serological tests available to confirm the diagnosis.

References

1. Bennett, M., Gaskell, C. J., Gaskell, R. M., Baxby D. and Gruffyd-Jones, T. J. (1986). Poxvirus infection in the domestic cat: Some clinical and epidemiological observations. *Veterinary Record*, **118**: 387–390.

2. Collins, R. R. (1987). Dermatologic Disorders of Common Small Nondomestic Animals. In: Nesbitt, G. H. (Ed.) *Contemporary Issues in Small Animal Practice, Dermatology*, pp. 235–294. Churchill Livingstone, New York.

3. Ferrer, L., Rabanal, R., Fondevila, D., Ramos, J. A. and Domingo, M. (1988). Skin lesions in canine leishmaniasis. *Journal of Small Animal Practice*, **29**: 381–388.

4. French, A. (1988). Canine ehrlichiosis. In: Grunsell, G. S. C., Raw, M-E. and Hill, F. W. G. (Eds.) *The Veterinary Annual 28 edition,* pp. 196–201. Scientechnica, London.

5. Ganière, J-P., Gourreau, J-M., Montabord, D., Rive, M. and Chantal, J. (1991). Myxomatosis of the depilated Angora rabbit. A preliminary study. *Veterinary Dermatology*, **2**: 11–15.

6. Green, C. E. (1986). Rocky Mountain spotted fever and ehrlichiosis. In: Kirk, R. W. (Ed.) *Current Veterinary Therapy, IX* pp. 1080–1084. W. B. Saunders, Philadelphia.

Chapter 7

Fungal skin diseases

Introduction

Fungal infections of the skin are classified according to the depth of the infection, in a similar fashion to the classification of pyoderma. Thus infections are described as superficial, sub-cutaneous and intermediate or systemic.

Superficial mycoses
The most important of these is dermatophytosis, or ringworm, but includes superficial infections with *Malassezia pachydermatis* and *Candida* spp.

Subcutaneous and Intermediate mycoses
Including eumycotic mycetoma, phaeohyphomycosis, prototheocosis and sporotrichosis.

Systemic mycoses
Including cryptococcosis.

In contrast to the causal organisms of pyoderma, some of the fungal organisms have the ability to behave as primary pathogens and can infect normal skin and hair in the absence of predisposing factors. Nevertheless, since humoral and cell-mediated immunity is responsible for the host defence and, ultimately, for limiting the infection, factors such as specie, age and health of the host will have an effect on the severity, clinical signs of and course of the disease. Thus, young animals are considered susceptible to dermatophytosis because of decreased immunological ability.

The species of pathogen is also important in that infection with less well host-adapted fungi, such as the geophilic *Microsporum gypseum* for example, is usually more inflammatory than infection with a relatively well host-adapted species such as *Microsporum canis*. For this reason, diseases are classified as much by causal organism as by depth of infection.

Many of the fungal infections have the ability to cause zoonotic infection and this should be borne in mind when handling infected animals. Although many cases of dermatophytosis will spontaneously resolve it is this potential for zoonotic infection that makes treatment mandatory.

Superficial mycoses

Dermatophytosis is an infection of the keratinised cells of the stratum corneum, the hair and the claws by fungi of the genera *Microsporum, Trichophyton* or *Epidermophyton*. The term 'ringworm' is often applied to infections in this category; it is not always descriptive of the lesions as they occur in animals. The vast majority of dermatophytosis in small animals is due to infection by one of three species of fungi; *Microsporum canis, Microsporum gypseum* and *Trichophyton mentagrophytes*. The incidence of dermatophyte infection is relatively low in cool, temperate climates, but is considerably higher in tropical and subtropical regions where there is also a higher incidence of florid forms of infection.

Infections with yeast such as *Malassezia pachydermatis* and *Candida albicans* are uncommon and, in contrast to dermatophytosis, usually found to be secondary to an underlying condition, atopy or defects in immunocompetence for example.

Diagnosis of the superficial fungal infections is suggested by consideration of the history and clinical examination and may be supported by the microscopic examination of skin scrapings. Histopathological examination of biopsy samples may support the diagnosis of dermatophytosis but definitive diagnosis and identification of the species can only be achieved by fungal culture and identification of colony characteristics and macroaleurospores.

283

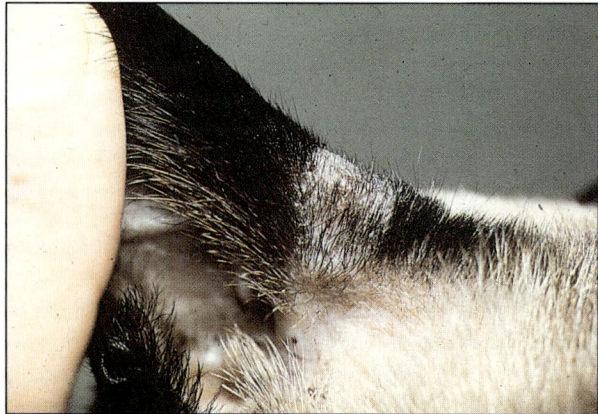

283 *Microsporum canis* infection. Classic appearance of dermatophytosis on a cat. Note the focal area of scale and alopecia. There is a central area of hyperpigmentation.

284

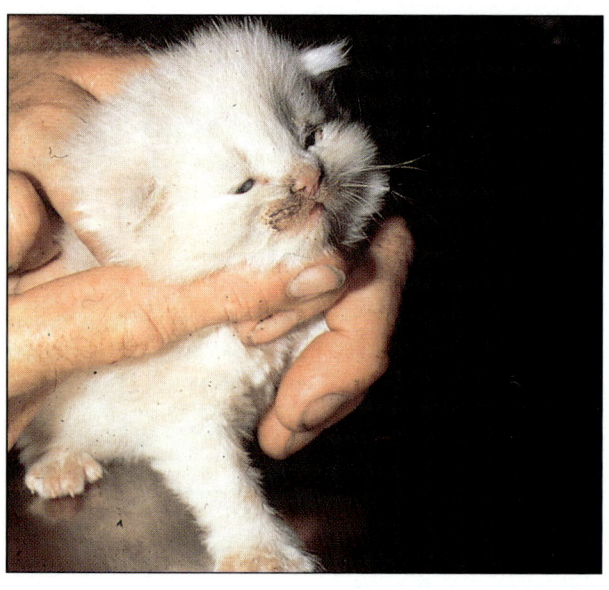

284 *M. canis* infection of muzzle and feet of a kitten. This infection was probably contracted during suckling. Note the singed appearance of lesions.

285

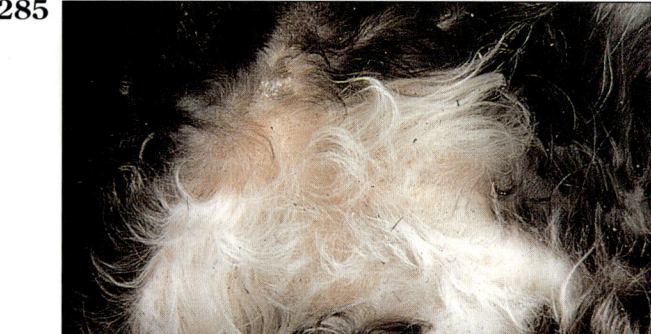

285 *M. canis* infection in a cat showing focal scaling ('cigarette ash') lesion.

Microsporum canis in cats

This organism is the principal cause of dermatophyte infection in dogs and cats[8], and the one most likely to cause zoonotic infections in people. It is best adapted to the cat and in many instances there is a minimal effort on the part of the host to reject the infection. In the cat lesions vary. The most frequent presentation is a focal collection of scale, the so-called 'cigarette ash' deposit, accompanied by stubbled, broken hairs (**283–285**). Other presentations include inapparent infection of individual hairs; areas of broken hair and zones of alopecia; mild discoloration of the skin; crusted papules; folliculitis or, occasionally, severely inflamed zones of acute dermatitis (**286** and **287**).

Lesions are most frequently found on the head and limbs but, occasionally, generalised infection involving the entire body surface occurs (**288** and **289**). Fluorescence, particularly noted with *M. canis* may provide the diagnosis (**290** and **291**)

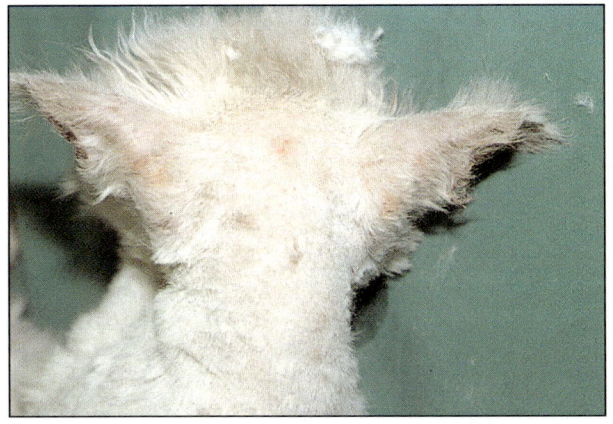

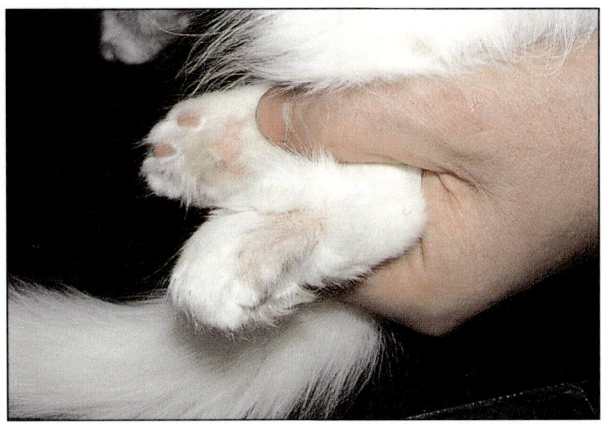

286   *M. canis* in a long-haired kitten. Hair has been clipped to show crusted papules.

287   *M. canis* infection on the feet of a cat. Alopecia with minimal inflammation.

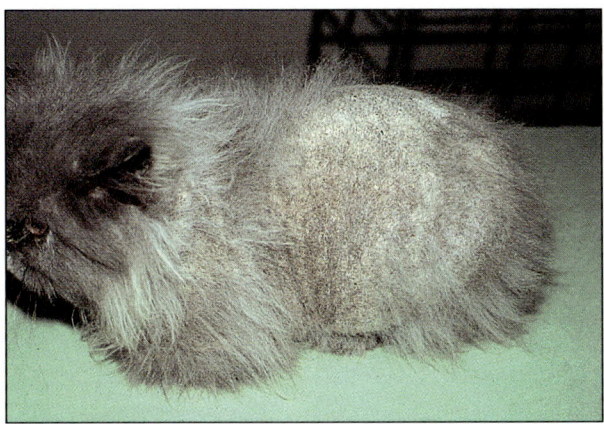

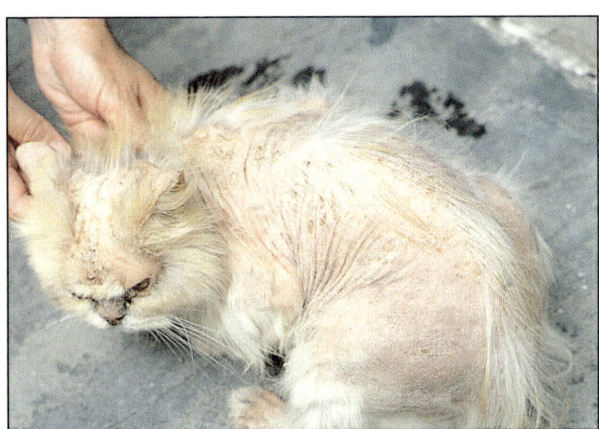

288   *M. canis* infection. Generalised infection in a long-haired cat showing extensive hair loss and profuse scaling.

289   *M. canis* infection. Severe generalised infection of 2 years duration showing almost total hair loss, erythema, scaling, thickening and corrugation of the skin.

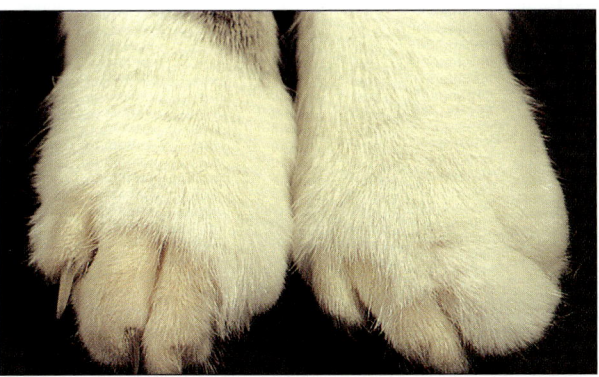

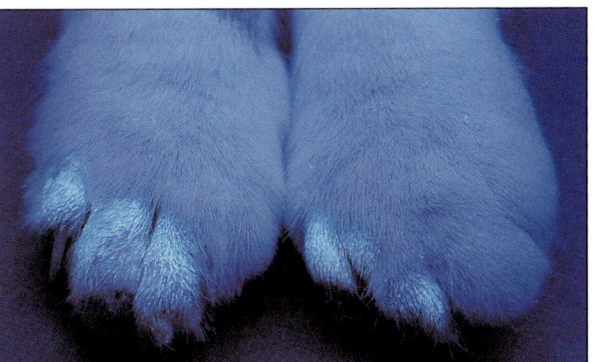

290 and 291   *M. canis* infection photographed in natural light and under Wood's light. Note the fluorescence under the ultraviolet light of the Wood's light. Fluorescence is a property of only a proportion (50–90%) of strains of *M. canis*.

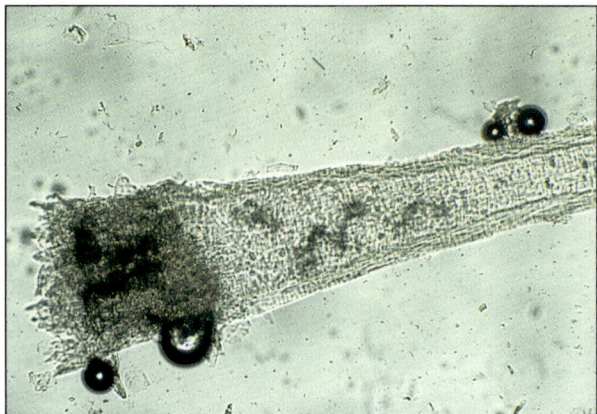
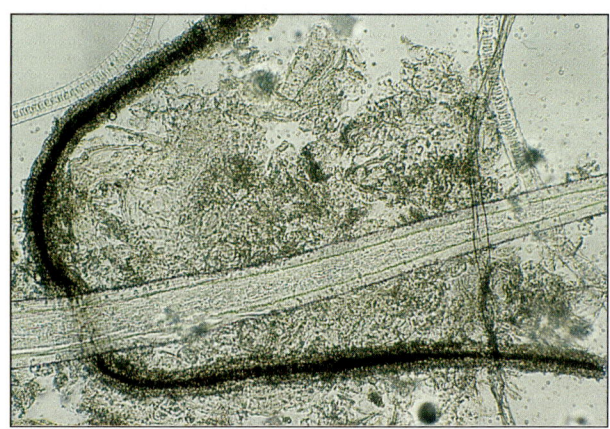

292 and 293 *M. canis* infection. KOH preparation of infected hair. Note the swollen, distorted appearance of the hair shaft with ectothrix spores clustered around it. In such preparations infected hairs are often brown in colour and appear thicker than normal hair shafts.

294

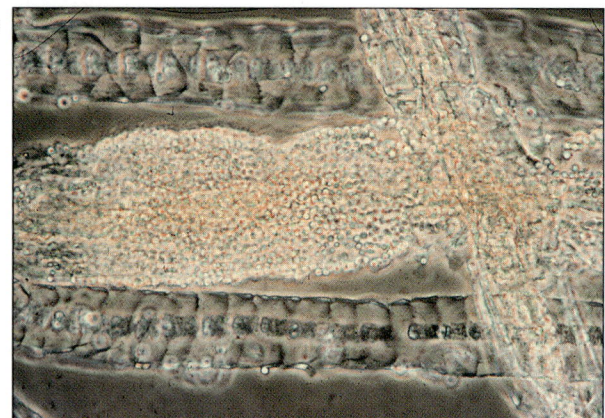

294 *M. canis* infection. Phase contrast photomicrograph showing an infected hair between two normal hairs. Another hair in the early stages of infection crosses all three. Note the numerous blue-green spores investing the infected hair shaft and the loss of the normal architecture of the latter.

and infected hairs may be found on microscopical examination of skin scrapings (**292–294**).

Problems of diagnosis may occur particularly in long-haired cats where the long, intrafollicular, portion of the hair and very narrow shaft make detection of individual infected hairs very difficult.[3,5,6,8] These factors combine to make some cats asymptomatic carriers in whom diagnosis can only be achieved by fungal culture.

Microsporum canis in dogs

In dogs the lesions are more obvious as parasite adaptation to the host is not so efficient as in the cat. Immunological reaction to the presence of the fungi causes inflammation and, ultimately, rejection, with fungal elements being 'washed out' in the growing hair shaft or stratum corneum. In some cases the fungal infection spreads laterally into adjacent normal tissue and a spreading zone of erythema ensues; giving rise to the term 'ringworm'. A major differential diagnosis is the epidermal collarette associated with superficial pyoderma. In the dog the distribution of the lesions is usually random with less tendency to concentrate about the head and face.

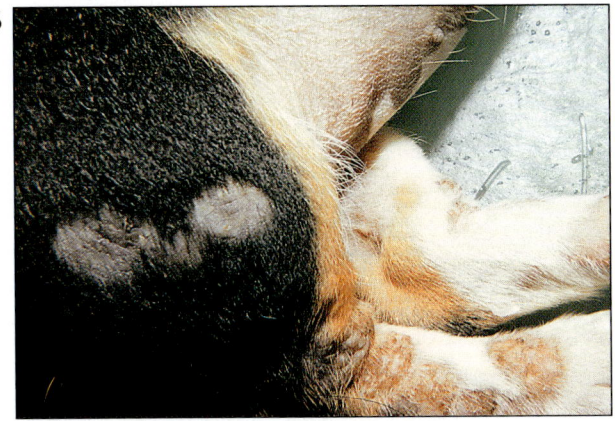

295 *M. canis* infection is not confined to the cat. This illustration shows classic ringworm lesions of peripheral scale and hyperpigmented, healing centres on a puppy.

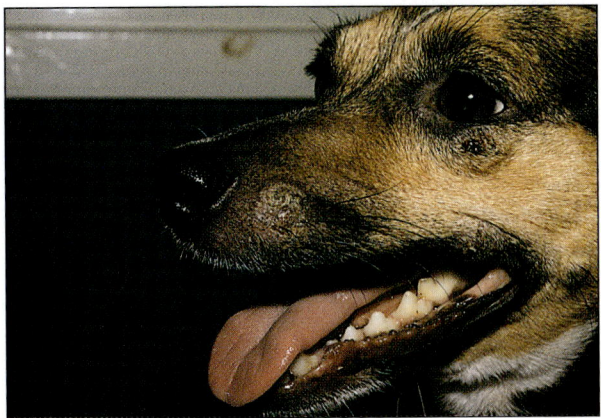

296 *M. canis* infection. Discrete area of inflammation on the muzzle.

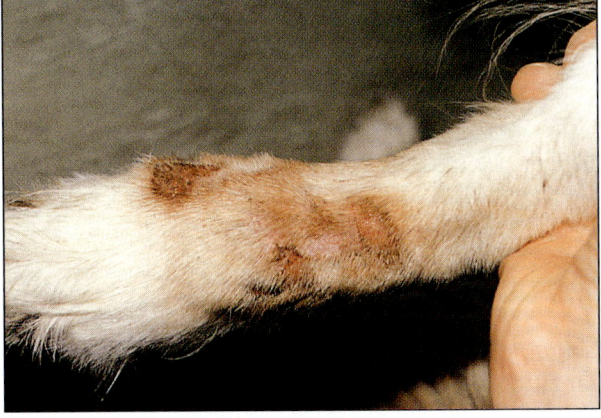

297 *M. canis* infection. A kerion is a highly inflamed focal lesion in which there is secondary bacterial infection. This kerion on a dog's leg is inflamed, erythematous and eroded. Note the saliva staining around lesions.

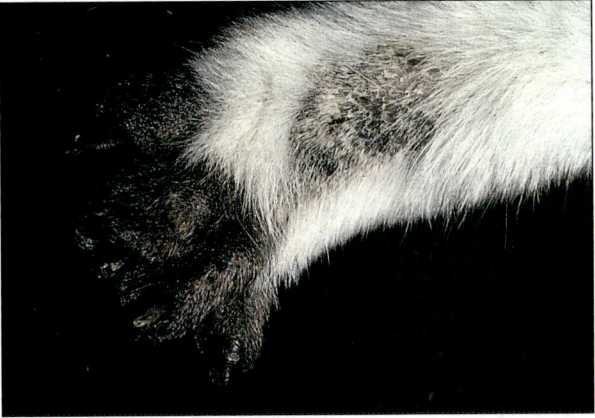

298 *M. canis* infection of the nails (onychomycosis) in a cat. Onychomycosis is often accompanied by abnormal nail growth. (Illustration courtesy J. M. Keep.)

The lesion may appear as a flat, circular area of total alopecia with a fine, pink, lightly scaling border or as an expanding zone of folliculitis with a well-defined erythematous border (**295** and **296**). However, occasionally, inflamed lesions may present with local thickening of the affected skin and even rather prominent tumour-like masses or granuloma.

Both dogs and cats may occasionally develop a lesion called a kerion; a localised area of suppurative folliculitis and furunculosis involving both a fungal and a bacterial infection. The lesion appears as a swollen, doughy area of acute inflammation oozing purulent material (**297**).

Onychomycosis may be very troublesome (**298**). It may occur in both dogs and cats but is more common in the dog. Affected nails exhibit abnormal growth and are frequently twisted, friable and prone to shedding. Management of onychomycosis can be very frustrating with long courses of therapy necessary.

Transmission of *Microsporum canis* is by infective material in the form of spores and hyphae on hairs and keratin fragments which may be free or attached to clothing or grooming implements. The incubation period is very variable but lesions may appear on in-contact animals within 14 days of contact. Individual lesions may show spontaneous resolution, particularly in the dog, unless complicated by bacterial infection, chemical dermatitis from topical medicaments, or self-inflicted trauma. In general the course of the whole disease is relatively short in the dog. On the other hand the course in the cat may be very long, the duration appearing to be directly proportional to the length of the hair coat and may extend for years.

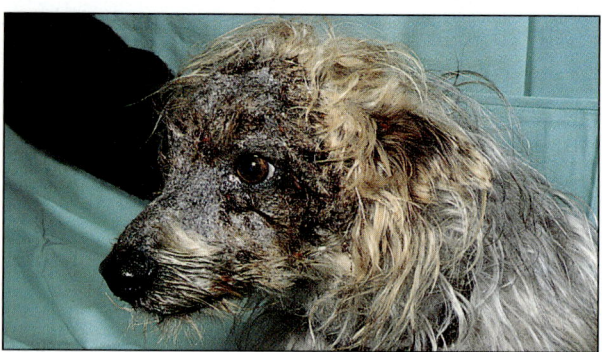

299

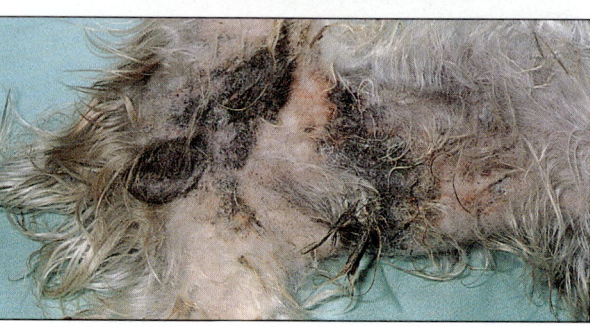

300

299 and 300   *Microsporum gypseum* infection. Sydney Silkie terrier showing lesions on the head and in the inguinal region. There is hyperpigmented, adherent thick crust overlying inflammatory reactions in the skin.

***M. canis* infection is characterised by:**
In the cat:
- Chronicity.
- Hair loss, scaling and crusting, often generalised.
- Little or no pruritus.

In the dog:
- More acute course.
- Typically focal or regional alopecia.
- Often a clearly defined, erythematous margin.

Major differential diagnoses are:
In the cat:
- Cheyletiellosis.
- Demodicosis.

In the dog:
- Superficial pyoderma.
- Demodicosis.

Diagnosis is made by:
- Fluorescence under Wood's light of hair and scales.
- Microscopic examination of potassium hydroxide (KOH) preparations.
- Fungal culture and identification of macro-aleurospores.

---

single, although a number of lesions may be found on any one patient. Typical predilection sites are on the ears, head and face, and the extremities.

***M. gypseum* infection is characterised by:**
- Chronicity.
- Well circumscribed areas of hair loss, heavy crusting and thickening of the skin, pruritus and local tenderness.

Major differential diagnoses are:
- Nasal pyoderma (in the dog).
- Demodicosis.
- Pemphigus foliaceus.

Diagnosis is made by:
- Microscopic examination of KOH preparations.
- Culture and identification of macroaleurospores.

Microsporum gypseum

This organism causes a small proportion of dermatophyte infections in cats but up to 50% of canine cases. Individual lesions tend to be well circumscribed, heavily crusted and associated with a distinct thickening of the skin (**299** and **300**). When this crust is removed haemorrhage is often seen in the exposed area which is tender to the touch. Lesions are often

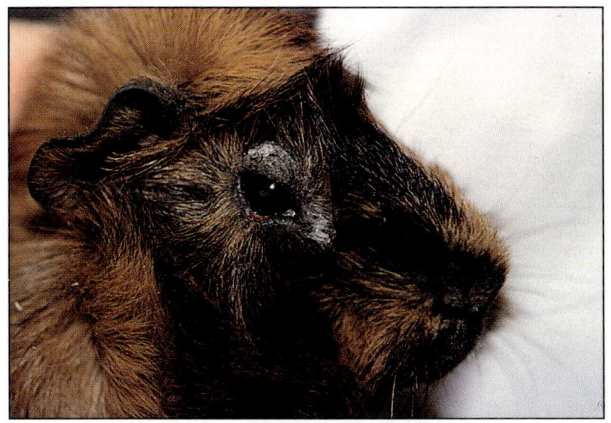 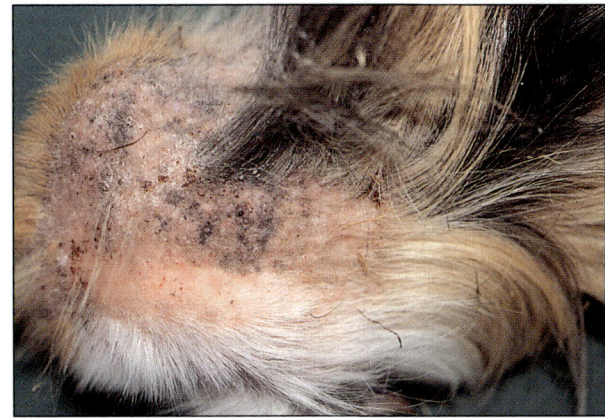

301 and 302 **Dermatophytosis** of small mammals is usually due to *Trichophyton mentagrophytes*. This guinea-pig (**301**) has a focal patch or alopecia and scale over the right eye whereas the other (**302**) has a large area of erythema and alopecia on the dorsal trunk which was highly pruritic.

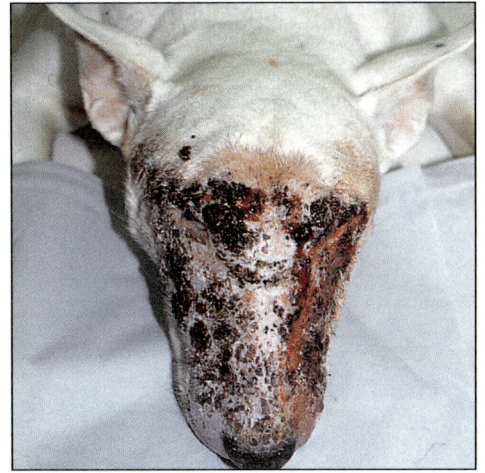

303 *T. mentagrophytes* infection, like *M. gypseum*, is often much more inflammatory than dermatophytosis due to *M. canis*. Dermatophytosis of the face of a Bull terrier. Note the acutely inflamed appearance of the lesion which covers a considerable portion of the face.

Trichophyton mentagrophytes

This fungus is responsible for a very small percentage of dermatophyte infections in cats and a variable proportion of those in dogs, dependent upon the locality.[8] This organism is the major dermatophyte of small mammals, in particular the rabbit and the guinea pig.[1] The infection tends to spread and may cover large areas of skin and from a small focus it may, in time, cover the entire animal (**301** and **302**). In dogs, spontaneous healing of the originally infected area does not occur, as it does with *Microsporum* infections, whereas in rabbits and guinea pigs spontaneous resolution of the lesions is the rule, although carrier states remain.

Lesions may be associated with a secondary bacterial infection.

The appearance is often suggestive of a dry, crusting folliculitis due to the severe involvement of many hair follicles. Distribution of the lesions is quite variable. The head and distal extremities appear to be predilection sites (**303**) but infection can begin virtually anywhere on the body. The infection may, for example, involve the face and the head and three of the limbs, or large areas of one side of the body, or several foci may be affected and gradually coalesce into considerable areas (**304–307**).

304

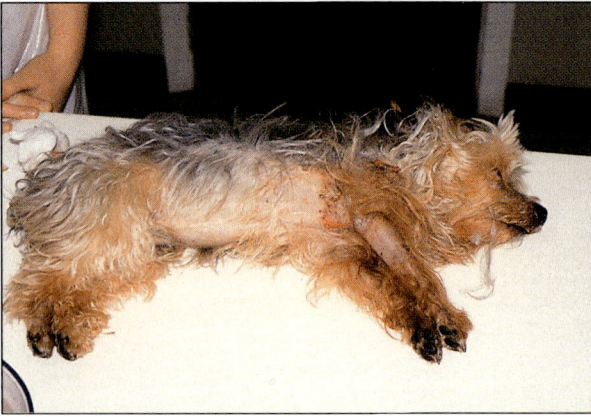

305

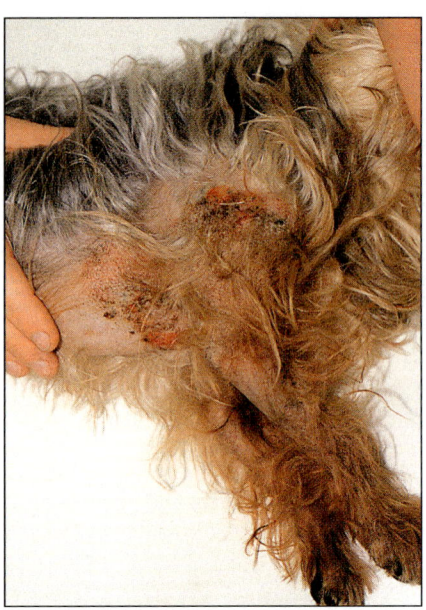

304 and 305 **T. mentagrophytes** infection on the foreleg of a Yorkshire terrier. Note clearly demarcated advancing edge of the affected region.

306

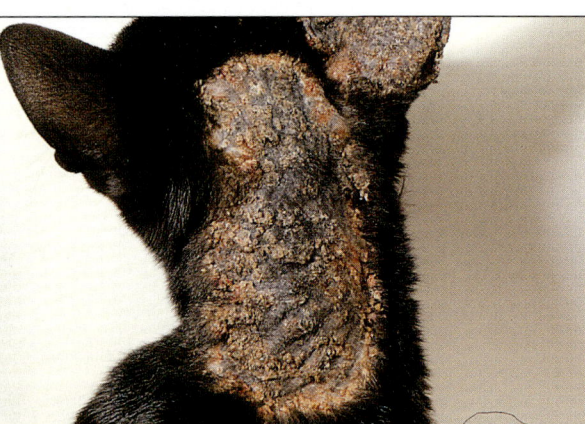

307

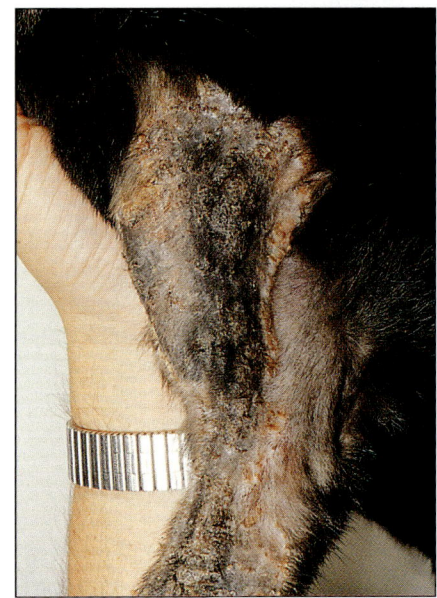

306 and 307 **T. mentagrophytes** infection of the back of the neck, shoulders, right ear and left foreleg of a cat. Note the extensive nature of the lesions and the marked crusting, pustulation and hyperpigmentation of the affected areas.

T. mentagrophytes **infection is characterised by:**
- Chronicity.
- Large areas of skin involved.
- No pruritus but may be painful.

Major differential diagnoses include
- Folliculitis.
- Canine demodicosis.

Diagnosis is made by
- Microscopic examination of KOH preparations (**309**).
- Fungal culture and identification of macro-aleurospores.

Local trauma to the skin seems to provide conditions conducive to the establishment of *Trichophyton mentagrophytes* infections and kerion formation may occur (**308**). The possibility of this infection being present should not be overlooked when dealing with a chronic dermatitis or folliculitis. In some individuals the infection may prove very refractory to treatment.

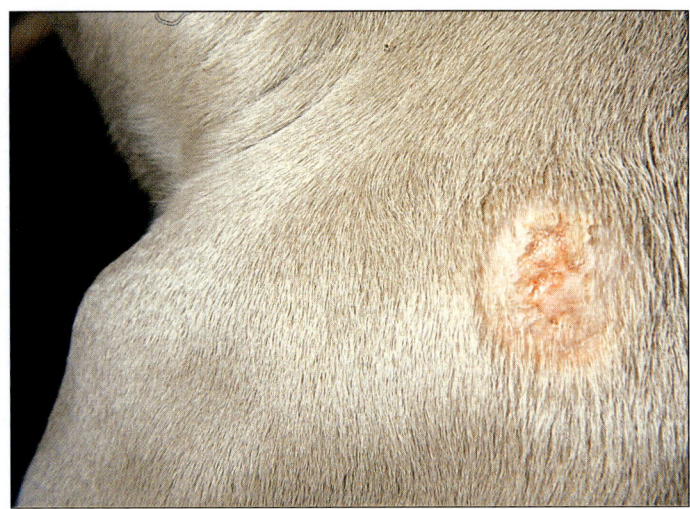

308 *T. mentagrophytes* infection. Kerion on the hip of a Weimaraner puppy.

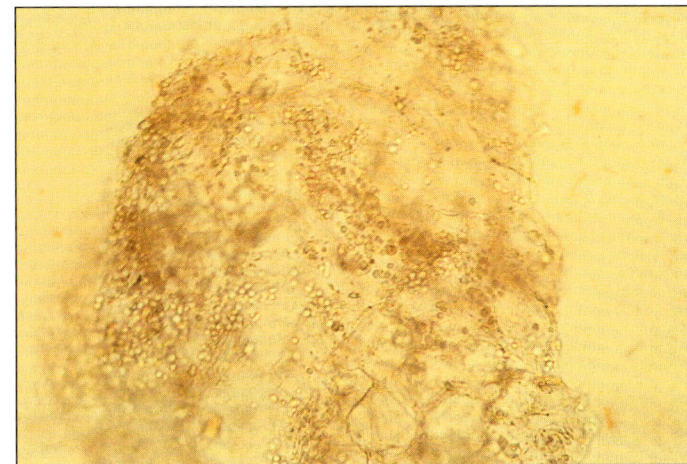

309 *T. mentagrophytes* infection. KOH preparation of infected scales. Note the larger size of the spores compared with those of *M. canis* (**292**) and their tendency to be arranged in chains along the hair shaft.

Other dermatophytes

Infection of the dog with the dermatophytes *Trichophyton erinacei,* derived from hedgehogs, and *Microsporum persicolor*, contracted from bank voles, has been reported occasionally in the United Kingdom and Europe.

Malassezia pachydermatis

Malassezia pachydermatis is a lipophilic non-mycelial yeast. It has an elongated, oval shape and exhibits unipolar budding. It is considered a normal inhabitant and opportunist pathogen of the external ear canal and may also be found in the rectum, anal sacs and vagina. Low numbers may be found on the inflamed skin that is associated with a number of conditions, for instance atopy or defects in keratinisation. Increased prevalence is also associated with previous antibacterial therapy and combinations of antibacterial and glucocorticoid therapy.[7]

The presence of the yeast has been associated with highly pruritic dermatoses, often exhibiting glucocorticoid-resistant pruritus.[4] In dogs the disease is associated with erythema, variable but

310

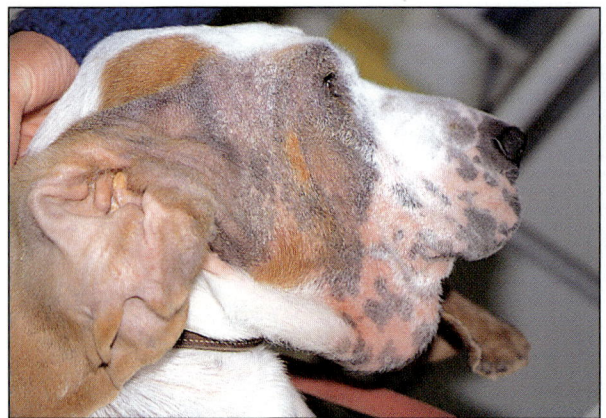

311

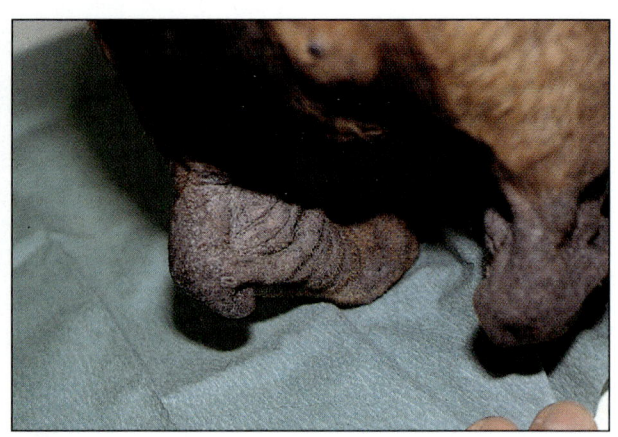

310 *Malassezia pachydermatis* infection in a Basset hound. Compare the normal colour on the ventral pinna to the hyperpigmented skin of the side of the head. Note the yellow/grey scale which is often found in association with this yeast.

311 *M. pachydermatis* infection in a miniature Dachshund. Thickened, hyperpigmented and alopecic skin on both hocks. This animal was very pruritic.

312

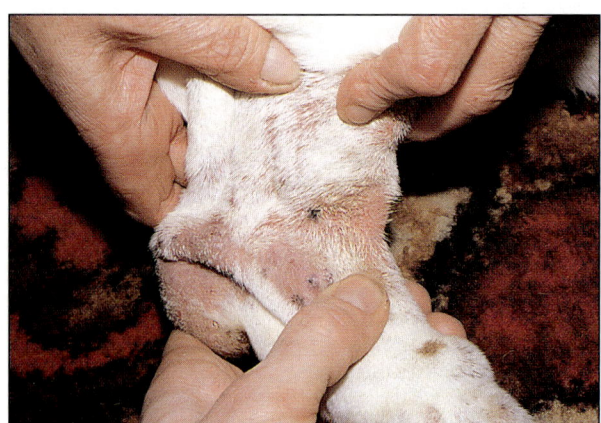

312 *M. pachydermatis* infection in the skin fold on the rear leg of a Basset hound. Erythema and inflammation are apparent.

often a yellowish/grey greasy scale, hyperpigmentation and alopecia (**310–312**). In the cat, otitis externa, acne and generalised exfoliative dermatitis have been associated with the organism. Although it may appear to act as a primary pathogen an underlying disease should always be suspected.

M. pachydermatis infection is characterised by:
- Pruritus and associated signs of chronic self-trauma.
- Erythema and greasy scale.
- Pruritus that is resistant to glucocorticoids.

Major differential diagnoses include:
- Atopy.
- Sarcoptic mange.
- Defects in keratinisation.

Diagnosis is made by:
- Examination of tape strips.
- Response to therapy.
- Histopathological examination of biopsy.
- Cultural characteristics.

Candida albicans

Candida albicans has been reported as a rare cause of lip fold pyoderma and mucocutaneous dermatitis in the dog.[3] Although the organism may form hyphae and appears rounder than *Malassezia pachydermatis* on tape strips, impression smears and in histopathological section, the distinction is best based on cultural characteristics. The prevalence and distribution of the organism on the normal dog is not known although it has been reported as a normal inhabitant of the gastro-intestinal tract of mammals. The disease is associated with severe pruritus and moist, erythematous, erosive, often crusting lesions. Underlying defects in immunity should be suspected in clinical cases.

C. albicans infection is characterised by:
- Erythema, erosions and crusting.
- Pruritus.

The major differentials are:
- *Malassezia pachydermatis* infection.
- Intertrigo.
- Neoplasia particularly mycosis fungoides and squamous cell carcinoma of the lip.

The diagnosis is made by
- Impression smears.
- Histopathological examination of biopsy material.
- Cultural characteristics.

Subcutaneous and intermediate mycoses

These infections are due to the traumatic implantation of (usually) fungal material into the skin and subcutis. Lesions are characterised by a chronic course and a tendency to remain localised. Fistula formation and serous, purulent or granular discharge is common. The host attempts to isolate the area of inflammation and a chronic granulomatous reaction occurs. Lesions often become tumefied. Occasionally pseudomycetomas may be diagnosed where infection is due to bacteria such as *Staphylococcus intermedius* or dermatophytes such as *M. canis*.

Suspicion of subcutaneous or intermediate mycosis should prompt investigation by biopsy. Samples should be taken both for routine histopathological preparation and also for submission for maceration and fungal culture.[2]

Suspicion may be aroused by the history and clinical signs. Examination of stained smears of exudate may be helpful in some of the conditions (Eumycotic mycetoma, Phaeohyphomycosis, Protothecosis). Definitive diagnosis is achieved by culture and histological features.

As a group the subcutaneous and intermediate mycoses are managed by:
- Accurate identification of the causal organism.
- Surgical excision.
- Adjunctive systemic therapy.

Subcutaneous and intermediate mycoses all present in a similar clinical fashion and major differential diagnoses common to all are:
- Foreign body granuloma.
- Deep pyoderma.
- Neoplasia.
- Atypical mycobacterial infections.

313

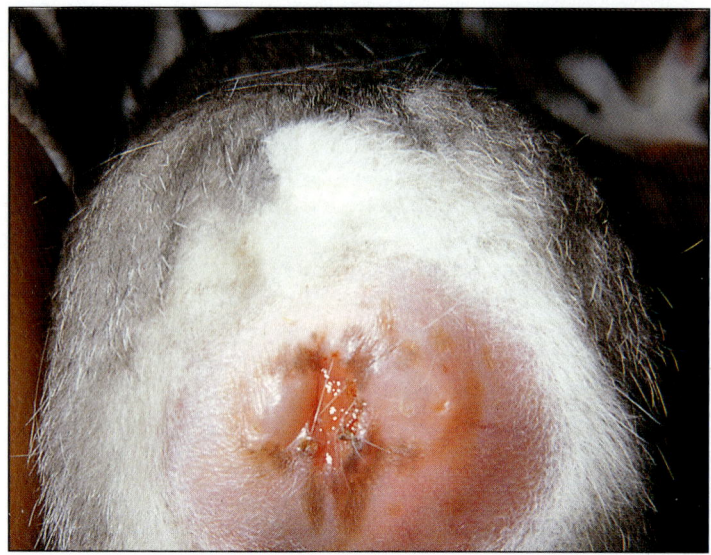

313 Eumycotic mycetoma. Infection occurred in the coccygeal vertebrae at the base of the tail in this cat. Despite radical surgery, including amputation of the tail, the condition recurred.

Eumycotic mycetoma

Eumycotic mycetoma is a rare condition in which the aetiological fungal agents form granules in the tissues. The lesions are granulomatous, often tumefied and are associated with the formation of draining sinuses and granules. The lesions are chronic, subcutaneous and are usually single and restricted to one area of the body, often to one foot (**313**).

Fungal species consistently isolated from myce-tomas in dogs and cats include *Allescheria boydii*, *Curvularia geniculata* and *Helminthosporium* spp.

Infection is via contaminated penetrating wounds involving the skin, subcutis, fascia and bone. In the early stages of the infection the affected area is swollen and painful and resembles an abscess. Later, draining sinuses form which discharge a serous or purulent exudate containing granules. The colour of the granules varies according to the particular fungus involved, e. g. *Curvularia geniculata* granules are black whereas *Allescheria boydii* is associated with white grains.

314 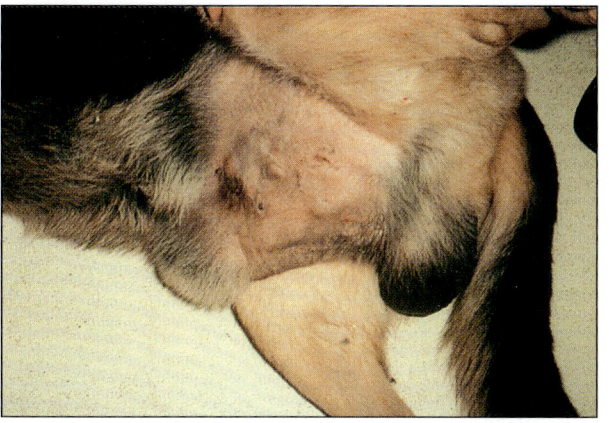 **315**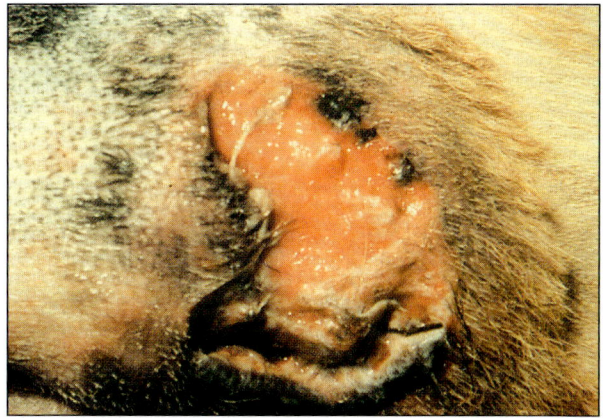

314 and 315 **Phaeohyphomycosis.** Granulomatous nodules with discharging fistulae in the perineal area of a German shepherd dog associated with *Phialophora verrucosa* infection.

316 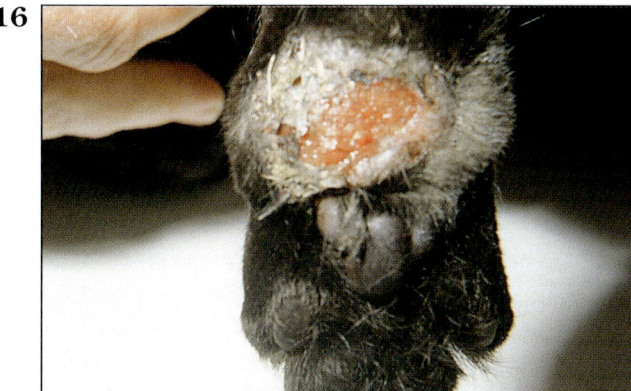 **317**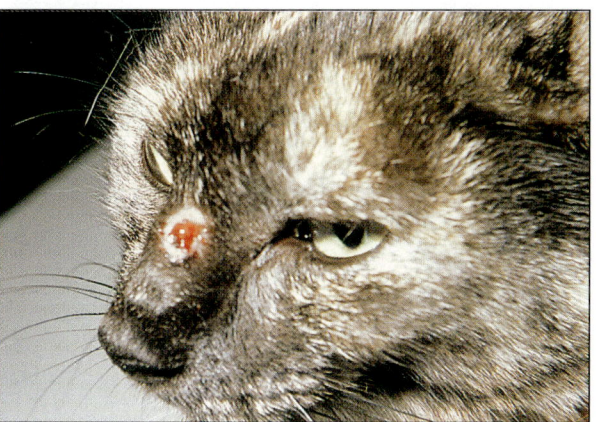

316 **Phaeohyphomycosis.** Chronic non-healing lesion on hind paw of cat associated with *Phialophora verrucosa* infection.

317 **Phaeohyphomycosis.** Sinus formation on nose of cat associated with *Exophiala spinifera* infection of nasal cavity.

Phaeohyphomycosis

Phaeohyphomycosis is a condition in which dematiaceous (pigmented) fungi grow in tissues as hyphae, pseudohyphae, yeast-like cells, or any combination of these. The disease can be classified as superficial, cutaneous, corneal, subcutaneous or systemic. Cutaneous and subcutaneous forms have, rarely, been reported in small animals, mainly in cats. The species of fungi involved include *Phialophora verrucosa*, *Bipolaris spicifera*, *Exophiala jeanselmei* and *Ex. spinifera*, *Moniliella suaveolens*, *Stemphylium* spp. and *Cladosporium* spp. Clinically the typical lesion is a subcutaneous nodule that gradually increases in size and develops fistulous tracts which discharge a yellow or watery, haemorrhagic exudate (**314–317**). Usually the lesion is not painful and may be soft and pultaceous to palpation. In other cases the cutaneous form presents as chronic, non-healing granulating areas.

318 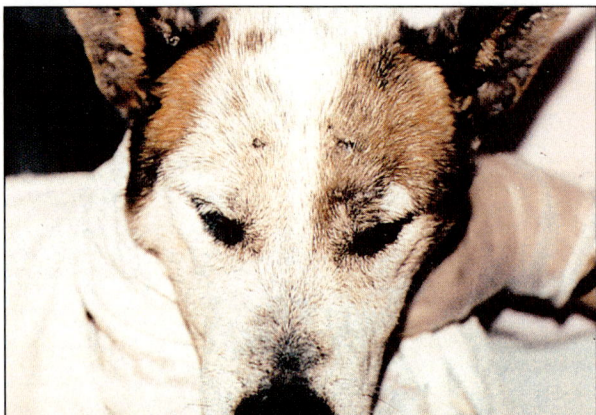 319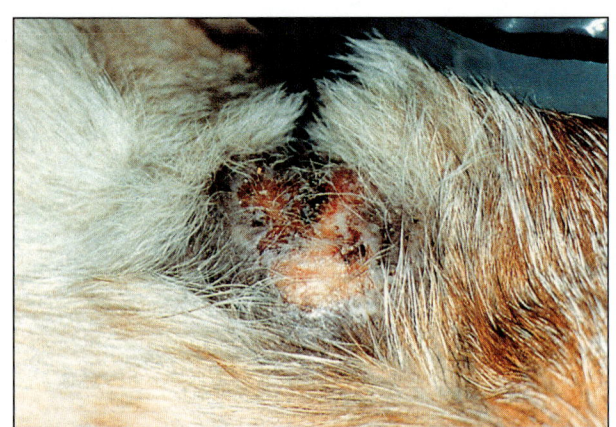

320 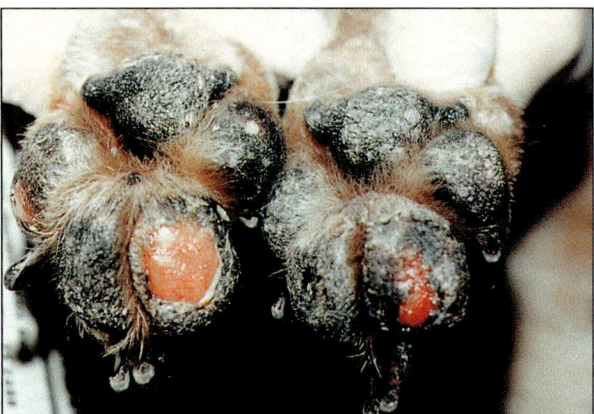 321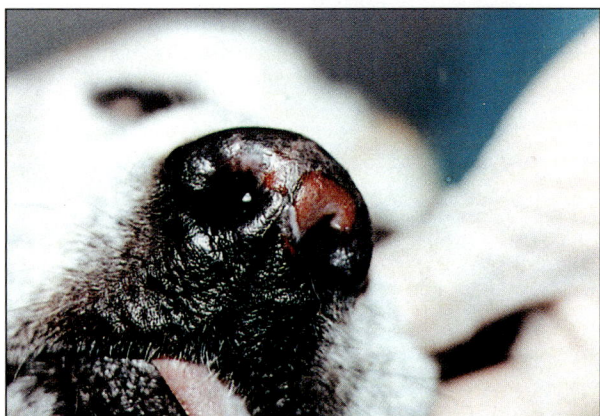

318–321   Protothecosis. Nodular lesions, some of which are ulcerated, on the face and over the tuber ischii of an Australian cattle dog infected with *Prototheca wickerhamii*. This dog showed signs of systemic infection in the form of colitis and chorioretinitis. The dog developed hyperkeratosis and ulceration of the pads and ulceration of the planum nasale (**320** and **321**) in the terminal stages of the disease. (Illustrations from Wilkinson, G. T and Leong, G. [1988]. Protothecosis in a dog. *Australian Veterinary Practitioner*, **18**: 47–49.)

Protothecosis

Protothecosis is a rare disease of animals and people caused by unicellular, colourless algae, which are ubiquitous in the environment and have been isolated from a wide variety of sources including tree sap, sludge, potato peelings, human fingernails and fresh and salt water. Although several species of *Prototheca* have been identified, only two, *Prototheca wickerhamii* and *P. zopfii*, have been proved to cause disease. In the cat the infection usually involves the subcutis in a chronic granulomatous process, whereas in the dog the majority of reported cases have been systemic infections, often with ocular, intestinal and nervous system involvement (**318–323**).

Sporotrichosis

Sporotrichosis is a disease caused by the dimorphic fungus *Sporothrix schenkii,* a soil saprophyte that has a world-wide distribution. Infection occurs by way of the contamination of wounds with soil. Three clinical manifestations of the disease have been reported; localised, cutaneous-lymphatic and disseminated. In the localised form the lesions occur as firm nodules that do not follow the course of the lymphatics. Cats often show such lesions on the face (**324** and **325**).

The cutaneous-lymphatic form is the most common in dogs, the lesions occurring as round firm nodules at the site where the infection was introduced and progressing from there to the subcutis and the lymphatics (**326**). The nodules and affected lymph nodes often ulcerate and discharge a

322 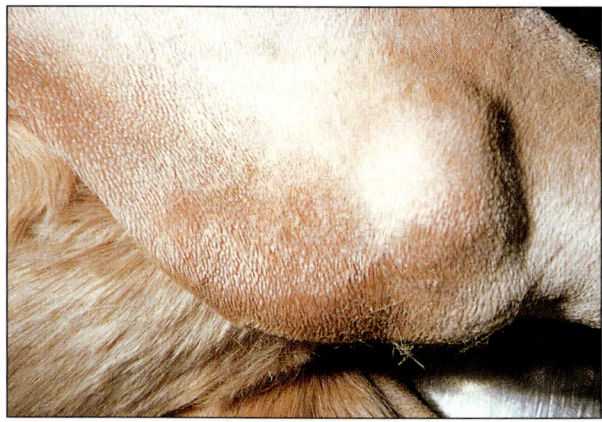 **323**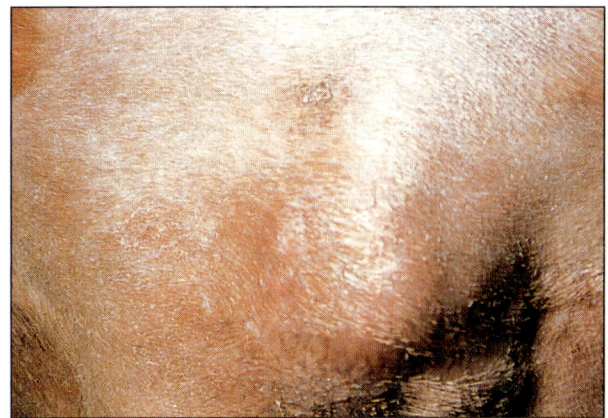

322 and 323   Protothecosis. Bursitis over the elbow and tuber ischii associated with *Prototheca zopfii* infection in a Cocker spaniel. This is the second most common presentation of the infection in people.

324 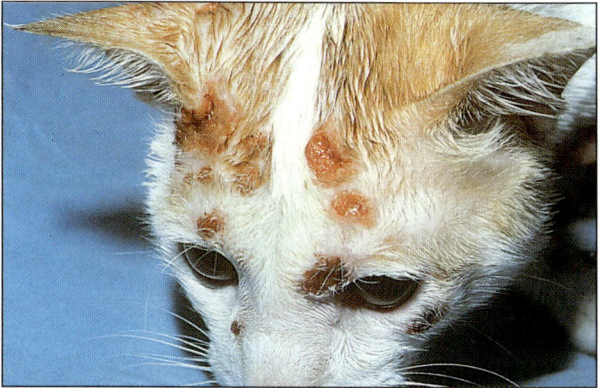 **325**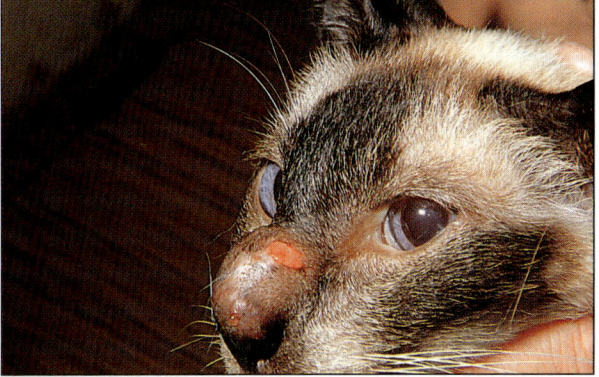

324   Sporotrichosis. Multiple erythematous, ulcerated nodules on the head of a cat. This condition is a zoonosis. The veterinarian handling this cat (G. H. Muller) became infected and developed a lesion on his thumb (see **809**). (Illustration courtesy G. H. Muller.)

325   Sporotrichosis. Localised discharging granulomatous lesion on the nose of a Siamese cat.

326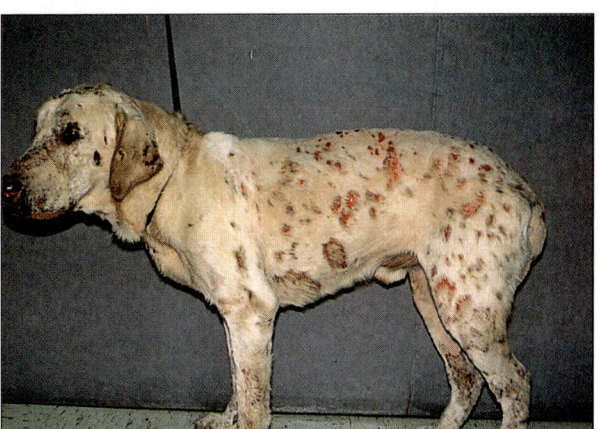

thick brown exudate. Either of these forms of the disease may be associated with the disseminated form in which widespread infection of the internal organs and tissues occurs. The disease is of major public health concern and affected animals, especially cats, should be handled only when wearing rubber gloves and hands should be washed thoroughly with fungicidal agents such as povidone-iodine or chlorhexidine.

326   Sporotrichosis. Generalised cutaneous-lymphatic form in a Labrador retriever showing multiple circular, ulcerated and depressed lesions. (Illustration courtesy K. A. Morello.)

This condition is characterised by:
- Formation of nodules often involving lymphatics.
- Occasional disseminated disease.

Systemic mycoses

Systemic mycoses are fungal infections which are predominantly respiratory in origin following inhalation of the spores. Causal organisms include *Blastomyces dermatitidis*, *Coccidioides immitis*, *Histoplasma capsulatum* and *Cryptococcus neoformans*. Blastomycosis, coccidioidomycosis and histoplasmosis are rare compared to cryptococcosis and also occur in limited geographical regions, principally the Southern and Southwestern United States.

Cutaneous signs of infection include discharging granulomas and abscess formation; erosive, ulcerative and proliferative lesions may also be seen. Local lymphadenopathy is present and there is usually a history of gradual onset accompanied by vague signs of malaise such as cough, weight loss and depression. The differential diagnosis of the cutaneous lesions includes foreign body granuloma, deep pyoderma, local neoplasia and the subcutaneous and intermediate mycoses discussed above.

Suspicion of the diagnosis may be based on local knowledge supported by clinical examination and consideration of the history. Support for the diagnosis may be gained by examination of stained smears of exudate and needle aspirates of lymph nodes where small, capsulate yeast-like organisms may be found. Definitive diagnosis is based on histopathological examination of biopsy samples and culture results. Abdominal and thoracic radiographs may demonstrate internal disease.

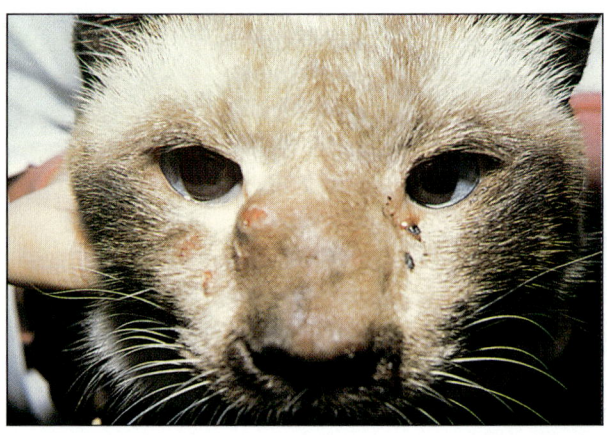

327   **Cryptococcosis.** Typical site for primary infection in the cat consisting of a hard, granulomatous swelling in the nasal passages distorting the shape of the nose. Note the bilateral nasal discharge, a common manifestation of the infection.

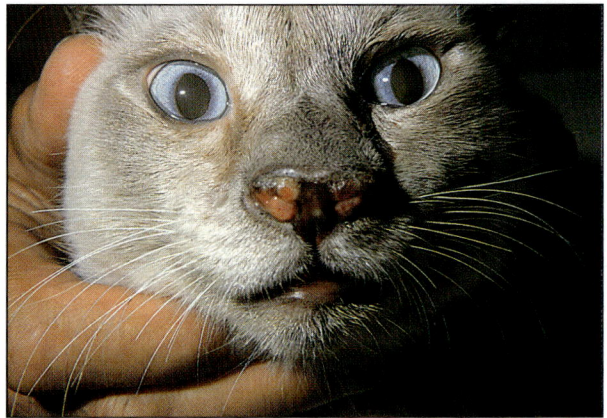

328   **Cryptococcosis.** Erosive granulomas obstructing the nostrils of a Siamese cat.

Cryptococcosis

Infection with the yeast-like fungus *Cryptococcus neoformans* occurs from sources in the environment, notably pigeon faeces. Infection is thought to be by inhalation with the primary site being the respiratory tract. In the cat the infection may remain localised to the nasal passages and overlying skin. In other cases the lower respiratory tract becomes infected and this is followed by dissemination throughout the body. In the cat there is a predilection for the central nervous system, the eye and the skin of the head and neck (**327–**

330). However, lesions may be distributed over much of the body surface, apparently the result of haematogenous or lymphogenous spread.

Lesions take the form of multiple, fairly rapidly growing, firm-to-hard, often flattened, painless nodules in the dermis and subcutis, ranging in size from 1 mm-1 cm in diameter. The nodules have a tendency to ulcerate, exposing a raw granular surface with a scanty sero-haemorrhagic exudate which fails to heal. More rarely there may be larger, primarily ulcerative lesions or

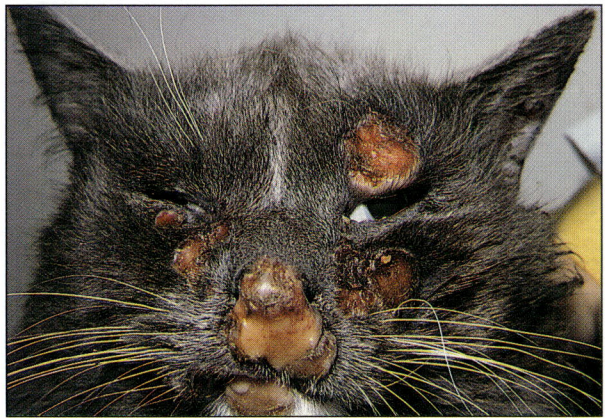

329   Cryptococcosis. Multiple, ulcerated granulomas on the head of a cat.

Cryptococcosis is characterised by:
- Chronicity.
- Formation of subcutaneous nodules which often ulcerate.
- Frequent systemic involvement.

Major differential diagnoses include:
- Other mycotic granulomatous disease.
- Atypical mycobacterial infections.
- Sporotrichosis.

Diagnosis is made by:
- Examination of stained smears for causal organism.
- Culture.
- Positive latex agglutination test.

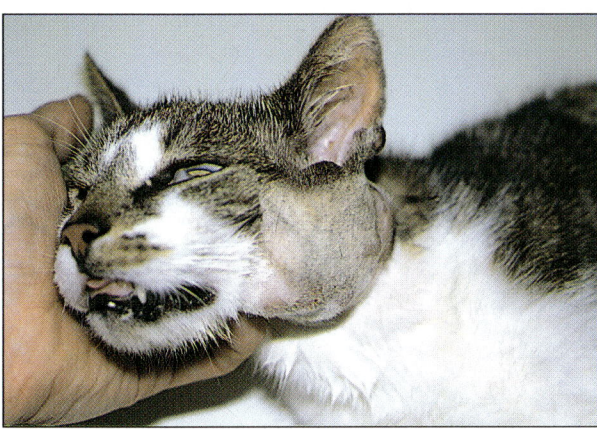

330   Cryptococcosis. Large nodule overlying the submandibular lymph node on a cat.

large fungating masses, the latter showing a predilection for the extremities.

With infection of the nasal turbinates in the cat there is usually a bilateral nasal discharge and a firm to hard swelling often appears over the bridge of the nose, sometimes with ulceration of the overlying skin. Occasionally, granulating lesions may protrude through and obstruct the nostrils, or erosive, crusted and exudative lesions may occur on the face. In most cases of systemic cryptococcosis the animal is in poor condition and there may be a peripheral lymphadenomegaly, particularly with the cutaneous form.

References

1. Collins, R. R. (1987). Dermatologic Disorders of Common Small Nondomestic Animals. In: Nesbitt, G. H. (Ed.) *Contemporary Issues in Small Animal Practice, Dermatology*, pp. 235–294. Churchill Livingstone, New York.

2. Fadok, V. A. (1985). Differential diagnoses of granulomatous dermatitis. In: *Proceedings of American Animal Hospital Association 52nd Meeting,* pp. 114–117.

3. Foil, C. S. (1897). Cutaneous fungal disease. In: Nesbitt, G. H. (Ed) *Contemporary Issues in Small Animal Practice, Dermatology,* pp. 123–158. Churchill Livingstone, New York.

4. Mason, K. V. and Evans, A. G. (1991). Dermatitis associated with *Malassezia pachydermatis* in 11 dogs. *Journal of American Animal Hospital Association,* **27**: 14–20.

5. Moriello, K. A. and Deboer, D. J. (1991). Fungal flora of the haircoat of cats with and without dermatophytosis. *Journal of Medical and Veterinary Mycology,* **29**: 285–292.

6. Moriello, K. A. and Deboer, D. J. (1991). Fungal flora of the haircoat of pet cats. *American Journal of Veterinary Research,* **52**: 602–606.

7. Plant, J. D., Rosenkrantz, W. S and Griffin, C. E. (1992). Factors associated with and prevalence of high *Malassezia pachydermatis* numbers on dog skin. *Journal of the American Veterinary Medical Association,* **201**: 879–882.

8. Wright, A. I. (1989). Ringworm in dogs and cats. *Journal of Small Animal Practice,* **30**: 242–249.

Chapter 8

Hypersensitivities

Introduction

As a group , the diseases covered in this chapter account for a very large proportion of the dermatological caseload. Flea bite hypersensitivity and atopy are by far the most common hypersensitivities seen in clinical practice. It should be remembered that hypersensitivities play a role in many dermatoses. For example, Type I hypersensitivity occurs in scabies and otodectic otitis where the pruritus may be seemingly out of proportion to the number of mites on the animal.

When dealing with the pruritus due to hypersensitivity it is important to remember the concepts of the pruritic threshold and the summation of itch. The pruritic threshold is the degree of irritation, from whatever cause, that the animal can tolerate without showing clinical signs.

Thus a dog with sub-clinical atopy or dietary hypersensitivity may show no signs of pruritus until a secondary superficial pyoderma or flea infection occurs. The pruritic threshold is now exceeded and typical signs of atopy are now manifest. Summation of itch is demonstrated by the dog showing clinical signs when fleas or pyoderma occur but not when they are absent, although the underlying hypersensitivity is present throughout. These features may greatly complicate diagnosis.

Flea bite hypersensitivity

Flea bite hypersensitivity (FBH) is a hypersensitivity reaction to components of flea saliva. It may involve both IgE-mediated (immediate or Type I hypersensitivity), cell-mediated (delayed or Type IV hypersensitivity) or cutaneous basophil hypersensitivity.[4] The primary lesion of delayed hypersensitivity is a papule and (if present) it erupts at the site of the bite. In most instances the papule encrusts, although it does not progress to an epidermal collarette as does the primary lesion of superficial pyoderma. In those cases mediated by other than delayed-type hypersensitivity there are no papules.

Pruritus, sometimes accompanied by erythema or alopecia is the presenting sign. The pruritus may be severe in some cases and may result in self-inflicted trauma, often complicated by acute pyotraumatic dermatitis. In temperate regions the condition is seen with equal frequency in the dog and the cat whereas in sub-tropical and tropical regions FBH constitutes the most frequent reason for presentation of dogs to veterinarians. It may prove difficult to convince the owner that FBH is the cause of the dermatosis, particularly if it is not possible to demonstrate fleas on the animal in question. Intradermal testing with aqueous flea allergen is useful in the dog but much less so in the cat. Support for a diagnosis of FBH may be drawn from the demonstration of fleas on in-contact animals, the presence of zoonotic lesions and the presence of *Dipylidium caninum*, of which the flea is an intermediate host.

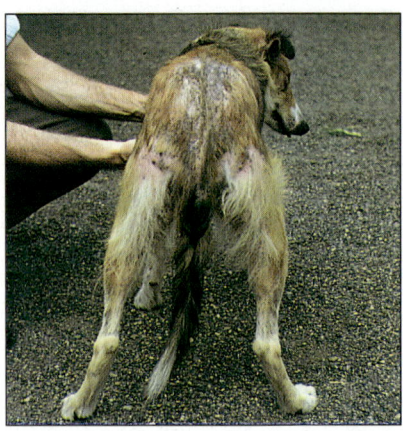

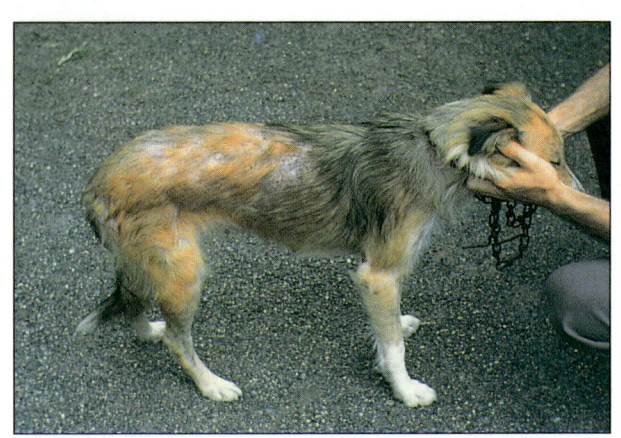

331 and 332 **Flea bite hypersensitivity in the dog.** Characteristic distribution of lesions of chronic flea allergy dermatitis in a collie cross bitch. The dorsolumbar region, base of the tail and posterior thighs are the areas of predilection.

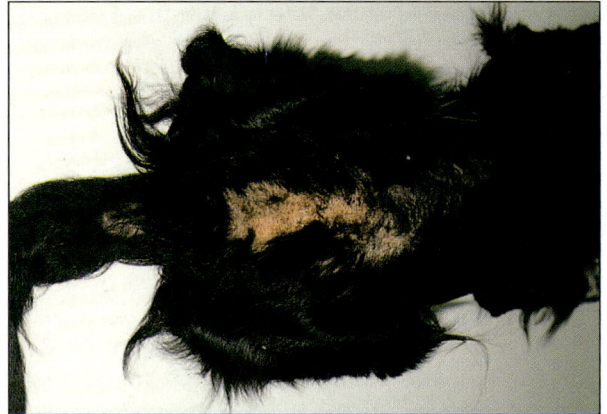

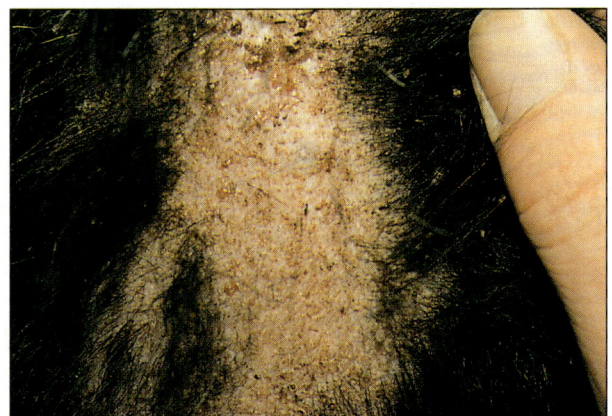

333 and 334 **Flea bite hypersensitivity in a cross collie** showing the characteristic papulocrustous dermatitis accompanied by alopecia over the dorsal lumbar region and the base of the tail.

In the dog

The lesions are most common at the root of the tail and extend rostrally along the dorsal surface of the trunk as far as the thoracolumbar junction (**331–334**). The affected area tends to form a triangle with the base situated at the tail root (the 'Florida triangle'). The caudal and medial aspects of the thighs usually are involved. The popliteal lymph nodes may be enlarged.

This distribution of secondary lesions conforms to the area that the dog can reach to nibble and lick and the majority of these lesions are the result of self trauma and consist of thickening and wrinkling of the skin, partial hair loss and either serum exudation or crust formation. In chronically affected animals the skin becomes thickened, lichenified and hyperpigmented. In very severe cases almost the whole of the skin of the trunk and hindquarters may be affected (**335** and **336**). Patches of pyotraumatic dermatitis appear as the lesions become secondarily infected (**337**).

335

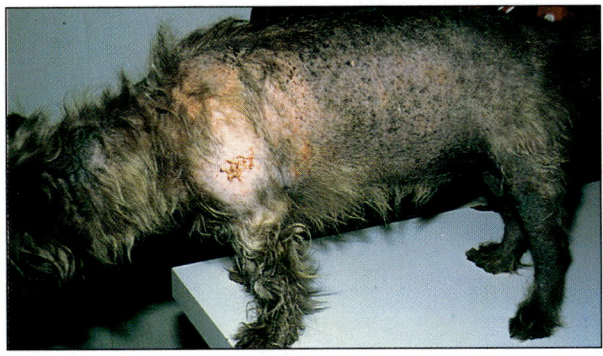

336

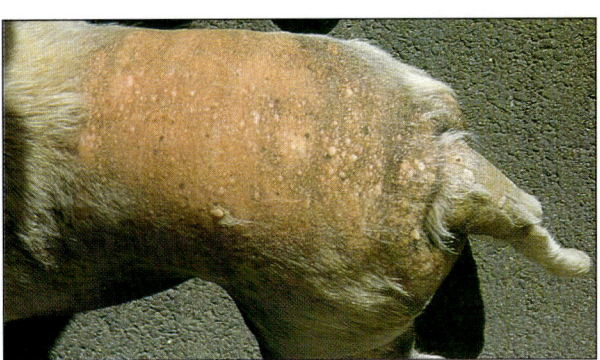

335 Flea bite hypersensitivity in the dog. Severe chronic flea allergy dermatitis in a Sydney Silkie terrier showing hair loss over trunk and hind legs, hyperpigmentation of the skin in the posterior portion of the body (readily accessible to chewing and biting) and erythema and excoriations around the shoulder area resulting from scratching with the hind feet.

336 Flea bite hypersensitivity in the dog. Chronic severe flea allergy dermatitis in a Bull terrier showing gross thickening of the dorsal pelvic area and tail.

337

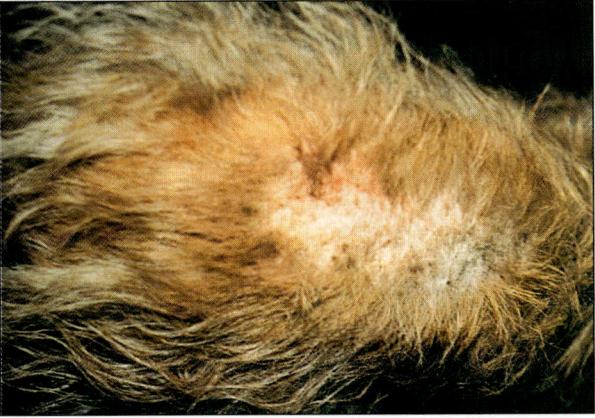

338

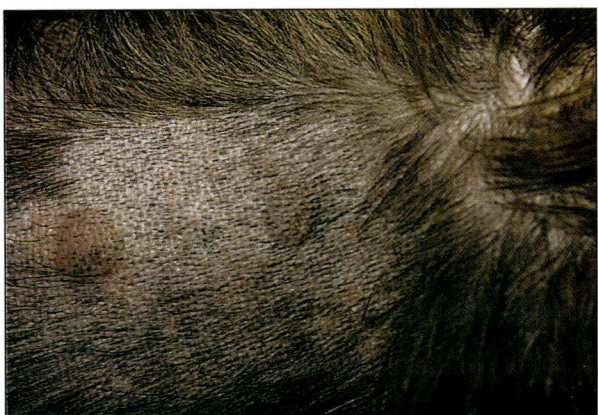

337 Flea bite hypersensitivity in the dog. Superficial excoriation and early lesions of pyotraumatic dermatitis resulting from self-inflicted trauma.

338 Positive immediate intradermal flea test. From left to right: positive and negative controls and a positive, immediate reaction to aqueous flea allergen.

FBH in the dog is characterised by:
- Ubiquity.
- Pruritus.

Differential diagnosis includes:
- Dietary intolerance.
- Atopy.
- Anal sac disorders.
- Other ectoparasite hypersensitivities.
- Drug eruption.

Diagnosis can be made by:
- Recognition of the primary lesion and distribution of the secondary lesions.
- Demonstration of the presence of fleas or flea faeces.
- Positive reaction to intradermal injection of aqueous flea allergen (**338**).

339

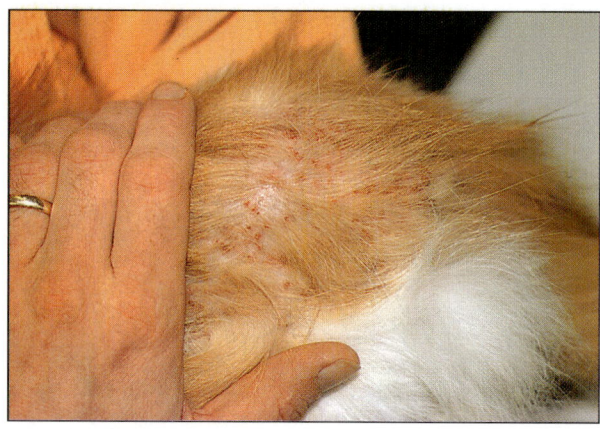

339   Flea bite hypersensitivity in the cat. A papulo-crustous dermatitis (miliary dermatitis) is a common cutaneous reaction in the cat. The condition is considered to be multifactorial in origin but 60-80% of cases are due to flea allergy.

340

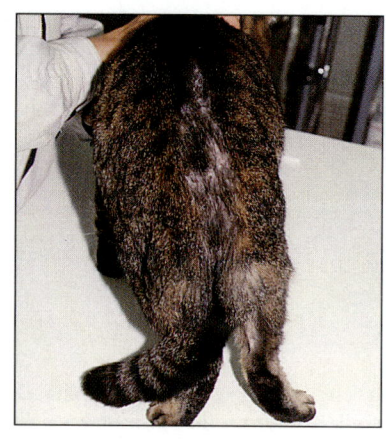

340   Flea bite hypersensitivity in the cat. Note that the lesions have a similar distribution to those in the dog.

341

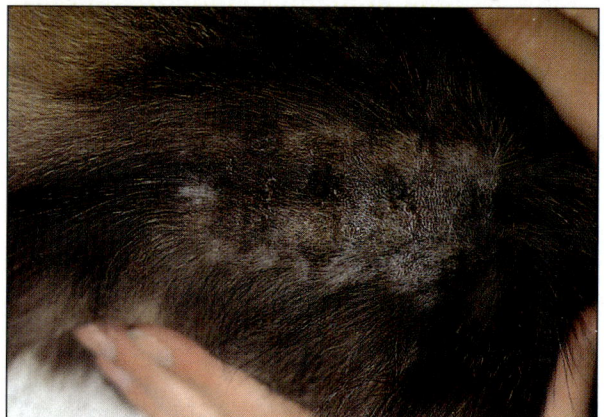

342

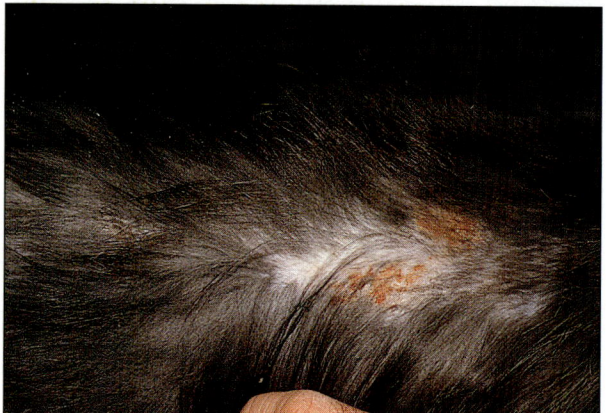

341 and 342   Flea bite hypersensitivity in a cat. Close-up of the dorsal lumbar region demonstrating crusted papules. Papulocrustous dermatitis can be palpated more easily than seen, particularly in long-haired cats.

In the cat

The crusted papule is by far the most common manifestation of FBH (**339**). Typically, these occur on the dorsum, but they may generalise. Crusted papules are commonly referred to as 'miliary dermatitis,' but this is not a diagnosis, merely a descriptive term. Crusted papules are features of many diseases such as atopy, dietary intolerance, other ectoparasites and dermatophytosis (**Table 5**), but FBH is by far the most common cause. Other manifestations of FBH in the cat are dorsal hyperaesthesia, stubbled alopecia on the dorsum, multifocal patchy alopecia, bilaterally symmetrical alopecia (**340–345**) and manifestations of the 'eosinophilic granuloma complex', particularly eosinophilic plaque (see Chapter 18).

343

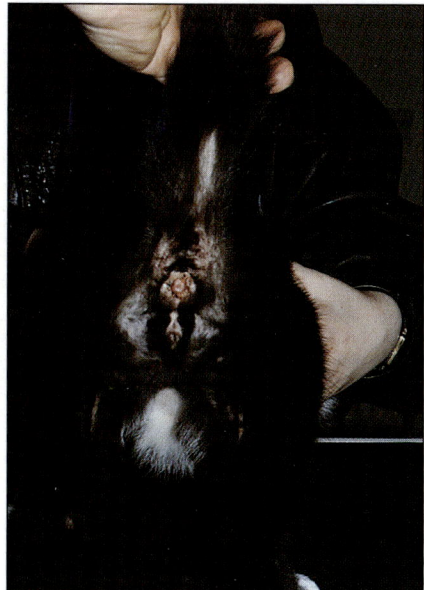

344

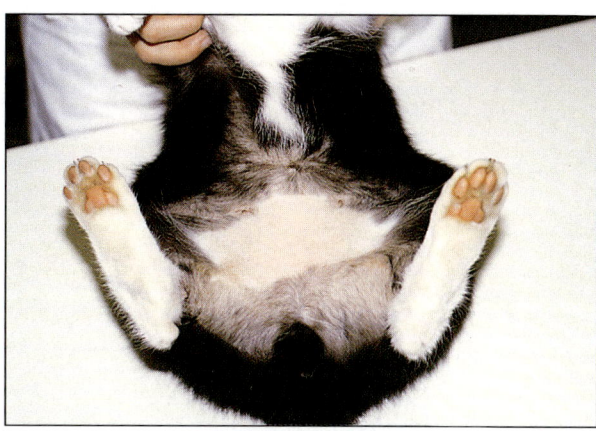

345

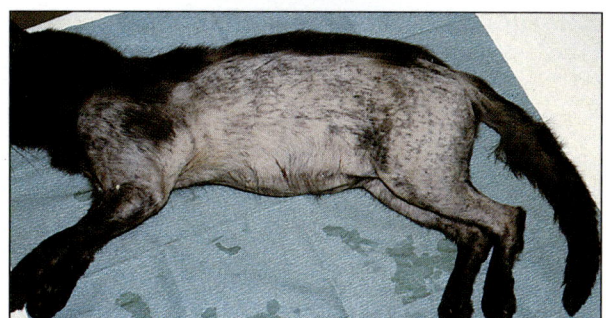

343–345   Flea bite hypersensitivity in the cat. Symmetrical alopecia is a common result of the increased grooming activity manifested by pruritic cats. As with crusted papules this presenting sign is characteristic of many diseases although flea allergy is the most common. Varying degrees of alopecia may be seen. In **343** the alopecia is limited to the caudal thighs and underside of the tail whereas in **344** there is symmetrical alopecia confined to the groin and ventral abdomen. An exceptional case with very extensive symmetrical alopecia is depicted in **345**.

FBH in the cat is characterised by:
- Ubiquity.
- Pruritus.

The differential diagnosis includes:
- Atopy.
- Dietary intolerance.
- Other ectoparasites.
- Dermatophytosis.
- Drug eruption.

Diagnosis can be made by:
- Recognition of the primary lesion and distribution of the secondary lesions.
- Demonstration of the presence of fleas or flea faeces.
- Positive response to the intradermal injection of aqueous flea allergen.
- Response to trial therapy with appropriate topical and environmental flea control.

Table 5 *The differential diagnosis of papulocrustous dermatitis ('miliary dermatitis') in the cat*

Hypersensitivities
  flea bite hypersensitivity
  atopy
  dietary intolerance
Ectoparasites
  cheyletiellosis
  trombiculidiasis
  pediculosis
  ectopic otodectic mange
  Lynxacarus radovsky infestation
Infectious dermatoses
  dermatophytosis
  bacterial folliculitis
Nutritional disorders
  biotin deficiency
  essential fatty acid deficiency
Miscellaneous dermatoses
  drug eruption
  hypereosinophilia

346
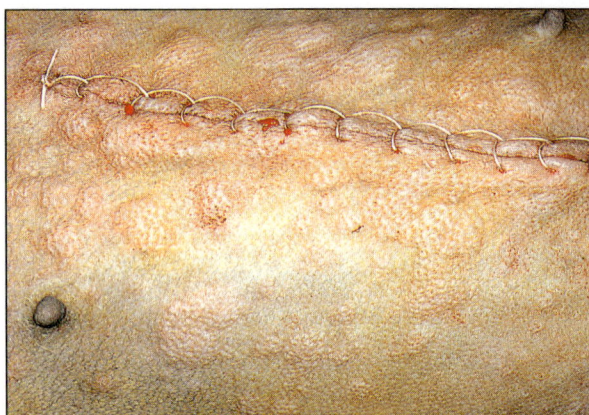

347
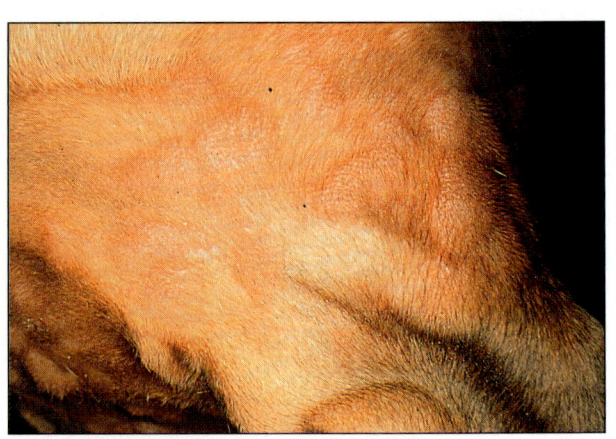

346 and 347   Urticaria. These large, flat-topped wheals appeared within minutes following the intravenous injection of neostigmine to counter a muscle relaxant used during a laparotomy in a dog.

348

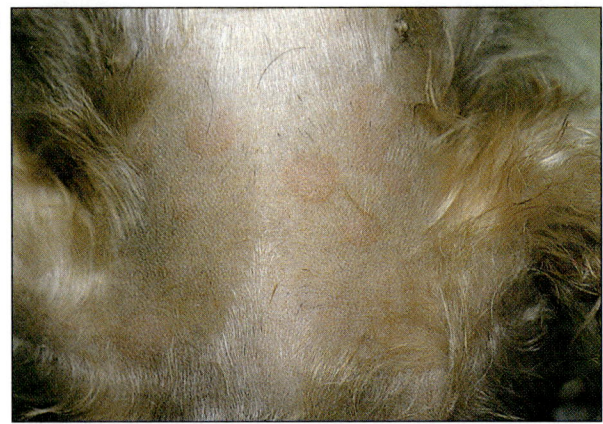

348   Urticaria. Wheals of unknown origin on the glabrous ventral skin of a collie cross.

Urticaria

A condition characterised by variably pruritic wheals which may be immunological or non-immunological in origin. The condition is uncommon in the dog and rare in the cat. Urticaria may result from insect bites and stings, plant stings, allergens in food, administration of antiserum, vaccines and drugs and many other factors.

Clinical signs are usually acute in onset, developing within a few minutes to a few hours. The lesions may be localised or generalised and consist of elevated, plaque-like areas which are oedematous to the touch. Wheals may be small and well-defined or large and poorly-circumscribed (**346–348**). In short-coated dogs the sites of the lesions are revealed by tufting of the overlying hair and bacterial folliculitis is a major differential diagnosis (**349**).

Occasionally there may be large, poorly defined oedema involving a region of the body such as the lips, muzzle, eyelids or pinna, a condition called angioedema (**350 and 351**). Insect bites and stings and plant stings tend to be pruritic or even tender, but otherwise the lesions appear to be painless and non-irritant. Urticarial lesions are not associated with exudation or haemorrhage and the lesions usually disappear within 24 hours. They may recur and have a cyclic nature and in rare instances they may be chronic.

349

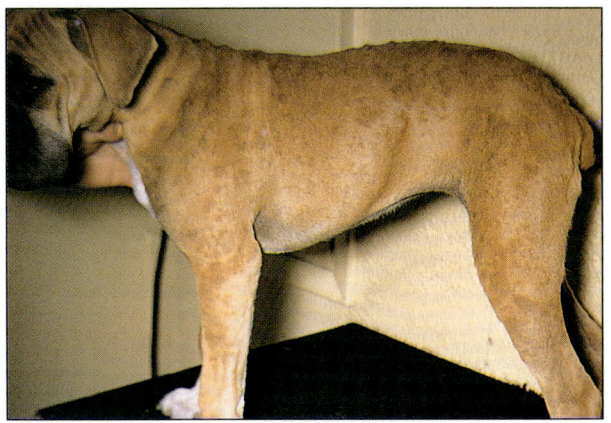

349 Urticaria. In short-coated dogs, such as this boxer, the urticarial wheals cause the appearance of small tufts of raised hair over the whole body surface which may be confused with superficial folliculitis (see Chapter 5). There may be an associated angioedema of the head and ears.

350

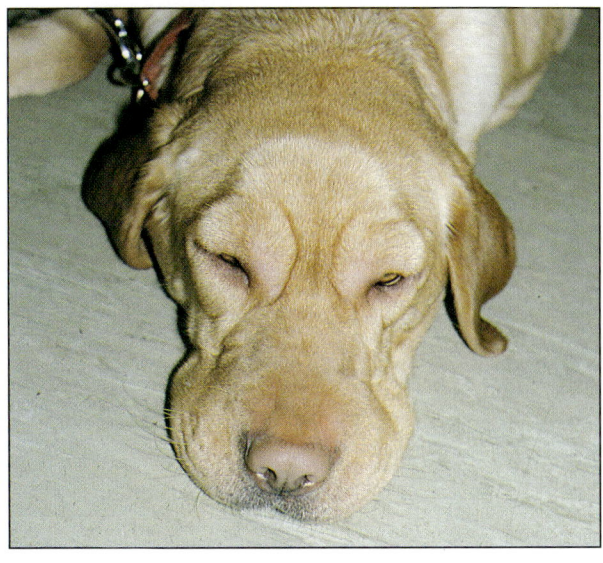

350 Urticaria. Angioedema of the face of a Labrador retriever caused by an insect sting.

Urticaria is characterised by:
- Acute onset.
- Variably sized, often poorly circumscribed, elevated wheals.

Differential diagnoses include:
- Staphylococcal folliculitis.
- Cutaneous neoplasia particularly mast cell and lymphoid neoplasia.

Diagnosis can be made by:
- Consideration of the history and clinical signs.
- Identification of the primary lesion.

351

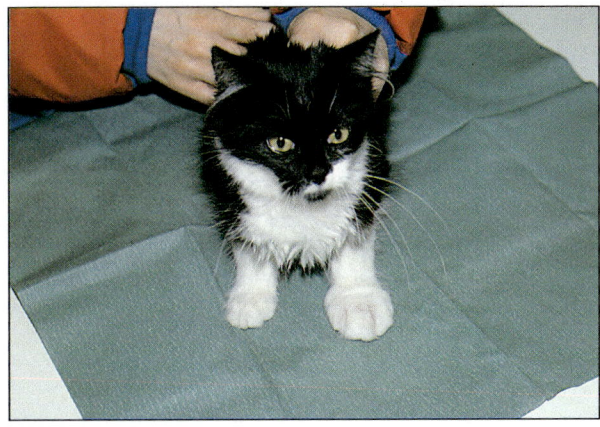

351 Urticaria. Angioedema of a cat's paw caused by an insect sting.

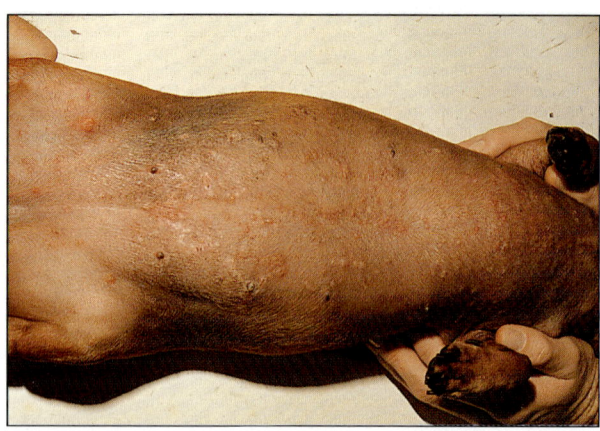

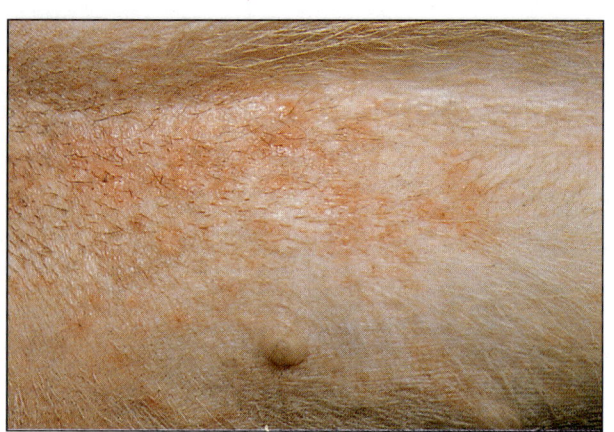

352 and 353   Allergic contact dermatitis. The primary lesions of this condition are erythematous papules. They are readily apparent on the ventral abdomen of these two dogs.

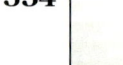

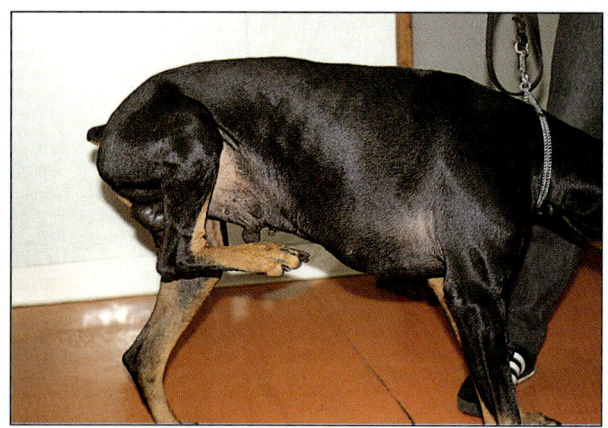

354   Allergic contact dermatitis. This Doberman pinscher has ventral pruritus. Note the enlarged nipples, a consequence of chronic inflammation and self-trauma.

Allergic contact dermatitis

Allergic contact dermatitis is rare in the dog. Naturally-occurring allergic contact dermatitis has yet to be reported in the cat, although experimental models suggest that cats can mount a cell-mediated response to topically applied chemical sensitisers.[14] Affected animals become sensitised to specific environmental allergens and they mount a cell-mediated (Type IV hypersensitivity) response to the allergen when it comes into contact with the skin. Most authorities agree that animals take a long time (years) to become sensitised.[16,18]

Allergens may be domestic (dyes, mordants, waxes, dry carpet shampoos), of vegetable origin (grass, *Tradescantia*) or result from exposure to medications (topical neomycin, povidone iodine).[3,10,18] These are substances to which most animals show no reaction. In contrast, in irritant contact dermatitis, sensitisation is not necessary, reaction is typically rapid (hours to days), allergens may be obviously caustic (cement powder, acids, strong detergents) and most animals coming into contact will react. It is, however, difficult, if not impossible, to distinguish between allergic and irritant contact dermatitis on clinical examination.

In order to elicit a reaction substances must contact the skin and initial signs of dermatitis occur those areas where the hair coat is sparse or absent such as the ventral abdomen and thorax,

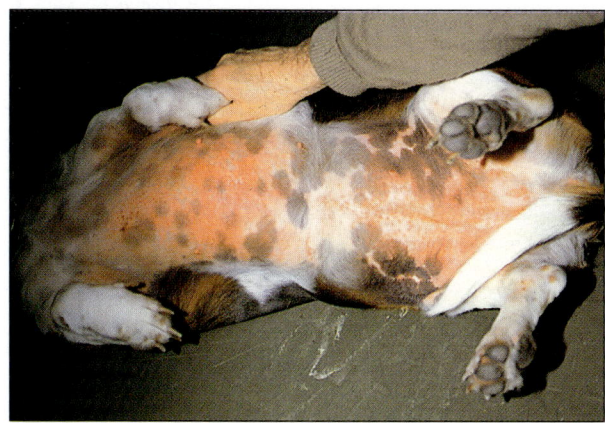

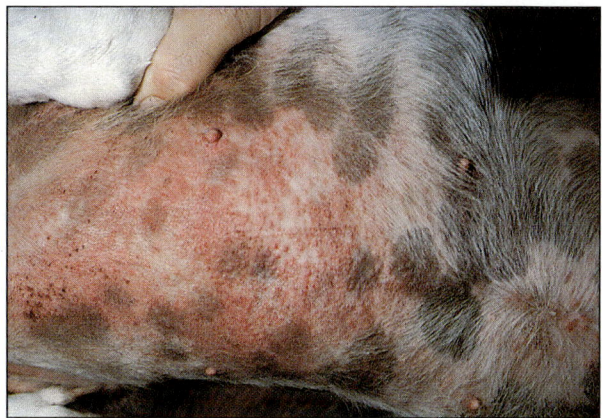

355 and 356   Allergic contact dermatitis. Severe reaction to grass pollen in a Basset hound bitch.

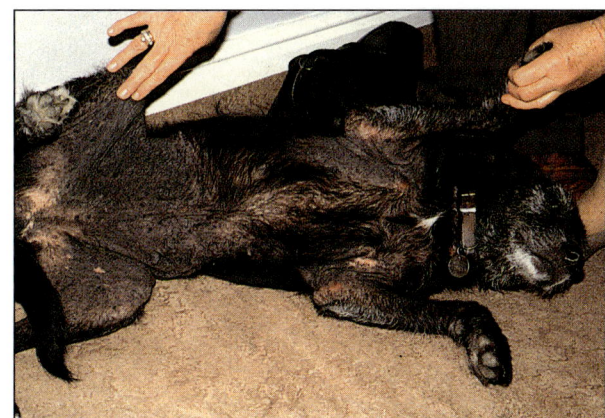

357   Allergic contact dermatits in a Labrador retriever. Note the extensive hyperpigmentation. Note the sharp demarcation between the affected area and the intertrigines, which are spared.

axillae, flanks, interdigital spaces, caudomedial aspects of the legs, perianal region, ventral pinnae and eyelids. It is only when the allergen is in liquid form, such as a shampoo, that hairy regions are involved. Allergic contact dermatitis may occur in very limited areas if topical medicants are responsible; for example the external ear canal in the case of otic preparations containing neomycin.

The primary lesion consists of erythematous papules[2,7,13] (**352 and 353**). Vesicles may occasionally be seen, although these have usually ruptured at the time of examination. The pruritus may result in chronic self trauma (**354**). Almost conflu-

ent areas of erythema may be seen in severe cases (**355** and **356**). As the condition progresses these primary lesions are obscured by secondary lesions such as hyperpigmentation, crusts and excoriations[9] (**357–359**).

However, close examination at the periphery of the affected areas will reveal a sharp demarcation between unaffected skin and skin displaying primary lesions. Seasonal recurrence may occur when the allergen is pollen or plants (**360** and **361**). Perioral allergic contact dermatitis has been reported in animals who react to plastics in the form of drinking and feeding bowls (**362**).

358

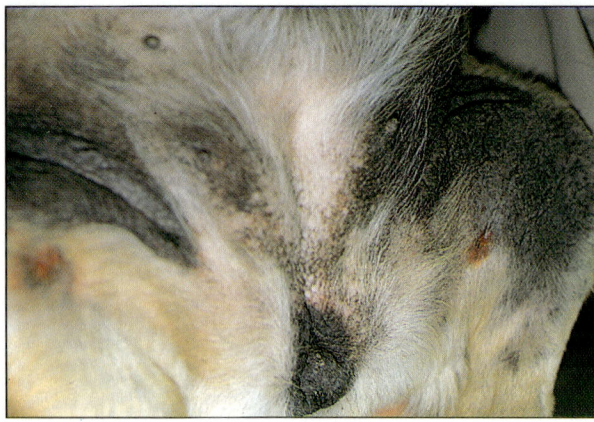

359

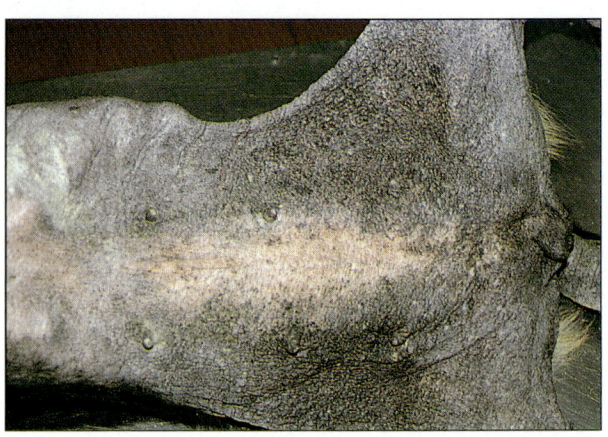

358 and 359   Allergic contact dermatitis. Overweight cross-breed with hyperpigmented, lichenified areas in the leg folds. The original diagnosis was intertrigo and a diet advised. The dog represented after 6 months with extensive lesions of alopecia, hyperpigmentation and lichenification. A cotton sheet was identified as the allergen.

360

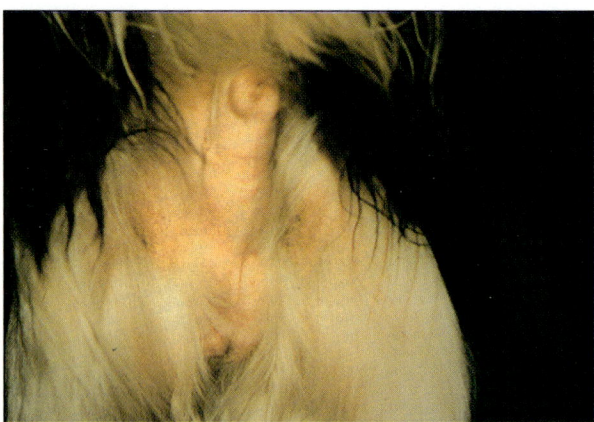

361

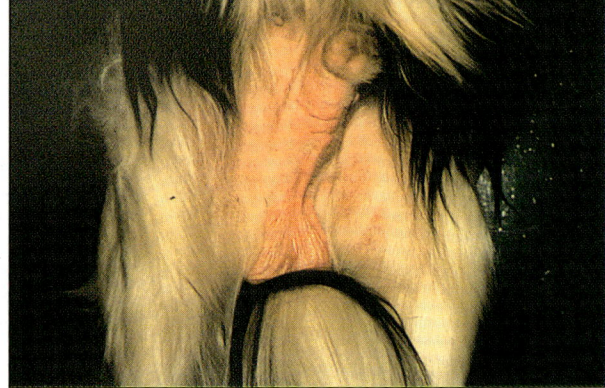

360 and 361   Seasonal reaction to grass in a Cavalier King Charles spaniel. In winter (**360**) the erythema and pruritus resolved, but the lichenification remained. In summer (**361**) erythema and pruritus returned.

Allergic contact dermatitis is characterised by:
- Rarity.
- Long refractory period before clinical signs are apparent.
- Poor response to therapy.

Differential diagnoses include:
- Irritant contact dermatitis.
- Dietary intolerance.
- Atopy.
- Sarcoptic mange.
- Staphylococcal folliculitis.

Diagnosis can be made by:
- Consideration of the history and clinical signs.
- Removal of patient from putative allergen and provocative challenge.
- Closed patch testing (**363–364**).

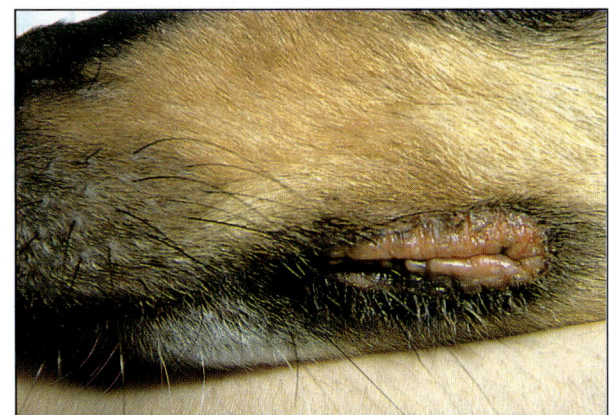

362

362 Perioral dermatitis due to allergic reaction to plastic feeding dish.

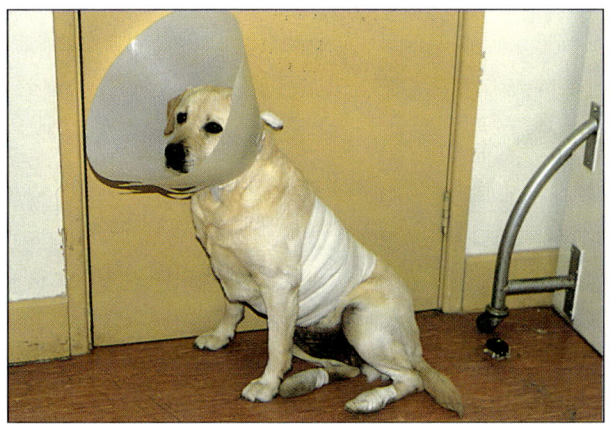

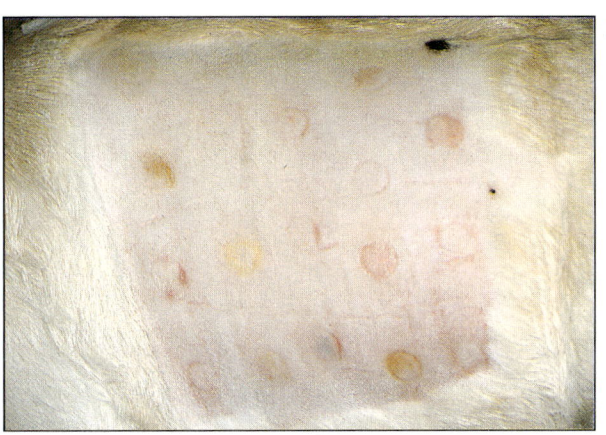

363

364

363 Allergic contact dermatitis. Diagnosis can be confirmed by exclusion and challenge or by closed patch testing. The allergens are placed in nickel cups affixed to tape. This is held in close apposition to the clipped skin for 48 hours. Kennelling, Elizabethan collars and footwraps may be necessary to prevent the dog removing the patches.

364 Allergic contact dermatitis. Close-up of a positive patch test. There is erythema and oedema at the second from top right and third from top in the adjacent panel.

365

366

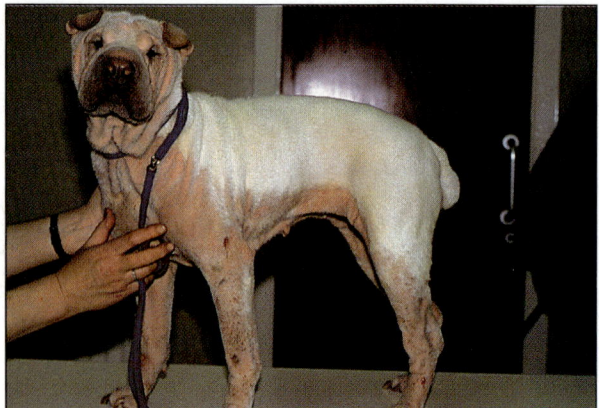
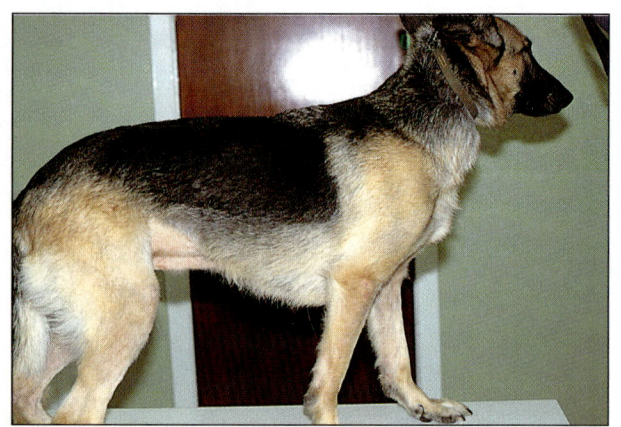

365 and 366   Atopy. Two extremes. The Shar pei has almost confluent ventral erythema, crusting, alopecia and secondary pyoderma whilst at first glance the German shepherd dog shows no lesions.

367

368

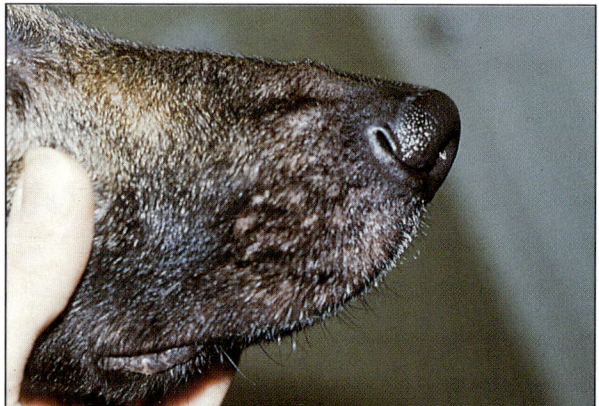
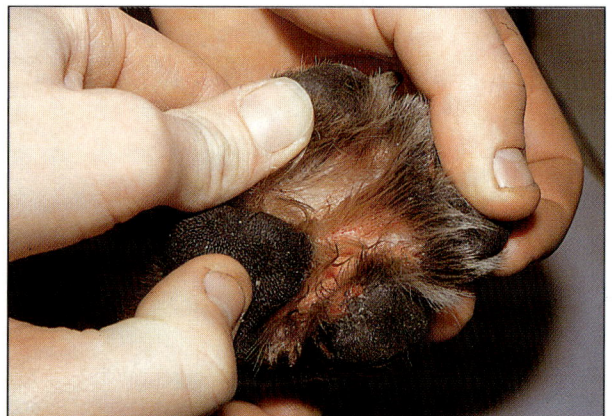

367–370   Atopy. Close-up photographs of the German shepherd dog in **366**. There is facial erythema (**367**), mild erythema of the external ear canals, a superficial folliculitis on the anterior aspects of the proximal fore-limb (**369**), interdigital erythema (**368**) and a superficial folliculitis in the groin (**370**).

Atopy

Atopy, atopic dermatitis or allergic inhalant dermatitis is a pruritic dermatitis occurring in genetically predisposed dogs and cats. Affected animals develop reaginic (IgE) antibody to environmental dusts and pollens and, on exposure, exhibit signs of pruritus. The most common allergens are house dust and food mites (particularly *Tyrophagus putresceantiae, Dermatophagoides pteronnyssinus, Dermatophagoides farinae, Acarus siro*), human dander, pollens (particularly ragweed and grass pollens), moulds and other environmental allergens such as kapok, wool, feathers and cat dander.[8,15,22]

Atopy is an IgE-mediated (immediate Type I) hypersensitivity in which allergen binds to mast cell-bound IgE within the skin. Cross-linking of bound IgE molecules results in mast cell degranulation, the release of preformed and the synthesis of nascent mediators which result in local inflammatory reactions and pruritus. Although experimental allergen challenge via the respiratory tract has been demonstrated to result in pruritus it is believed currently that most allergen exposure is via the percutaneous route. This would be consistent with the typical distribution of clinical signs in the dog.

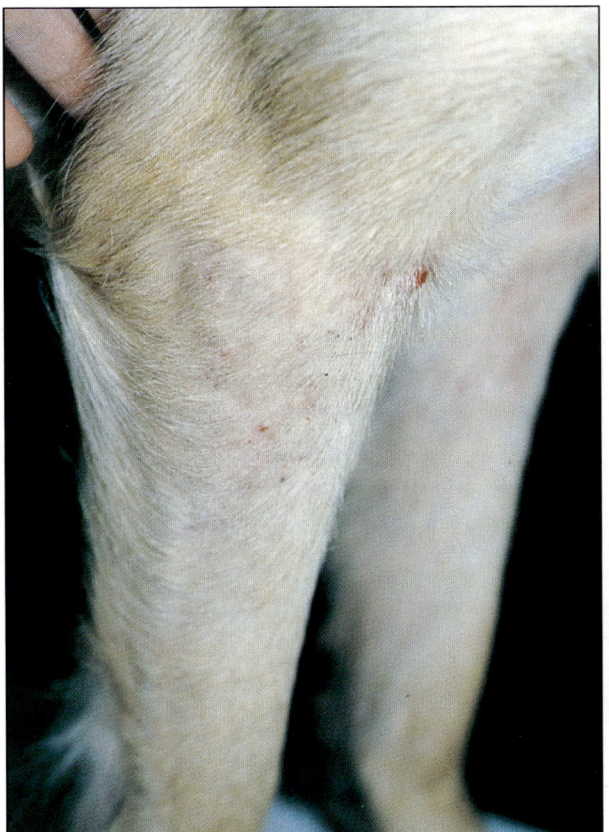

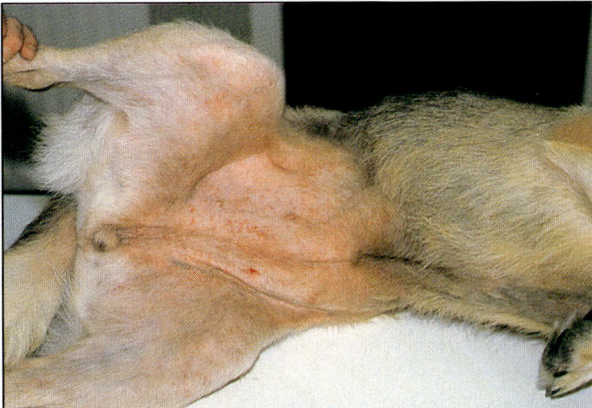

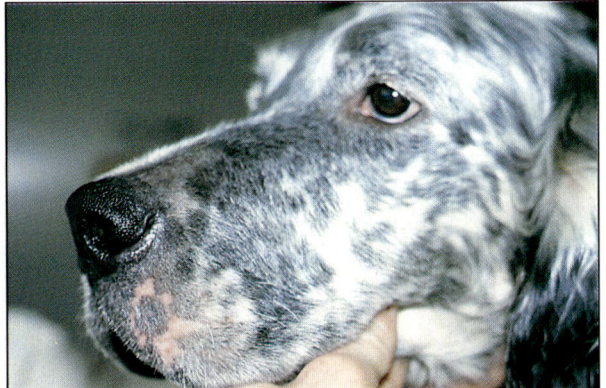

371 **Atopy.** Erythema of the muzzle. Erythema is the earliest lesion and is often masked by secondary lesions.

Canine atopy

It has been estimated that in some canine populations 10% of dogs suffer from atopy. Certain breeds, and lines within a breed, show a high incidence of atopy and these include the Scottish breeds of terriers, wire-haired Fox terriers, Staffordshire bull terriers, Dalmatians, Irish setters, Lhasa apsos, Boxers, German shepherd dogs and Labrador retrievers. Patently, different gene pools in different countries will result in a differing breed predisposition. Atopy affects females more frequently than males.[8,15] Atopy is unusual in dogs less than six months of age but 75% of cases are showing clinical signs of disease before they are three years of age.[15]

Although a number of dogs show seasonal signs (when the allergen is a pollen or a mould) most become perennially affected, illustrating the importance of house mites and human dander as major allergens, particularly in Northern Europe. Even in the United States, where pollens are major allergens, the majority of dogs exhibit non-seasonal signs.[8,13,15]

Clinical signs result from the self-inflicted trauma induced by the pruritus (**365** and **366**). The predilection sites for such damage are the face, the feet and the ventral surface of the trunk[8,15,21], hence the descriptive 'foot licker and face rubber' (**367–370**). The lower limbs, particularly in the

372

373

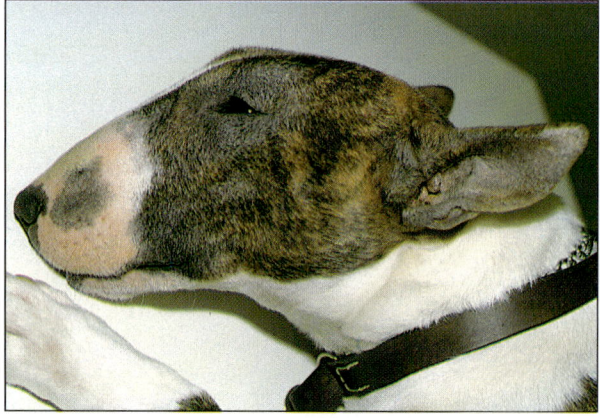

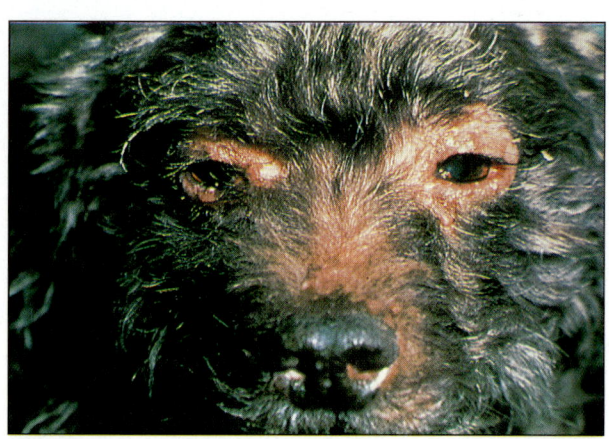

372 Atopy. Periorbital dermatitis due to face rubbing. Note the hyperpigmentation on the ventral aspect of the pinna.

373 and 374 Poodle showing effects of face rubbing and feet licking. (Illustrations courtesy J. A. Yager.)

374

375

376

377

378

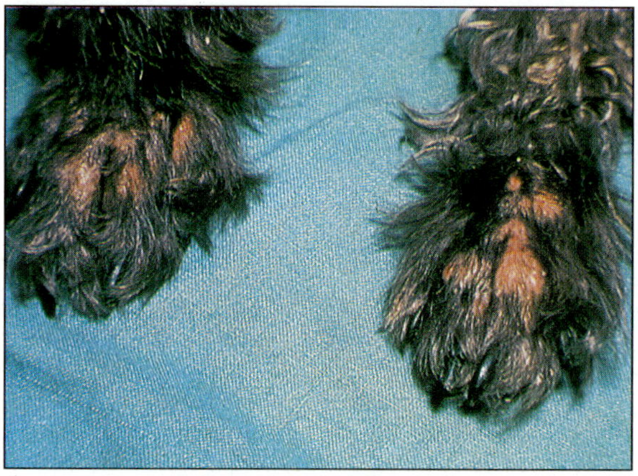

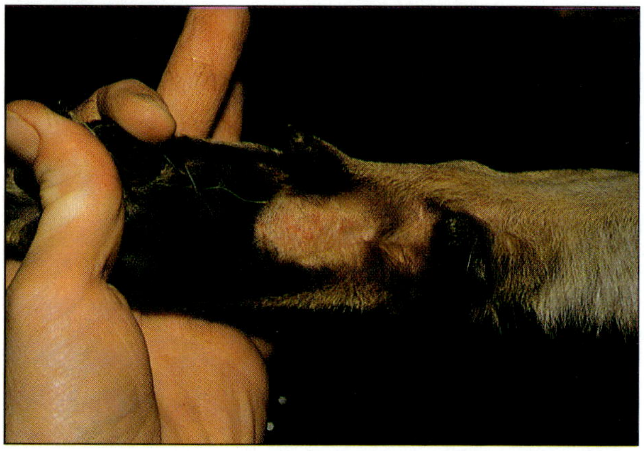

375–378 Atopy. Pedal lesions may include saliva staining (**375**), interdigital erythema and hyperpigmentation of the dorsal aspect of the foot (**376**), interdigital erythema of the ventral foot (**377**) or discrete alopecia between the accessory carpal pad and the main digital pad (**378**).

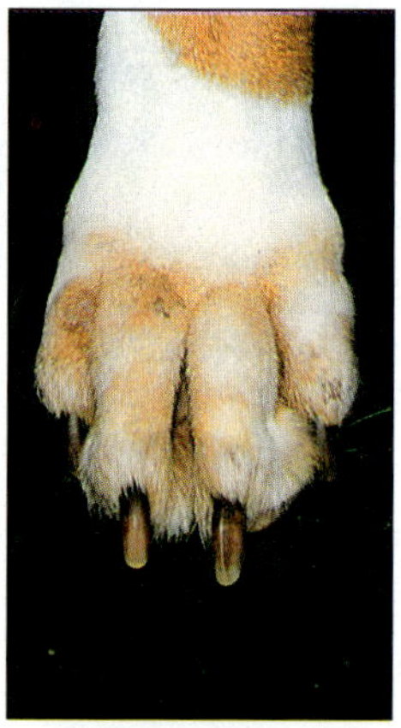

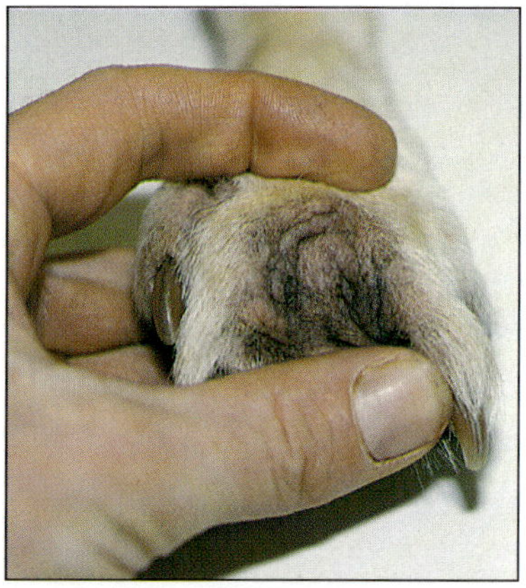

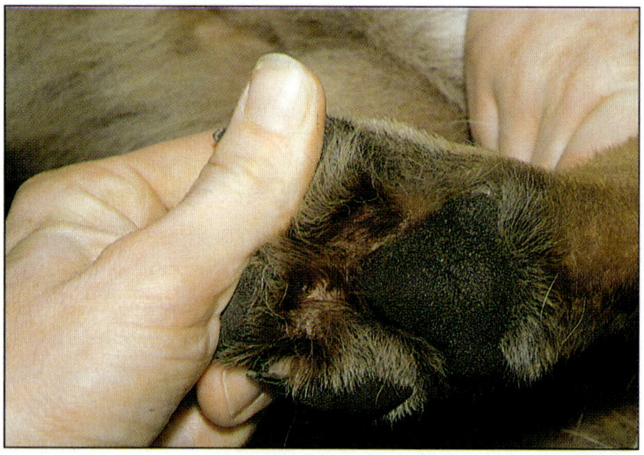

379

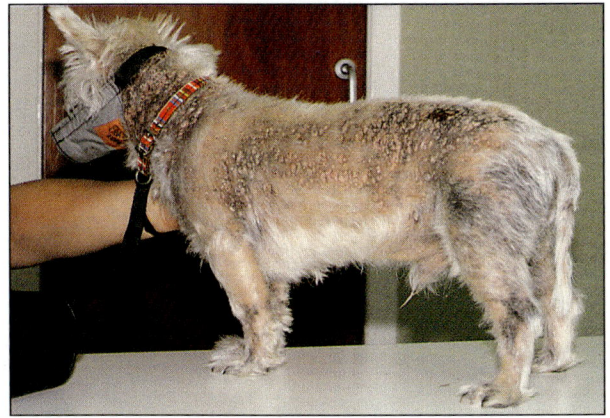

380

379 Atopy. Generalised alopecia, lichenification and hyperpigmentation of the skin and saliva staining of the remaining hair coat in a chronically affected West Highland White terrier bitch. This is almost 'end-stage skin'. The dog could equally well be suffering from demodicosis, *Malassezia pachydermatis*, dietary intolerance or an idiopathic defect in keratinisation and a complete investigation is warranted.

380 Atopy. Very extensive erythema, alopecia and excoriations in a terrier dog.

381

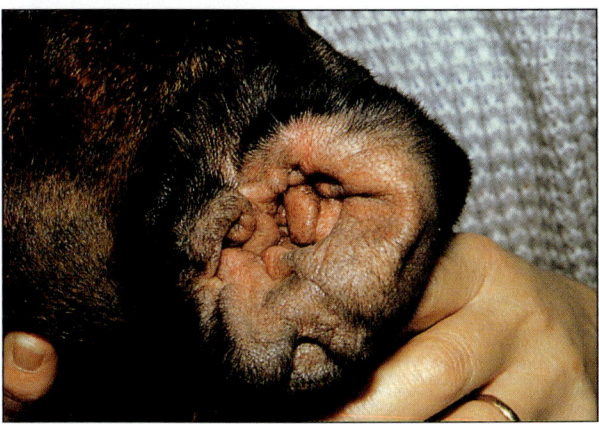

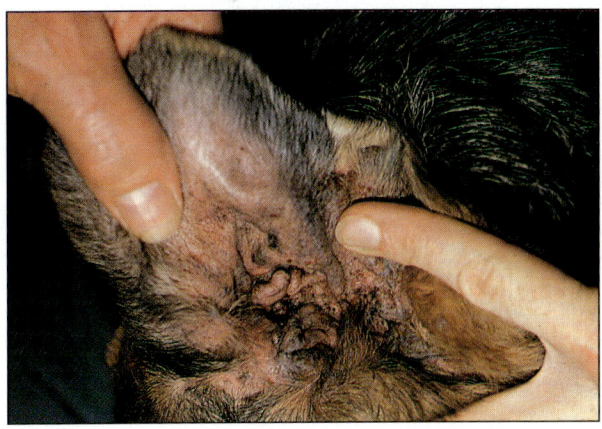

382

381 and 382 Atopy. Chronic bilateral otitis externa is a common feature of the disease. The vertical ear canals are usually erythematous as are the ventral surfaces of the pinnae. The ear of the German shepherd dog in **382** was subjected to lateral wall resection in an attempt to resolve the otitis externa. Unless hypersensitivity is recognised and attended to then resolution cannot be expected.

regions of the carpal and tarsal joints are often sites of pruritus.[21,22] These signs are sometimes accompanied by conjunctivitis and rhinitis. More commonly, most of the body (with the exception of the dorsum) becomes involved. The earliest clinical sign is erythema (**371**).

Chronic inflammation leads to saliva staining of the coat, alopecia, secondary pyoderma, hyperpigmentation and lichenification (**372–380**). Otitis externa is a feature of many cases and in a minority may be the only sign[15] (**381 and 382**). Hyperhidrosis, detectable as the appearance of tiny droplets of water on the skin, is a frequent accompaniment. Dogs with atopy are predisposed to secondary superficial pyoderma, *Malassezia pachydermatis* dermatitis, otitis externa and flea bite hypersensitivity.

383

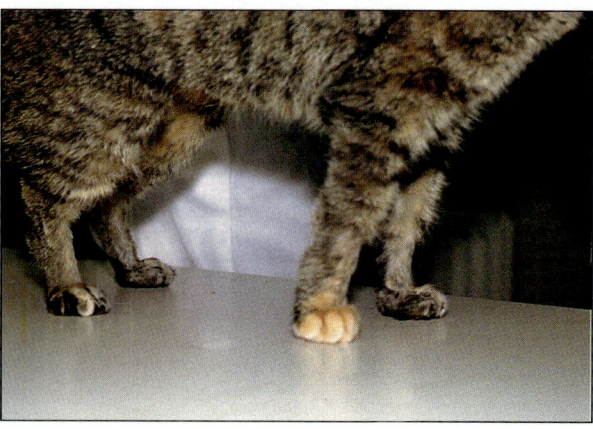

384

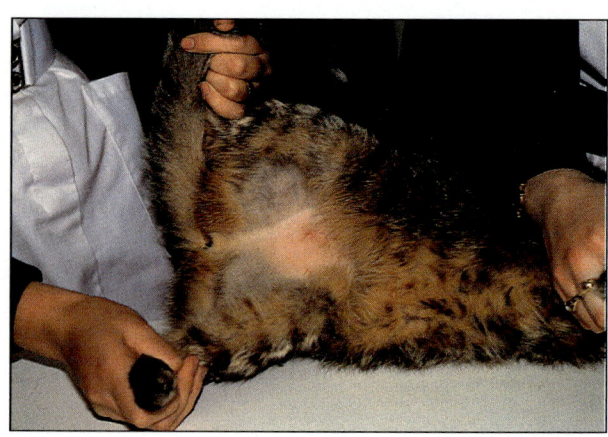

383 and 384   Feline atopy demonstrating pedal alopecia and alopecia of the groin. This cat exhibited seasonal pruritus.

385

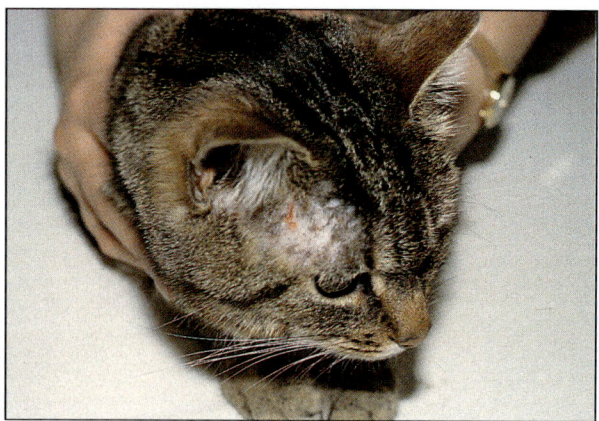

385   Feline atopy is a common cause of facial pruritus in cats.

386

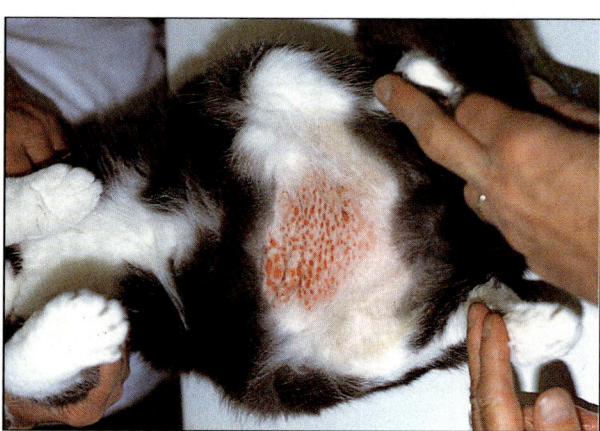

386   Atopy is one of the causes of eosinophilic plaque in cats. In this case there are multiple, discrete areas of plaque associated with alopecia.

Feline atopy

Although it is generally accepted that feline atopy occurs, definitive laboratory evidence has not yet been forthcoming, and it is not known at the present time whether the reaginic antibody is IgE or a sub-class of IgG. The predominant feature of feline atopy is the great variability in its clinical manifestations. Clinical findings may include papulocrustous dermatitis, manifestations of the 'eosinophilic granuloma complex', symmetrical feline alopecia (formerly called feline endocrine alopecia), and pruritus with or without lesions affecting the face, the ears or the whole body (**383–386**).

Atopy is characterised by:
- Ubiquity.
- Pruritus.

Differential diagnoses include:
- Flea bite hypersensitivity.
- Dietary intolerance.
- Sarcoptic or notoedric mange.

Diagnosis can be made by:
- Consideration of the history and clinical signs.
- Rule out of differential diagnoses.
- Intradermal skin testing (**89 and 90**), RAST or ELISA testing.

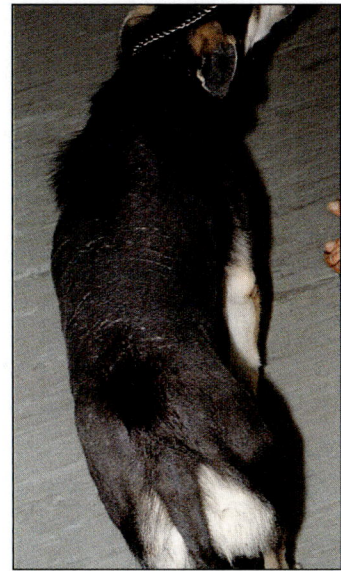

387 **Dietary intolerance.** Cross-bred dog with almost total alopecia as a consequence of continued licking. Restricted diets and challenge identified beef as the offending allergen.

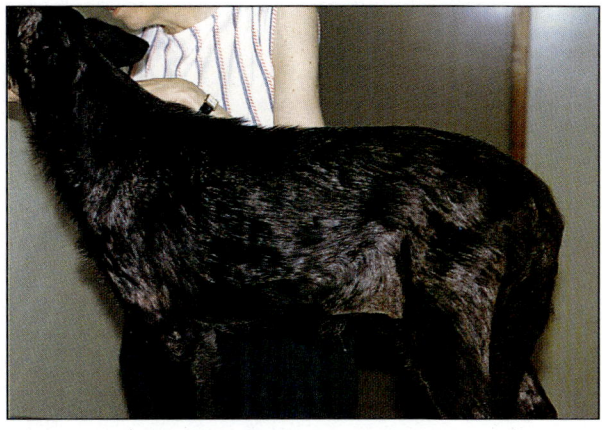

388 **Dietary intolerance.** Generalised crusting and patchy alopecia in a dog with intolerance to egg.

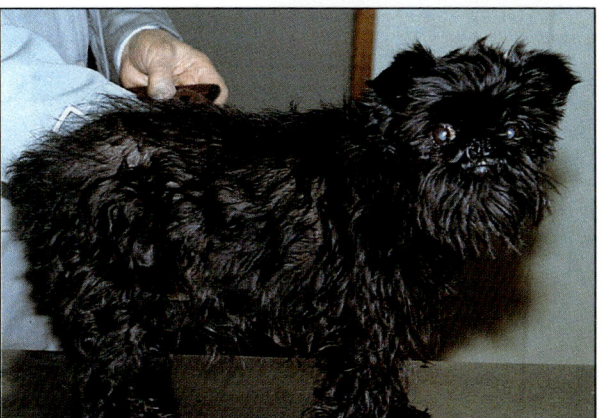

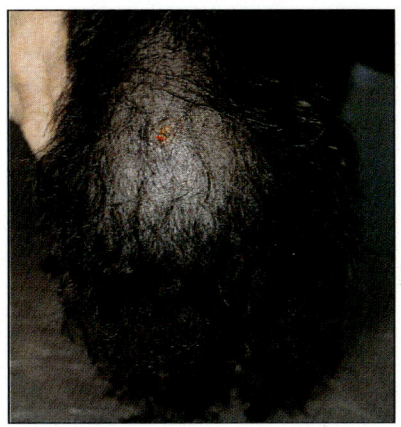

389 and 390 **Dietary intolerance.** An area of pruritus and alopecia on the dorsal lumbar region of this dog. Although the area of alopecia is suggestive of flea bite hypersensitivity, there are no primary lesions and no crusted papules. Dietary intolerance to a component of chocolate biscuit was identified.

Dietary intolerance

Dietary intolerance is an uncommon, non-seasonal, pruritic dermatitis affecting both dogs and cats. There is some controversy about the frequency with which the condition occurs—some workers consider it to be the third most common hypersensitivity skin disease in small animals after flea bite hypersensitivity and atopy, while others think it is a much over-diagnosed condition. There is no breed, age or sex predisposition.

Dietary intolerance cannot be ruled out of any differential diagnosis without the use of restricted diets and provocative feeding, as *in vitro* and intradermal tests are not reliable.[6] The most commonly implicated components are beef, milk (and other dairy products) and cereal products, although any dietary component may be implicated.[2,5,17]

There is no characteristic distribution of lesions and associated clinical signs include papules, urticarial wheals, erythema, scales, crusts, excoriations and even ulceration[1,2,5,19] (**387–392**). There may be bilateral external otitis, seborrhoeic dermatitis and pyoderma. The response to systemic glucocorticoids is usually good in most cases.[5,12] In the cat, as with so many conditions, the condition may be manifested as papulocrustous dermatitis, symmetrical alopecia, 'eosinophilic granuloma complex' or just marked pruritus with the main self-inflicted lesions occurring on the head and neck[2, 20] (**393–398**). There may be signs of gastrointestinal disturbances with diarrhoea and occasionally vomiting although these are not common.

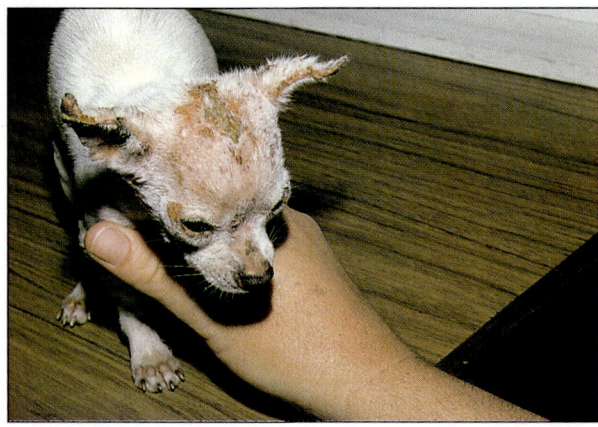

391   **Dietary intolerance.** Severe self-inflicted lesions on the head and ears of a young Chihuahua dog with an intolerance to chicken meat. There was an associated chronic enteritis.

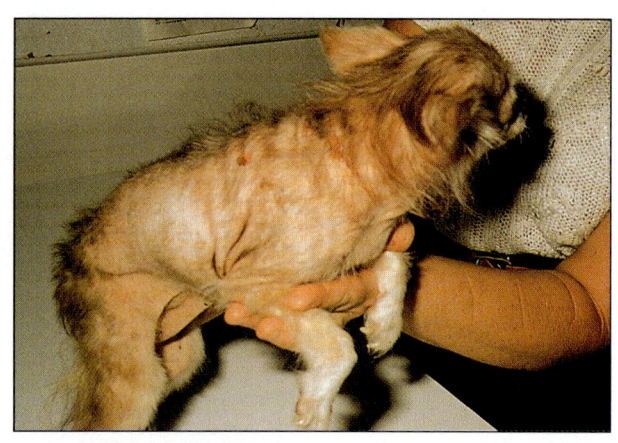

392   **Dietary intolerance.** Chihuahua bitch with generalised hair loss, lichenification and excoriations.

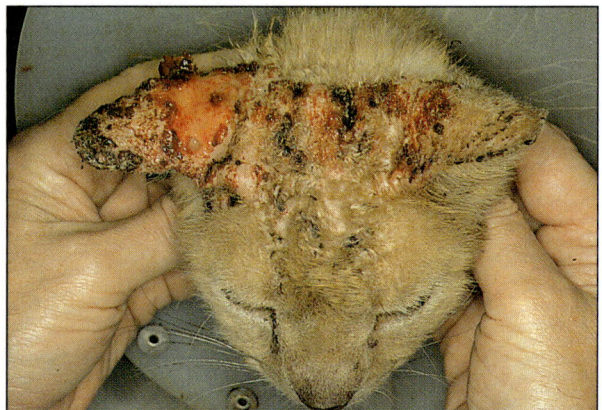

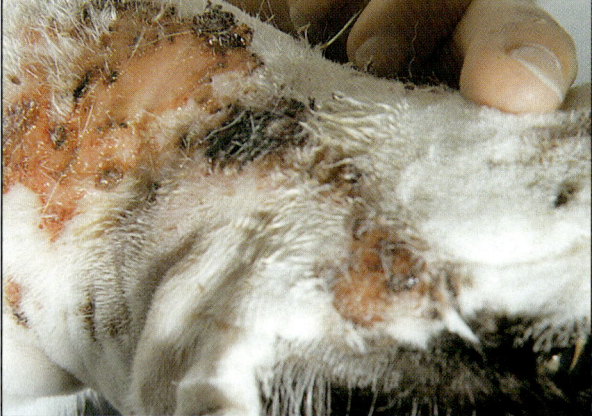

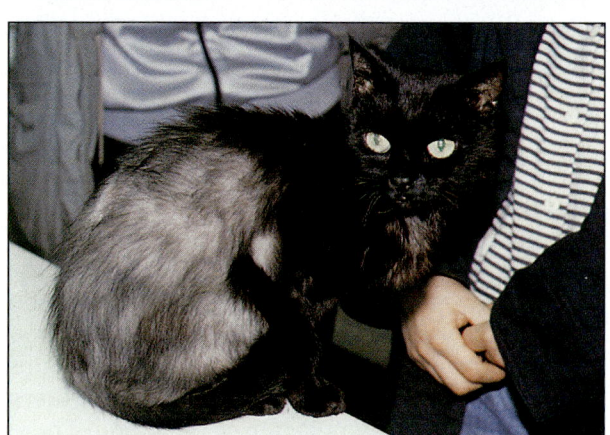

393–395   **Dietary intolerance.** Various degrees of damage due to self-inflicted trauma on the head and neck of three cats.

396   **Dietary intolerance.** Symmetrical alopecia in a cat due to the self trauma associated with allergy to a component in canned tuna.

397

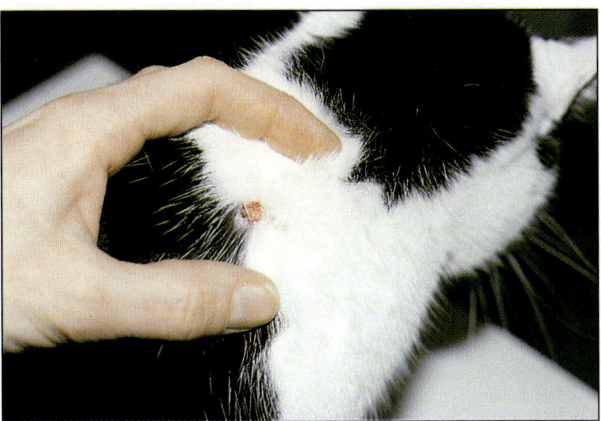

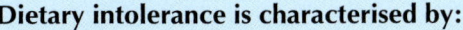

398

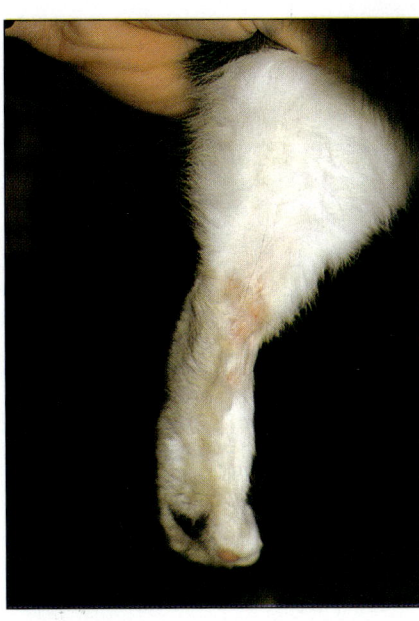

397 Dietary intolerance. Focal crusting on the head of a cat. Intolerance to a component of dried cat food.

398 Dietary intolerance Crusting and alopecia on the medial aspect of the hock of a cat with intolerance to cereal.

Dietary intolerance is characterised by:
- Non-seasonal pruritus.
- Variable response to systemic glucocorticoid therapy.

Differential diagnoses include:
- Flea bite hypersensitivity.
- Atopy.
- Sarcoptic and notoedric mange.

Diagnosis can be made by:
- Restrictive diet and provocative challenge.

399

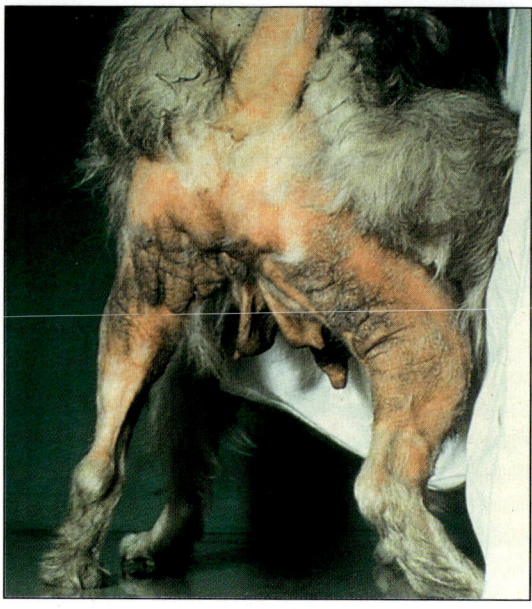

399   Hormonal hypersensitivity. Cross-bred bitch with signs of pruritic alopecia and secondary changes of hyperpigmentation and lichenification, particularly on the perineum and caudomedial thighs. Note the tumefied vulva.

Hormonal hypersensitivity

A rare hypersensitivity reaction to gonadal hormones. The condition has not been reported in the cat. The vast majority of cases have been reported in intact bitches with a history of irregular oestrous cycles or repeated episodes of pseudocyesis. The hypersensitivity is thought to be a Type I or IV reaction and may occur to progesterone, oestrogen or testosterone.

Cutaneous signs are of a pruritic, bilaterally symmetrical alopecia accompanied by erythema, hyperpigmentation and lichenification (**399**). The lesions often begin in the perineum and caudomedial thighs but the changes advance rostrally to involve the face, ears and feet. In bitches the lesions may be cyclic, in synchronisation with endocrine fluctuations of the oestrous cycle. In males the clinical signs are not cyclic.

Hormonal hypersensitivity is characterised by:
- Pruritic, bilaterally symmetrical, alopecia.
- Papulocrustous dermatitis in affected areas.
- Signs in phase with oestrous cycle.

Differential diagnoses include:
- Hyperoestrogenism.
- Flea bite hypersensitivity.
- Atopy.
- Dietary intolerance.
- Drug eruption.

Diagnosis can be made by:
- Consideration of the history and clinical signs.
- Intradermal testing with aqueous solutions of gonadal hormones (if Type I reaction).

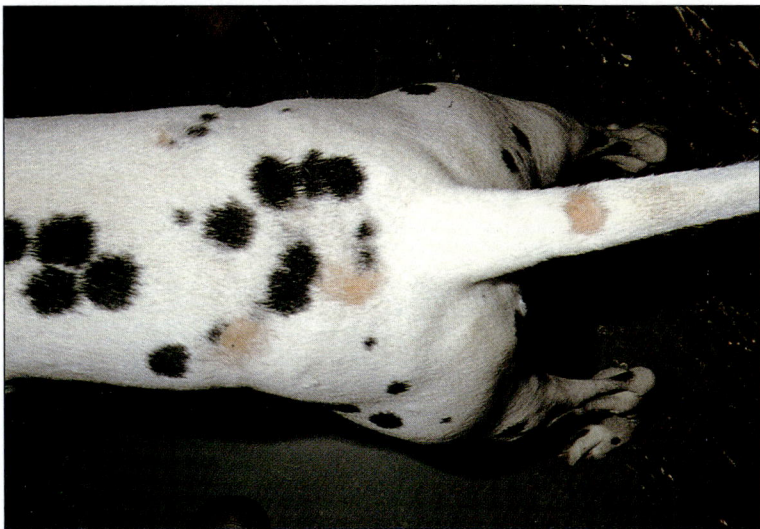

400

400 **Drug eruption.** Exfoliative dermatitis. Focal hair loss and exfoliation without pruritus associated with the topical administration of fenthion for flea control in a Dalmatian dog.

401

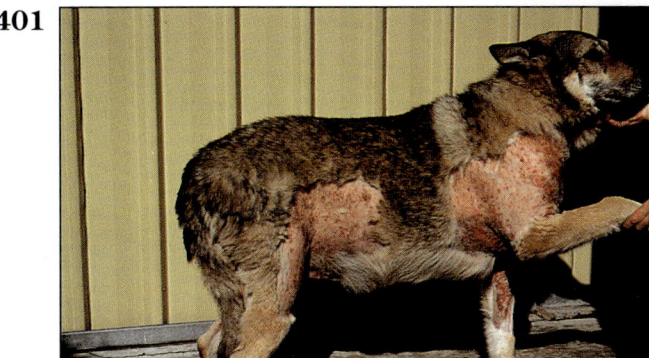

402

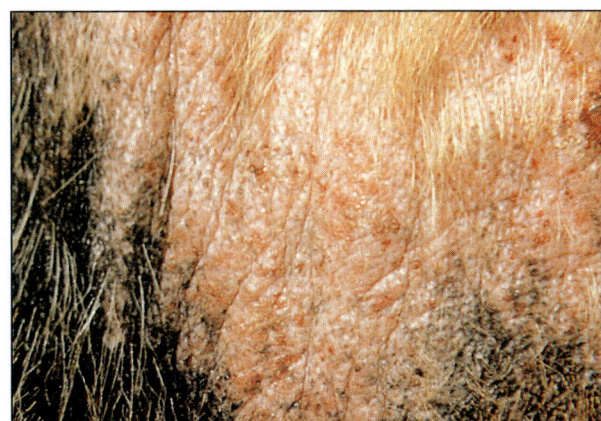

401 and 402 **Drug eruption.** Exfoliative dermatitis. Widespread and severe dermatitis lesions in a German shepherd bitch associated with the administration of levamisole for heartworm therapy. Note the hair loss and erythema, hyperpigmentation and lichenification of the skin (**402**).

Drug eruption

Hypersensitivity to drugs is usually the result of the formation of either specific antibodies or sensitised lymphocytes which produce a reaction upon re-exposure to the offending drug or to related compounds. Drug eruptions may not be immunological in nature as some drugs apparently have the ability to initiate the complement cascade without the formation of antigen-antibody complexes. This alternative pathway which amplifies C3 cleavage and the later part of the effector sequence is not immune-mediated. In such cases an induction period is not necessary and the reaction occurs within a short time after initial exposure to the drug.

Drug eruptions can mimic virtually any dermatosis with the exception of most genetic dermatoses and tumours. Clinical signs include exfoliative dermatitis, erythroderma, toxic epidermal necrolysis, urticaria and vesiculobullous dermatitis[7,11] (**400–409**). Because of the multiplicity of clinical signs the disease is often missed and it is likely that drug eruption is more common than published reports would lead one to suppose.[7]

403 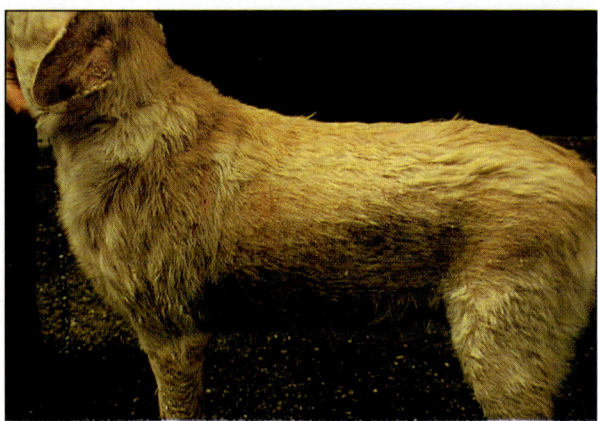 **404**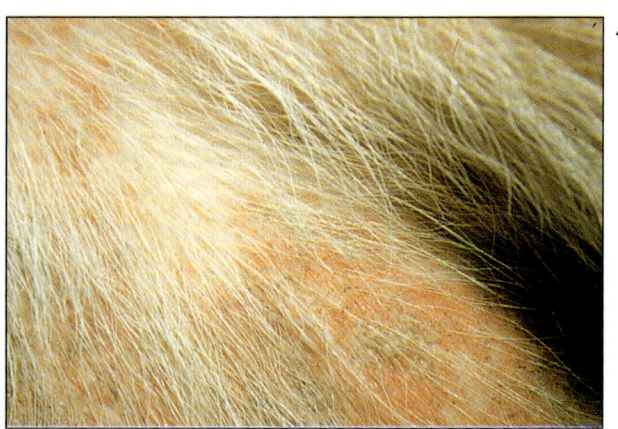

403 and 404   Drug eruption. Erythroderma. Generalised erythema with scaling and mild hair loss in a Labrador retriever bitch following topical application of fenthion for flea control.

405 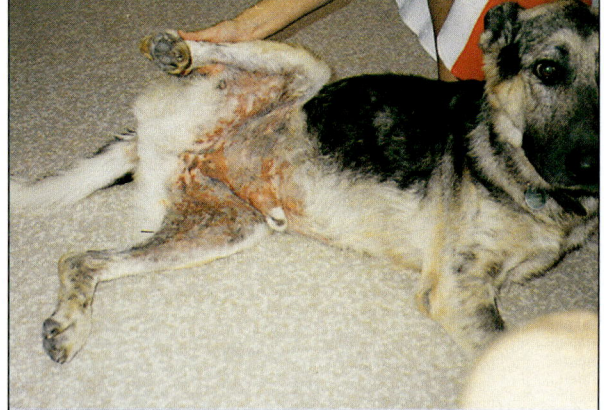 **406**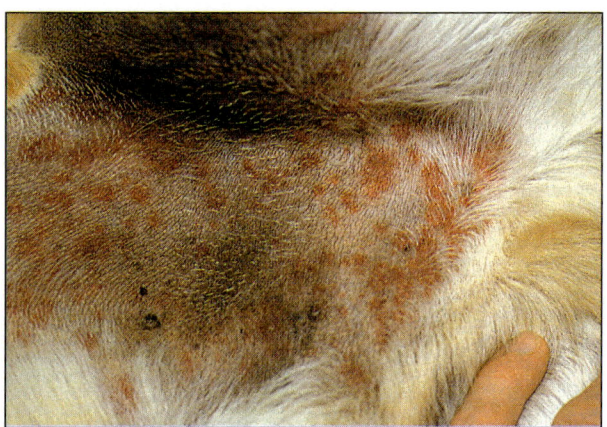

405   Drug eruption. Vesicobullous dermatitis. This German shepherd dog was receiving levamisole for the treatment of heartworm infection when it developed vesicles and subsequently erosive lesions in the inguinal and ventral abdominal areas. The lesions resemble those seen in pemphigus vulgaris and bullous pemphigoid.

406   Drug eruption. Haemorrhagic patches in the groin of a Labrador retriever following the administration of immodium.

407 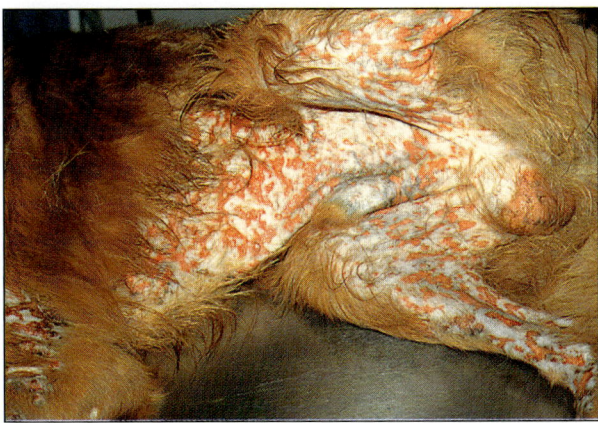 **408**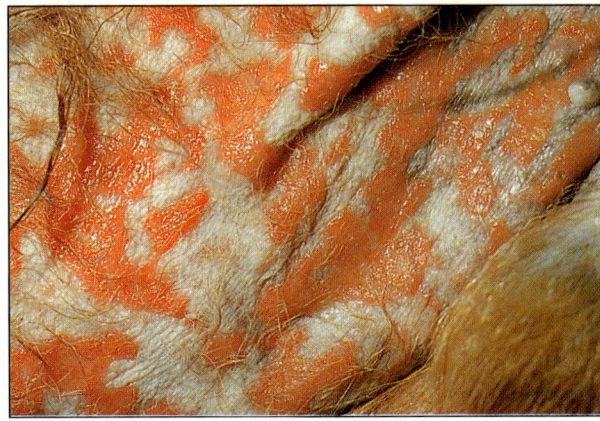

407–409 **Drug eruption.** Toxic epidermal necrolysis. These lesions appeared in this Irish setter during a course of levamisole for the treatment of heartworm infestation. Ten days after withdrawal of the medication the lesions had completely healed.

409 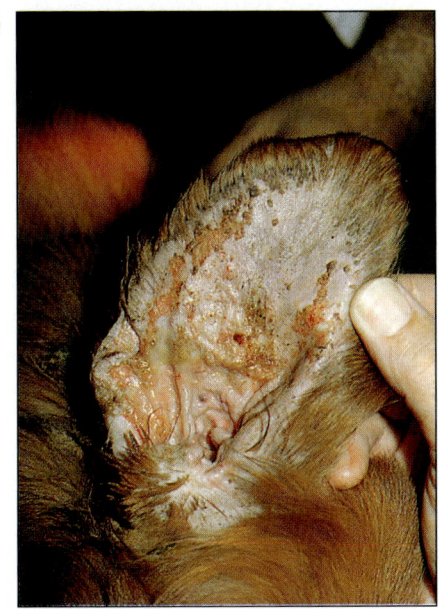 **410**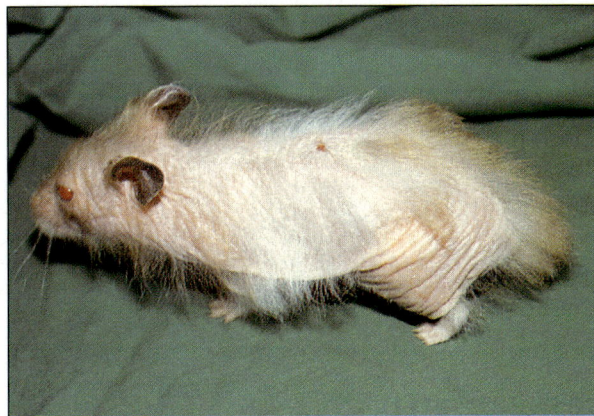

410 **Unidentified hypersensitivity resulted in a pruritic exfoliative dermatitis in this mouse.** The diagnosis was confirmed by histopathological examination of cutaneous biopsy material.

Hypersensitivities in small mammals

The diagnosis of hypersensitivities in small mammals is made by the exclusion of differentials such as ectoparasites and, if necessary, by histopathological examination of biopsy material. Management may be difficult unless the allergen is identified. The mouse in **410** was such a case. Attempts to identify the allergen proved unsuccessful and systemic glucocorticoids were necessary.

References

1. August, J. R. (1985). Dietary hypersensitivity in dogs: cutaneous manifestations, diagnosis and management. *Compendium on Continuing Education,* **7**: 469–477.

2. Carlotti, D. N., Remy, I and Prost, C. (1990). Food allergy in dogs and cats. A review and report of 43 cases. *Veterinary Dermatology,* **1**: 55–62.

3. Grant, D. I. and Thoday, K. L. (1980). Canine allergic contact dermatitis: a clinical review. *Journal of Small Animal Practice,* **21**: 17–27.

4. Halliwell, R. E. W., Preston, J. F. and Nesbitt, J. G. (1987). Aspects of the immunopathogenesis of flea allergy dermatitis in dogs. *Veterinary Immunology and Immunopathology,* **17**: 483–494.

5. Harvey, R. G. (1993). Food allergy and dietary intolerance in dogs: a report of 25 cases. *Journal of Small Animal Practice,* **34**: 175–179.

6. Jeffers, J. G., Shanley, K. J. and Meyer, E. K. (1991). Diagnostic testing of dogs for food hypersensitivity. *Journal of the American Veterinary Medical Association,* **198**: 245–250.

7. Mason, K. V. (1990). Cutaneous drug eruptions. In: DeBoer, D. J. (Ed.) *The Veterinary Clinics of North America, Advances in Veterinary Dermatology,* **20**: 1633–1653.

8. Nesbitt, G. H., Kedan, G. S. and Caciolo, P. (1984). Canine atopy Part 1. Etiology and diagnosis. *Compendium on Continuing Education,* **6**: 73–84.

9. Nesbitt, G. H. and Schmitz, J. A. (1977). Contact dermatitis in the dog: a review of 35 cases. *Journal of the American Animal Hospital Association,* **13**: 155–163.

10. Olivry, T., Prélaud, P., Héripret, D. and Atlee, B. A. (1990). Allergic contact dermatitis in the dog. In: Deboer, D. J. (Ed.). *Veterinary Clinics of North America, Advances in Veterinary Dermatology,* **20**: 1443–1456.

11. Rachofsky, M. A., Chester, D. K. and Read, W. K. (1989). Toxic epidermal necrosis. *Compendium on Continuing Education,* **11**: 840–845.

12. Rosser, E. J. (1990). Food allergy in the dog: a prospective study of 51 dogs. *Proceedings 6th Annual Meeting of the American Association of Veterinary Dermatologists,* p. 47.

13. Schick, R. O. and Fadok, V. A. (1986). Responses of atopic dogs to regional allergens: 268 cases (1981–1984). *Journal of the American Veterinary Medical Association,* **189**: 1493–1496.

14. Schultz, K. T. and Maguire, H. C. (1982). Chemically-induced delayed hypersensitivity in the cat. *Veterinary Immunology and Immunopathology,* **3**: 585–590.

15. Scott, D. W. (1981). Observations on canine atopy. *Journal of the American Animal Hospital Association,* **17**: 91–100.

16. Thomsen, M. K. and Kristensen, F. (1986). Contact dermatitis in the dog. *Nordisk Veterinær Medicine,* **38**: 129–147.

17. Walton, G. S. (1977). Allergic responses to ingested allergens. In: Kirk, R. W. (Ed.), *Current Veterinary Therapy VI,* pp. 576–579.

18. Walton, G. S. (1977). Allergic contact dermatitis. In: Kirk, R. W. (Ed.), *Current Veterinary Therapy VI,* pp. 571–575.

19. White, S. D. (1986). Food hypersensitivity in 30 dogs. *Journal of the American Veterinary Medical Association,* **188**: 695–698.

20. White, S. D and Sequoia, D. (1989). Food hypersensitivity in cats: 14 cases (1982–1987). *Journal of the American Veterinary Medical Association,* **194**: 692–695.

21. Willemse, A. (1986). Atopic skin disease: a review and a reconsideration of diagnostic criteria. *Journal of Small Animal Practice,* **27**: 771–778.

22. Willemse, A. and van den Brom, W. E. (1983). Investigations of the symptomatology and the significance of immediate skin test reactivity in canine atopic dermatitis. *Research in Veterinary Science,* **34**: 261–265.

Chapter 9

Autoimmune dermatoses

Introduction

Autoimmune skin diseases comprise a group of rare dermatoses in which auto-antibodies are formed that are directed against some component of the skin, mucosae or other body system. Inflammation and tissue damage may result from a number of causes such as the activation of complement by antibodies attached to their ligand *in situ* or by the deposition of antigen/antibody complexes at sites remote from their binding.

The most frequently-reported diseases can be divided into two groups. Firstly, the pemphigus and pemphigoid (or blistering) group, in which antibody is directed against either the intercellular components of the epidermis or antigen at the basement membrane zone of the skin or mucosa. Secondly, lupus erythematosus in which an antinuclear and other antibodies are formed, resulting in multisystemic involvement with clinical syndromes such as polyarthritis, haemolytic anaemia, glomerulonephritis and pyrexia in addition to the skin changes.

Pemphigus/pemphigoid complex

This group of diseases includes pemphigus foliaceus, pemphigus vulgaris, pemphigus vegetans, pemphigus erythematosus and bullous pemphigoid, all of which have been reported in the dog and, except for pemphigus vegetans and bullous pemphigoid, also in the cat. In the pemphigus diseases antibody is formed against proteins bound to plakoglobin, a component of both desmosomes and adherans junctions.[5]

These are the main intercellular bridges between the keratinocytes and are responsible for cell to cell cohesion. The assembly and function of these intercellular connections is defective, as a result of antibody binding to ligand, and there is a loss of cohesion between the keratinocytes. This results in acantholysis (rounding up) and subsequent vesicle formation. The acantholytic cells are present in the vesicles and bullae associated with pemphigus foliaceus and cytological examination of needle aspirates taken from these primary lesions will often reveal them, the Tzank test. The loss of cohesion between the keratinocytes may be demonstrated by the Nikolsky test in which erosions are formed by exerting a shearing force to the skin surface. The application and interpretation of these tests may give valuable clues on which a diagnosis may be based (see Chapter 3).

In bullous pemphigoid the antibody is directed toward elements of the basement membrane. Deposition of antibody results in a separation of the dermoepidermal junction and vesicle formation. Acanthocytes, however, are not found. In general, these conditions are characterised by transient blister formation accompanied by widespread, often symmetrical erosions, ulcerations, crusting, scaling and depigmentation. The diagnosis of the pemphigus diseases can be made by consideration of the history and physical examination and laboratory tests such as histopathological or immunofluorescent examination of biopsy material.

411

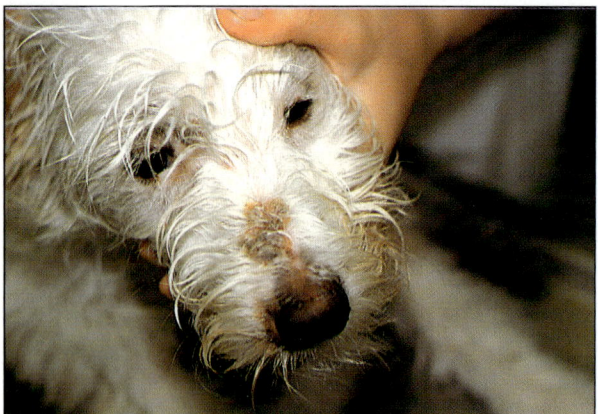

412

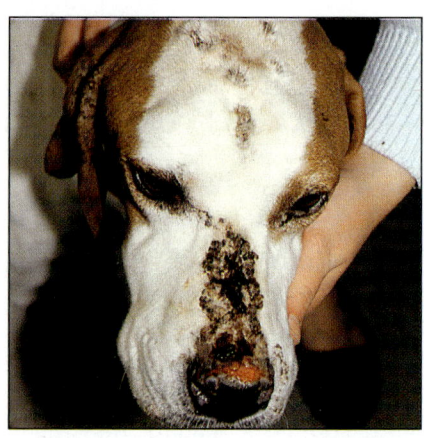

411 Pemphigus foliaceus. Most cases of pemphigus foliaceus involve facial lesions. This collie cross exhibits very localised lesions confined to the muzzle.

412 Pemphigus foliaceus. Short-haired pointer with a more inflammatory lesion. Note the erythematous planum nasale and the depigmentation that has occurred.

413

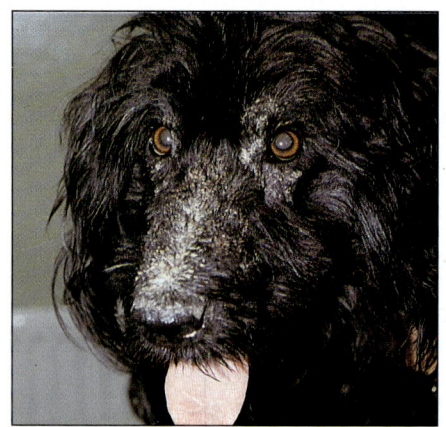

414

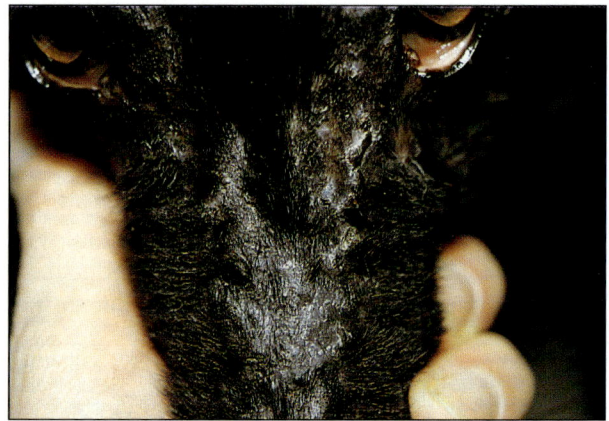

413 and 414 Pemphigus foliaceus. More extensive lesions of pemphigus foliaceus are often symmetrical in distribution. A Briard dog with symmetrical lesions on the face and extending to the periorbital regions.

Pemphigus foliaceus

This is the most common of the pemphigus disorders.[1,3] Acantholysis occurs in the subcorneal region of the epidermis resulting in vesicle formation. These primary lesions are often transient and the disease typically presents as a vesicobullous or pustular dermatitis with secondary erythema, scale, erosion and crust formation. Alopecia may occur. Secondary bacterial infection is frequent. The presence of epidermal collarettes may be associated with the pyoderma or may represent a manifestation of the underlying autoimmune disease. Usually, only the skin is affected and lesions on the mucocutaneous junctions and in the oral cavity are rare. Generally, lesions are symmetrical in distribution and usually commence on the face and pinnae (**411–416**). The footpads may be involved and become hyperkeratotic. The epidermis may separate and slough. Pedal lesions may be the only clinical manifestation of the disease in some individuals.[3] Lesions may be localised to small areas of the body, such as the pinnae (**417**). The ventral surfaces of the pinnae are good sites to find primary lesions (**418**). Pemphigus foliaceus is usually a disease of gradual onset and is rarely accompanied by systemic signs in the dog, even though generalised lesions may occur (**419– 421**). The disease is rare in the cat (**422–424**) and, in this species, anorexia and pyrexia may be noted.[3]

415
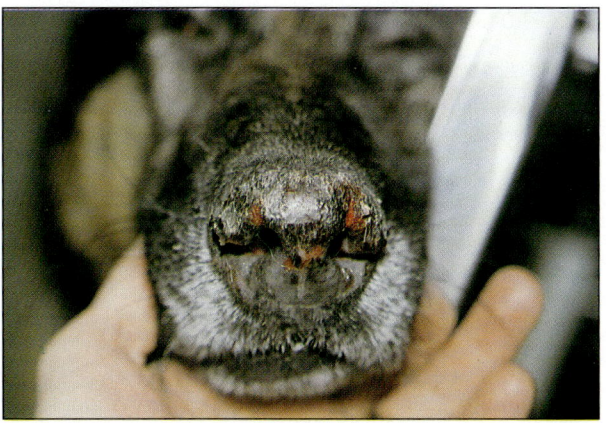

416
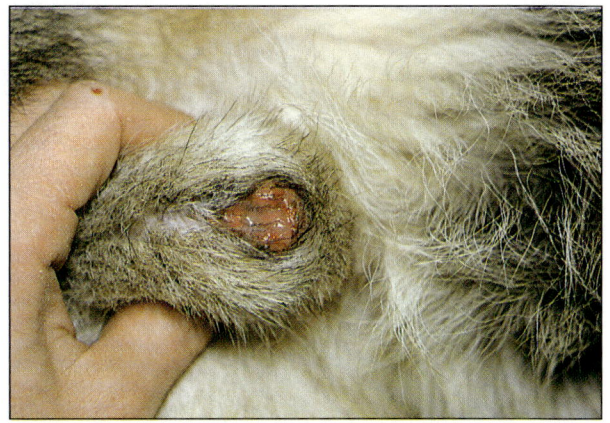

415 and 416   Pemphigus foliaceus. Ulcerated, crusted and depigmented planum nasale and nares in a German shepherd dog accompanied by an ulcerated mucocutaneous region on the sheath.

417
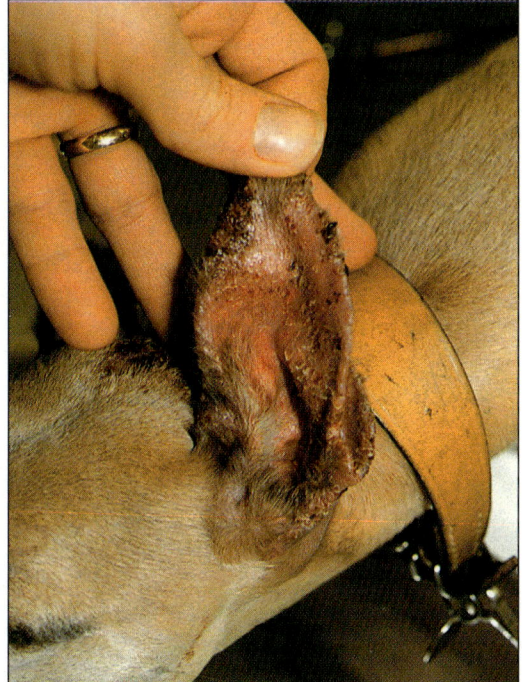

418
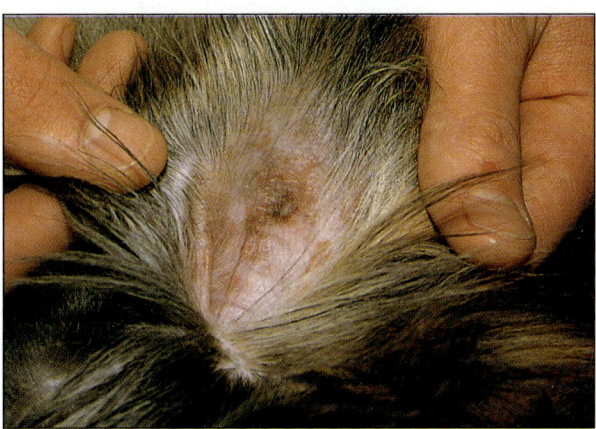

418   Pemphigus foliaceus. Primary lesions of pemphigus foliaceus are fragile and are most likely to be found in areas not easily subject to self trauma, such as the concave surface of the pinna and the interdigital areas of the footpads. This illustration depicts primary lesions on the pinna of a dog.

417   Pemphigus foliaceus. Lesions may be confined to the pinna, as in this whippet. Extensive crust formation is a common sequel to vesicle formation.

419

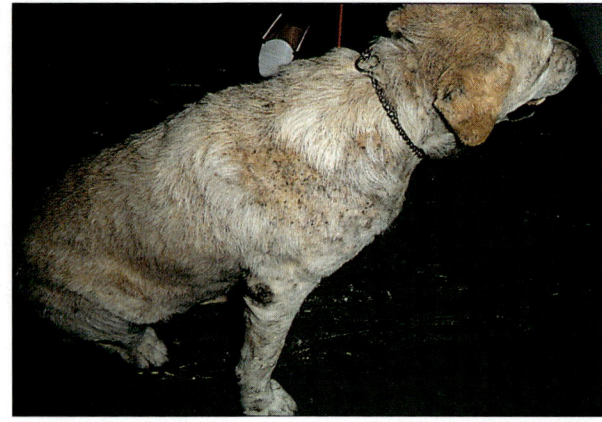

419   Pemphigus foliaceus. Labrador retriever showing generalised alopecia, scale and crust formation.

420

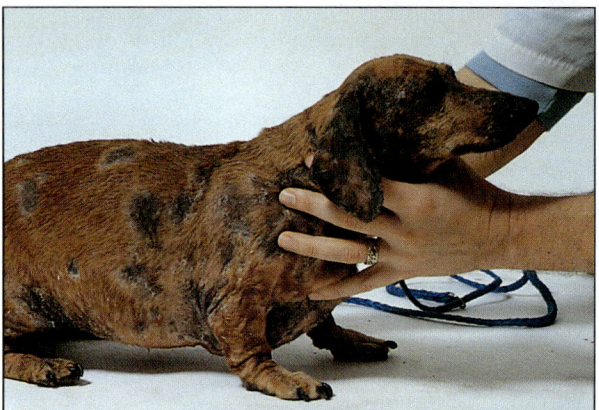

421

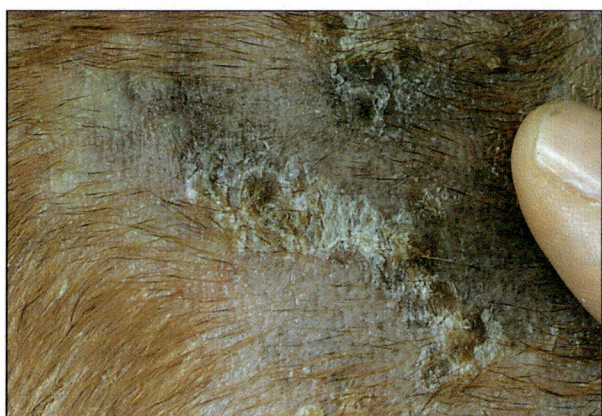

420 and 421   Pemphigus foliaceus. Dachshund showing multiple alopecic foci associated with hyperpigmentation and crust formation. Close-up (**421**) illustrating erythematous foci accompanied by alopecia crusting. (Illustrations courtesy D. W. Scott.)

422

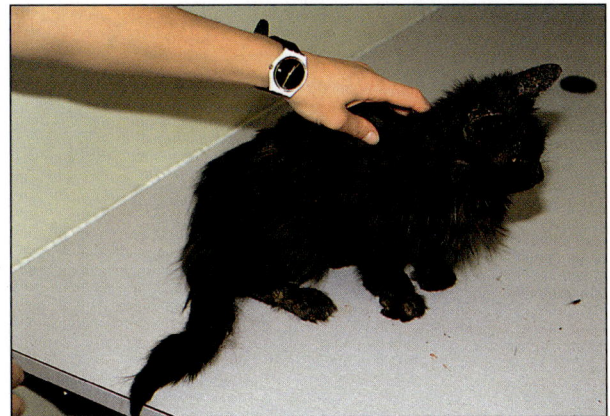

423

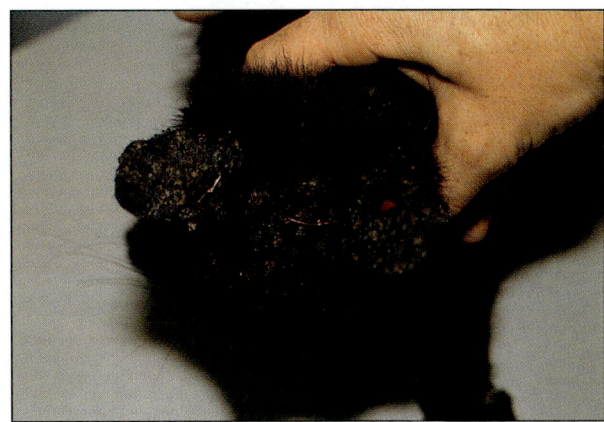

424

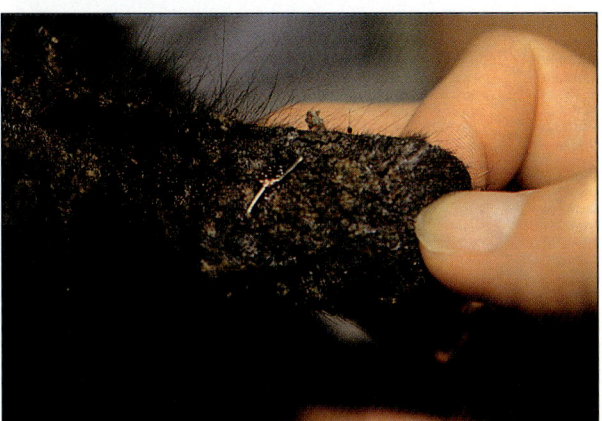

422–424 Generalised crust and alopecia in a juvenile domestic long-haired cat due to pemphigus foliaceus. Note the symmetrical pattern on the dorsal surfaces of the pinna and the heavily crusted forelimb. There is a suture at the site of punch biopsy.

Pemphigus foliaceus is characterised by:
- Gradual onset and lack of systemic signs.
- The presence of a transient primary lesion, a vesicle.
- Extensive secondary changes.

Differential diagnoses include:
- Demodicosis.
- Superficial pyoderma.
- Subcorneal pustular dermatosis.
- Zinc responsive dermatosis.
- Dermatophytosis.
- Actinic dermatosis.
- Mycosis fungoides.

Diagnosis is made by:
- Consideration of history and clinical signs.
- The presence of a vesicle.
- A positive Tzank test.
- A positive Nikolsky sign.
- Histopathological examination of biopsy material.
- Direct immunofluorescence or peroxidase/immunoperoxidase staining.

425

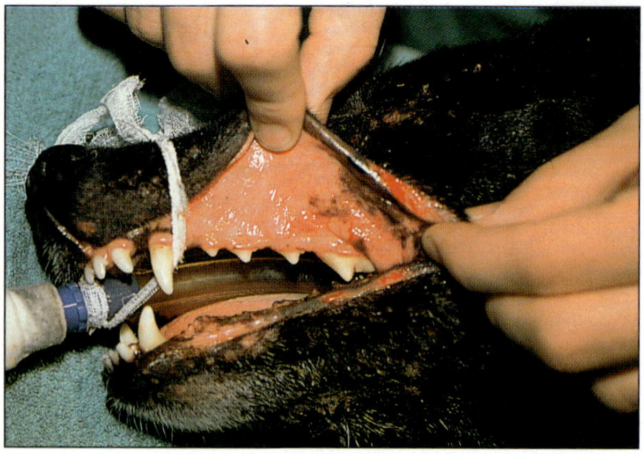

426

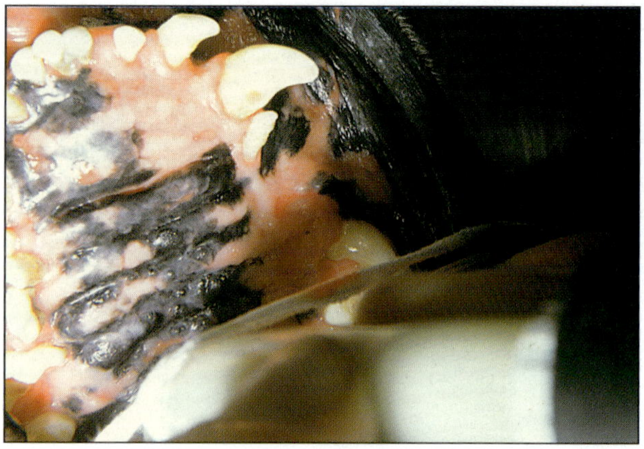

425 Pemphigus vulgaris. Nearly all cases of pemphigus vulgaris exhibit oral lesions. Note the erosions at the mucocutaneous junctions and on the oral mucosae. (Illustration courtesy D. W. Scott.)

426–429 Pemphigus vulgaris. This Boxer has extensive lesions on the oral, nasal, preputial and scrotal skin.

427

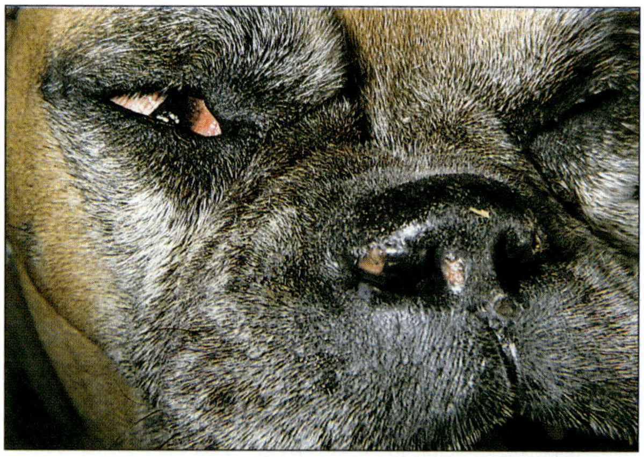

428

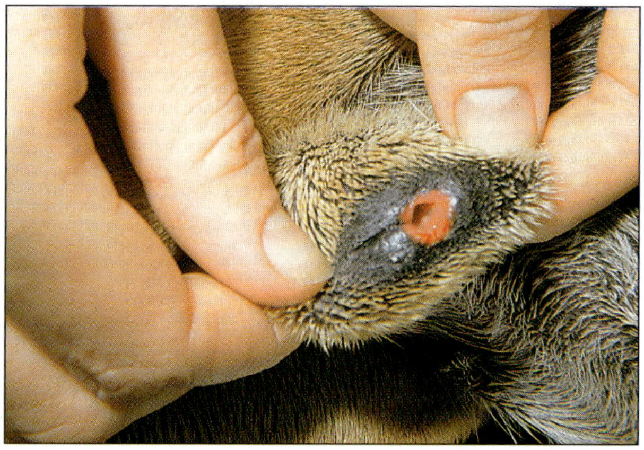

429

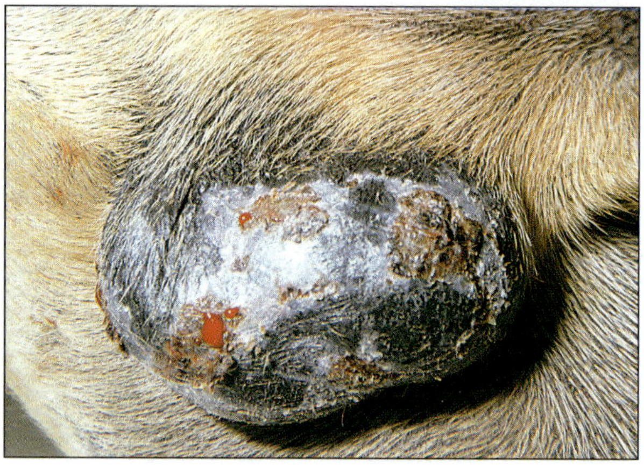

Pemphigus vulgaris

clinically indistinguishable from BULLOUS PEMPHIGO

This is the most serious disease of the pemphigus group and is a vesicobullous, erosive, ulcerative disease affecting the buccal cavity, the skin and the mucocutaneous junctions. Oral lesions are seen in about 90% of canine cases (**425**) and virtually all the feline cases that have been reported.[1,3] This is in direct contrast to pemphigus foliaceus. The mucocutaneous junctions are commonly affected and painful lesions are found around the lips, nose, prepuce, anus and vulva (**426–429**). In addition, lesions may occur in the axillae, groins and on the nailbeds. However, primary lesions are very rarely found in these sites as they rapidly become erosive, ulcerated and crusted (**430–432**). The disease is often acute in onset and is frequently associated with systemic signs such as pyrexia, anorexia and depression, again in contrast to pemphigus foliaceus.

430

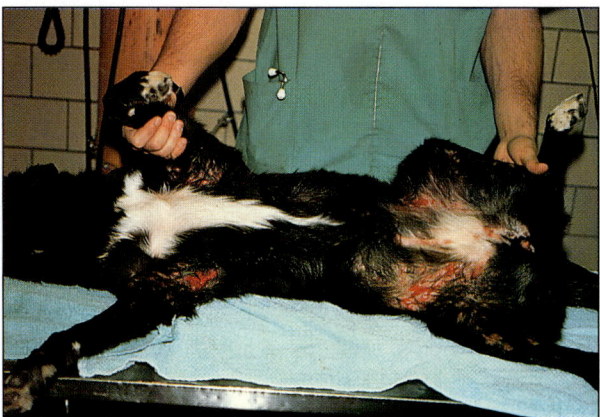

431

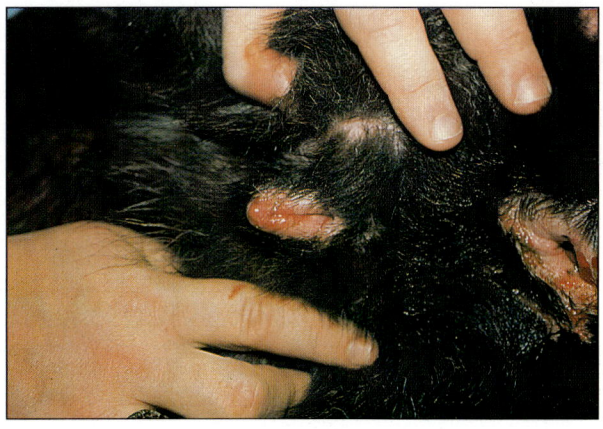

430 and 431 Pemphigus vulgaris. Oedema, erythema and erosions on the mucocutaneous junctions of the vulva and anus. Lesions on the skin are commonly found in the intertriginous region. Because of this they are usually erosions rather than vesicles. **430** illustrates large erosions and ulcerations in the axillae and inguinal region. (Illustration courtesy of D.W. Scott.)

432

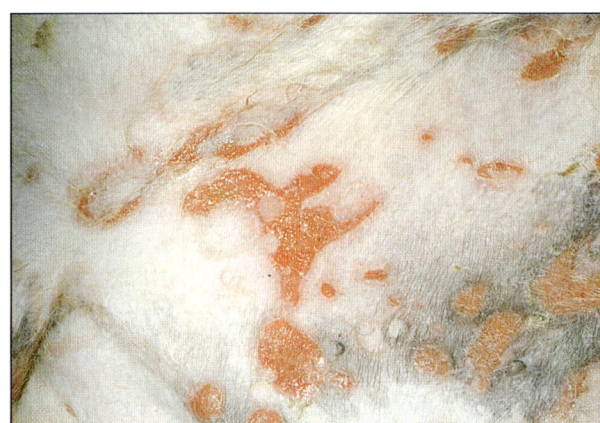

432 Pemphigus vulgaris. Erosive lesions in the inguinal region of a Cardigan corgi.

Pemphigis vulgaris is characterised by:
- Rarity.
- Acute onset in association with systemic signs.
- Oral lesions.

Differential diagnoses include:
- Bullous pemphigoid.
- Drug eruption.
- Mucocutaneous candidiasis.
- Systemic lupus erythematosus.
- Mycoses fungoides.

The diagnosis is made by:
- Consideration of history and clinical signs.
- Positive Nikolsky sign.
- Histopathological examination of biopsy material.
- Direct immunofluorescence or peroxidase/ immunoperoxidase staining.

433

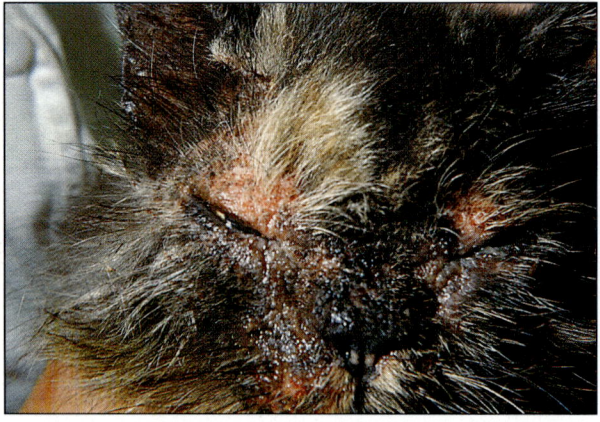

433 Pemphigus erythematosus. A rare disease, again presenting with secondary lesions due to the fragile nature of the primary eruption. Typically presenting with erythema, erosions, scale and crust. This tortoiseshell cat exhibits the characteristic 'butterfly' pattern of lesions on the face.

Pemphigus vegetans

This is an extremely rare condition in the dog and has not been reported in the cat. It commences as a vesiculopustular disorder, similar to other pemphigus diseases, but then develops into neoplastic-like vegetations and proliferations which are studded with pustules. Lesions tend to be generalised, exudative and are often crusted, although a localised distribution has been reported. The differential diagnoses include neoplasia, bacterial granulomas and mycotic granulomas. The diagnosis is made on the basis of characteristic histopathological findings and full thickness intercellular epidermal direct immunofluorescence, similar to that seen in the other pemphigus diseases described above.

Pemphigus erythematosus

In this condition the lesions are very similar to those of pemphigus foliaceus. There is subcorneal acantholysis and lesions are symmetrically distributed on the face, periorbitally and on the pinnae (**433**). The disease is exacerbated by sunlight and there may be depigmentation, particularly of the nasal region and this may lead to a misdiagnosis of 'collie nose'. There may be a variable degree of pruritus and pain. Some cases show a moderate antinuclear antibody titre, suggesting that the condition represents a cross-over syndrome between pemphigus and lupus erythematosus.

Differential diagnoses are as for pemphigus foliaceus and diagnosis is based on histopathological findings, antinuclear antibody titre and direct immunofluorescence. In pemphigus erythematosus there is fluorescence along the dermo-epidermal junction in addition to the epidermal pattern described above.

434

435

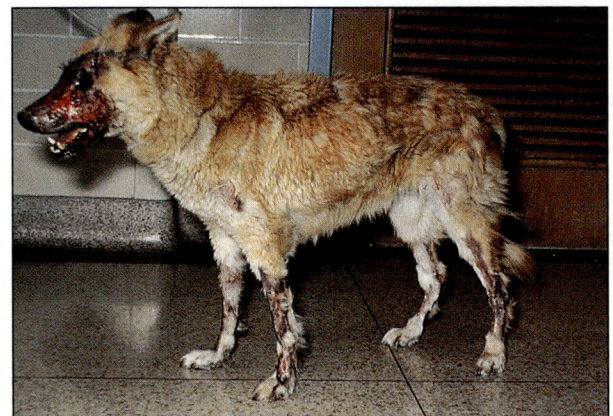
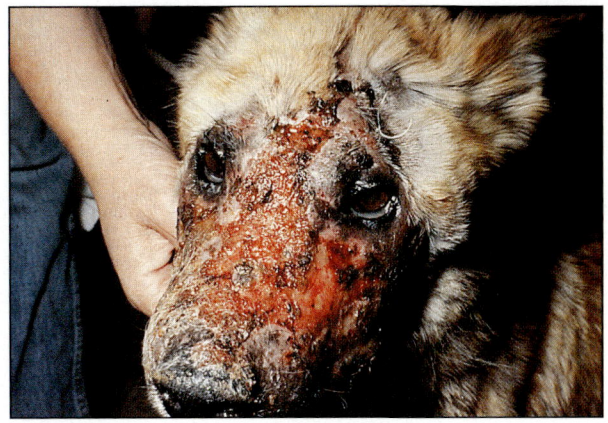

434 and 435   Bullous pemphigoid. German shepherd dog with extensive, symmetrical ulcerated lesions on the face and limbs. As with pemphigus vulgaris, lesions are also frequently found in the axillae, groins and perineal regions. (Illustrations courtesy of J. A. Yager.)

Bullous pemphigoid *Clinically indistinguishable from pemphigus vulgaris.*

Bullous pemphigoid is a rare, vesicobullous and ulcerative condition affecting the skin and oral mucosa which has been reported in the dog but not in the cat.[3] In this condition an auto-antibody directed against antigen at the basement membrane zone of the skin and the mucosa is formed, causing disruption of dermoepidermal cohesion and separation, and subsequently subepidermal vesicle formation. There is no acantholysis and the Nikolsky sign is rare.

Predilection sites are the axillae and groin and most cases have oral cavity involvement (**434** and **435**). The similarity between the appearance and distribution of the lesions in bullous pemphigoid and pemphigus vulgaris renders the two diseases clinically indistinguishable. Pain and pruritus are variable and severe cases may show systemic signs with pyrexia, anorexia and depression.

436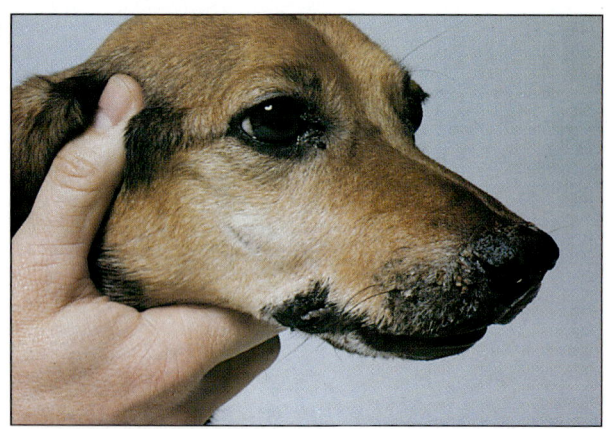

437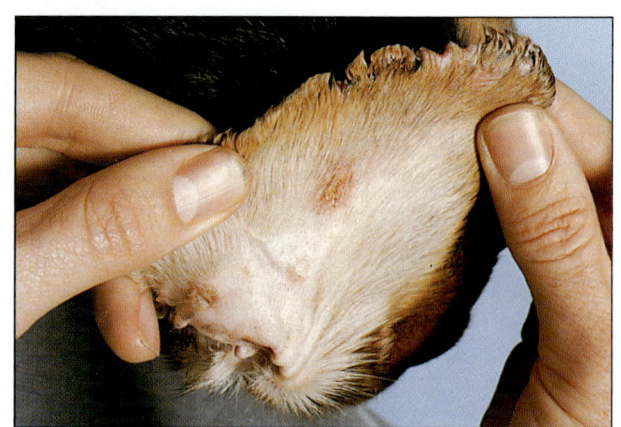

438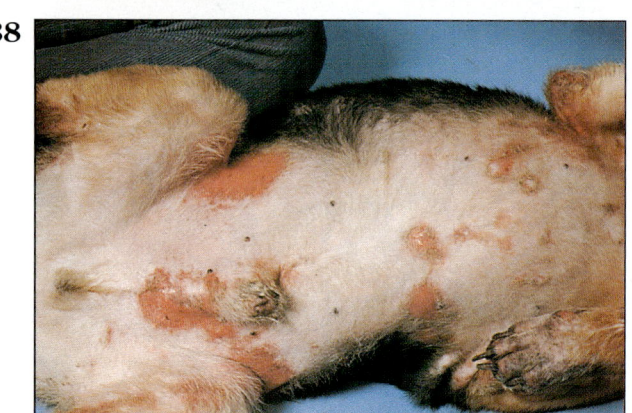

439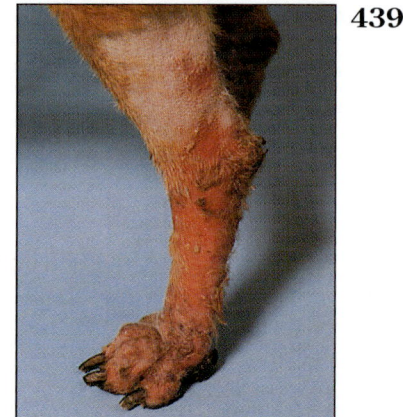

440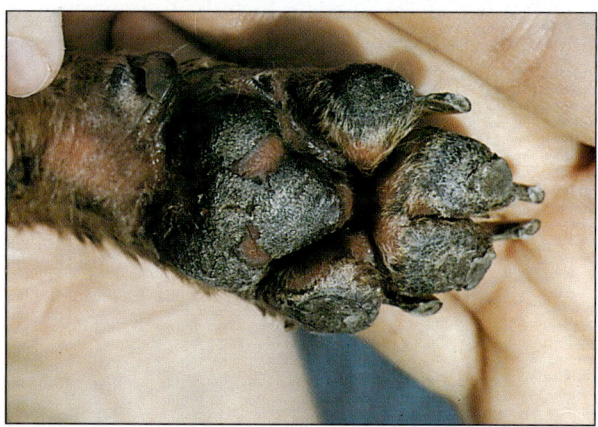

436–440   Systemic lupus erythematosus. This is a multisystemic disorder. Cutaneous lesions vary from focal erythema, alopecia, scale and crusting to haemorrhagic macules or patches and erosions or 'punched out' ulcers. These illustrations from the same dog demonstrate a number of these features. (Illustrations courtesy D. W. Scott.)

Systemic and discoid lupus erythematosus

Systemic lupus erythematosus

Systemic lupus erythematosus (SLE) is a rare, multisystemic, immunological disorder which occurs in both the dog and cat. The cause of the disease is not yet clear but it is considered to be multifactorial, in which genetic predisposition, viral infections, immunological disorder, ultraviolet light, hormonal imbalance or drug reactions all play a part.[3,4] The lesions result from the effects of auto-antibody and the precipitation of immune complexes resulting in inflammatory lesions in the renal glomerulus, walls of blood vessels and at the dermoepidermal junction.

Owing to the number of organ systems that may be involved a wide variety of clinical signs may occur such as dermatoses, pyrexia, polyarthritis, haemolytic anaemia, neutropaenia, myositis and glomerulonephritis.[3,4,6] These disorders may appear

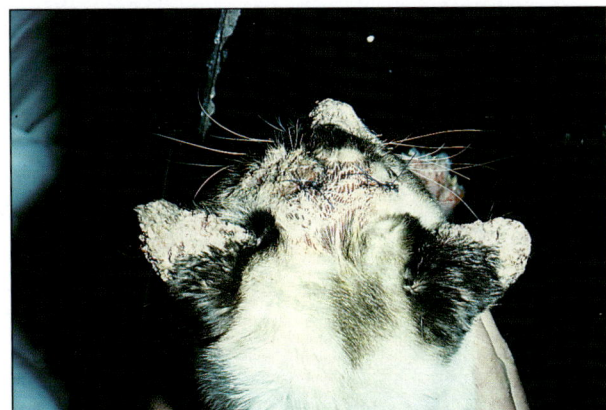

441

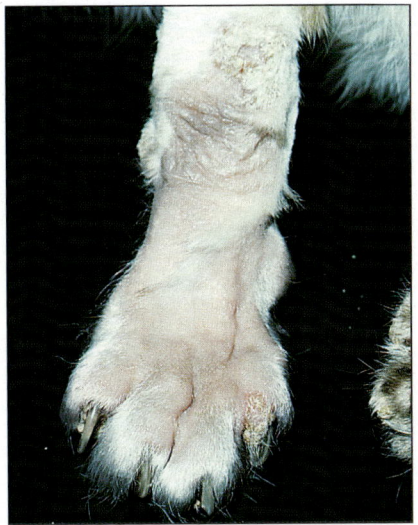

442

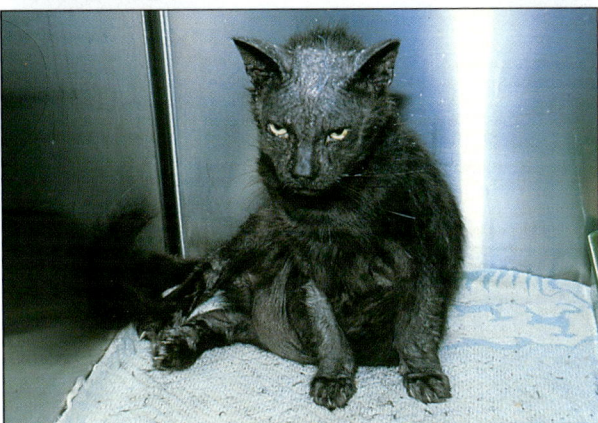

443

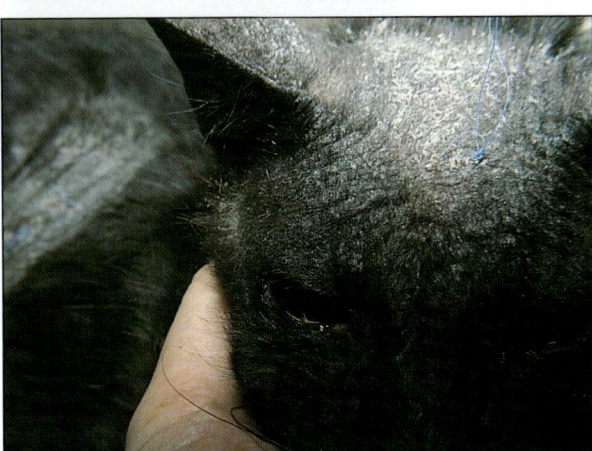

444

441–444   Systemic lupus erythematosus. The cutaneous lesions are similar in the cat, as depicted in these illustrations.

in various combinations which makes for great difficulty in establishing a definitive diagnosis. A number of authorities have advocated the use of clinical scores as a useful diagnostic technique in attempting to establish a diagnosis.[4]

The dermatological changes seen with SLE may be very varied with symmetrical cutaneous and mucocutaneous vesicobullous eruptions, alopecia, erythema, erosions, ulcerations, scale, crust, depigmentation and hyperpigmentation. Lesions in the dog frequently involve the face, ears and distal limbs, although they may be generalised (**436–440**). Hyperkeratosis of the footpads may be noted. Discharging fistulae may result from subcutaneous panniculitis. The cutaneous lesions are exacerbated by exposure to solar ultraviolet light. Feline lesions show a similar spectrum (**441– 444**).

SLE is characterised by:
- Symmetrical distribution of cutaneous lesions in association with systemic signs.

Differential diagnoses include:
- Pemphigus vulgaris and bullous pemphigoid.
- Drug eruption.
- Dermatomyositis.
- Discoid lupus erythematosus.

Diagnosis can be made by:
- Consideration of the history and clinical signs.
- Positive antinuclear antibody or platelet factor 3 (PF3) test.
- Positive lupus erythematosus (LE) cell test.
- Histopathological examination of biopsy material.
- Direct immunofluorescence or peroxidase/immunoperoxidase staining.

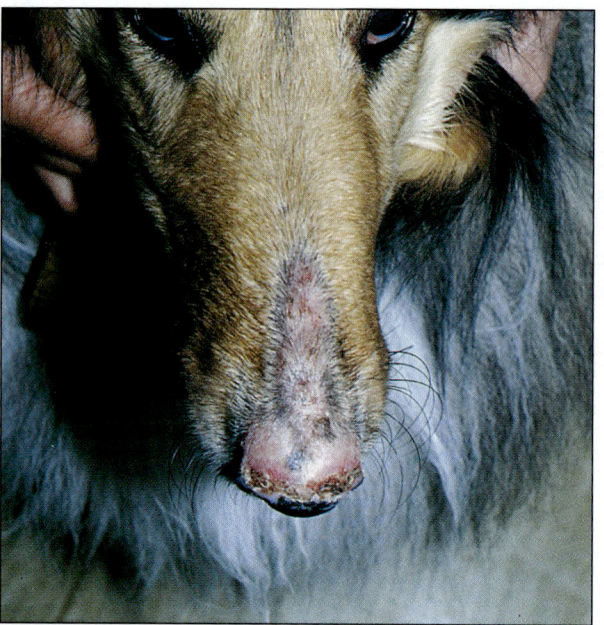 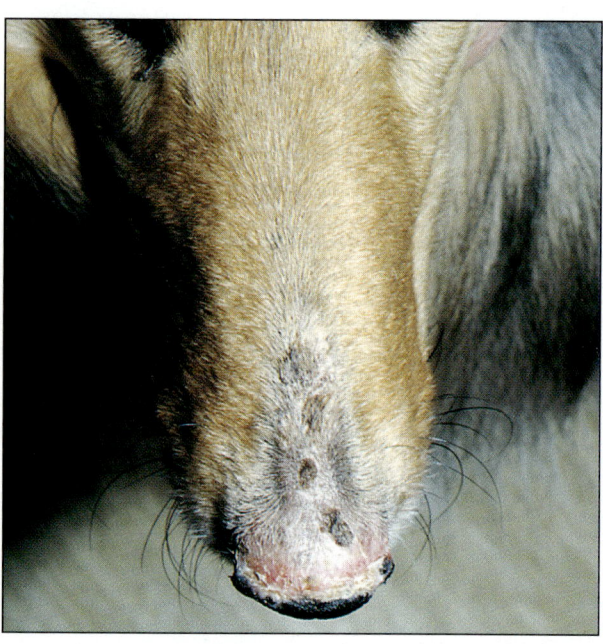

445 and 446   Discoid lupus erythematosus. This disorder is much more common than systemic lupus erythematosus. Most cases present with erythematous, scaling or crusting, and often depigmented, lesions on the planum nasale. Lesions are exacerbated by sunlight: **445** was taken during the summer months and **446** during the late winter.

Discoid lupus erythematosus

Discoid lupus erythematosus (DLE) is considered to be a form of SLE that is confined to the skin and in which there is no systemic involvement.[4,6] The condition has been documented in the dog but appears to be extremely rare in the cat. Lesions are often confined to the planum nasale and adjacent skin and consist initially of erythema and depigmentation.[8] Secondary lesions such as erosion, ulceration, scale and crust follow and the lesions tend to be slowly progressive. The lesions are exacerbated by exposure to the ultraviolet rays of sunlight (**445** and **446**) and it now seems probable that the condition has been misdiagnosed as 'collie nose' in the past.[3] Occasionally lesions may appear on the ears, around the eyes, the lower limbs and nail beds and commissures of the lips (**447–449**). Feline lesions are similar (**450**). Oral involvement is rare and consists of small mouth ulcers. Systemic signs are not seen. Haematological and serological tests such as LE, ANA, PF3 are negative.[4]

DLE is characterised by:
- Focal, depigmented erosions and crust typically confined to the nose.

Differential diagnoses include:
- The facial dermatoses.

Diagnosis can be made by:
- Consideration of the history and clinical signs.
- Histopathological examination of biopsy material.
- Direct immunofluorescence or peroxidase/immunoperoxidase staining.

447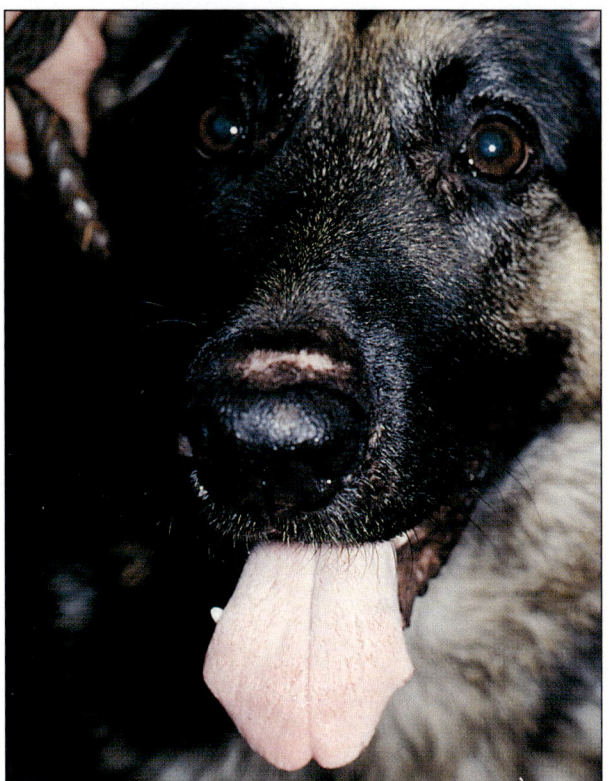

448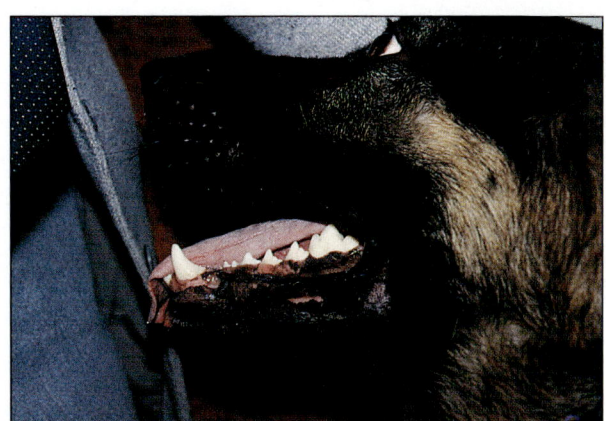

449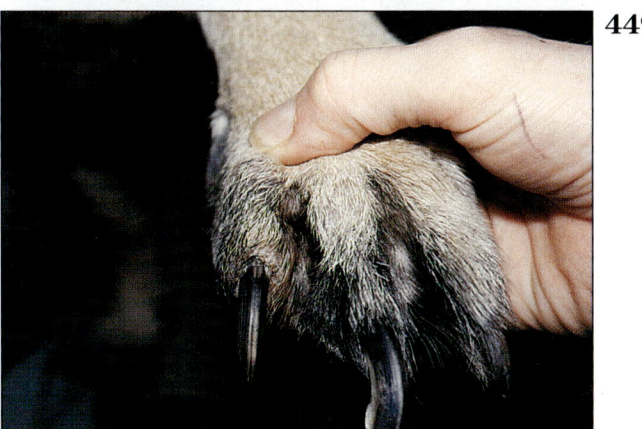

447–449   Discoid lupus erythematosus. German shepherd with depigmentation of the planum nasale and erythematous erosions at the medial canthi (**447**), erythematous crusting on the lower lips (**448**) and erythematous erosions on the nail beds (**449**).

450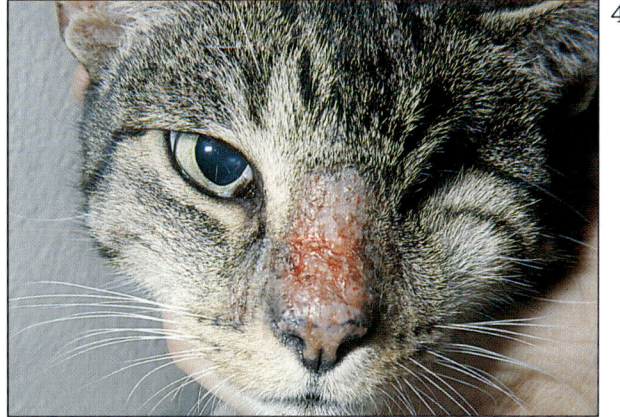

450   Discoid lupus erythematosus. This is a rare condition in the cat. This figure illustrates the typical presenting signs of alopecia, depigmentation, erosions and ulceration of the planum nasale and adjacent regions of the face.

References

1. Ackerman, L. A. (1985). Canine and feline pemphigus and pemphigoid, part 1. Pemphigus. *Compendium on Continuing Education*, **7**: 89–94.

2. Ackerman, L. A. (1985). Canine and feline pemphigus and pemphigoid, part 11. Pemphigoid. *Compendium on Continuing Education*, **7**: 281–285.

3. Angarano, D. W. (1987). Autoimmune Dermatoses. In: Nesbitt, G. H. (Ed.) *Contemporary Issues in Small Animal Practice*, **8**: 79–94. Churchill Livingstone, New York.

4. Halliwell, R. E. W. and Gorman, N. T. (1989). In: Halliwell, R. E. W. and Gorman, N. T. (Eds.). *Veterinary Clinical Immunology*, pp. 285–307. W. B. Saunders, Philadelphia.

5. Norman, N. J. (1990). Pemphigus. *Dermatology Clinics*, **84**: 689–700.

6. Scott, D. W., Walton, D. K., Manning, T. O., Smith, C. A. and Lewis, R. M. (1983). Canine lupus erythematosus. 1. Systemic lupus erythematosus. *Journal of the American Animal Hospital Association*, **19**: 461–479.

7. Scott, D. W., Walton, D. K., Manning, T. O., Smith, C. A. and Lewis, R. M. (1983). Canine lupus erythematosus. 2. Discoid lupus erythematosus. *Journal of the American Animal Hospital Association*, **19**: 481–488.

8. Walton, D. K., Scott, D. W., Smith, C. A. and Lewis, R. M. (1981). Canine discoid lupus erythematosus. *Journal of the American Animal Hospital Association*, **17**: 851–858.

Chapter 10

Endocrine dermatoses

Introduction

Hair growth occurs in a definite cycle of anagen (growth stage), catagen (intermediate stage) and telogen (resting stage). Each hair follicle appears to have an intrinsic rhythm but the relative length of each component is dependent on, and influenced by, other factors such as breed, age, sex, the region of the body involved and the interaction of the endocrine system with the follicle.[19]

For example, in the cocker spaniel, the hair on the face is short whereas hair on the ears and the hind legs is quite long, yet hairs from these three regions undergo the same hair cycle and are under the same hormonal control. The hair cycle itself is under the additional influence of external factors such as day length and nutritional status.[1]

Hair replacement occurs in different patterns which are characteristic for the species of animal. For example, rodents have a moulting wave where the hair is shed and replaced in clear-cut waves passing from the ventral midline to the dorsum.[4] In contrast, man, dog, cat and guinea pig have a mosaic form of replacement where the stage of hair cycle varies from one area of the body to another.[4,19]

Thus, in one follicle the cycle may be in anagen whereas in a neighbouring follicle it may be in telogen. The mosaic pattern can be altered by hormonal changes, such as occur during pregnancy, and by daylength, disease and nutrition. Hair cycles in quite large areas of skin, and even over the entire body surface, may become synchronised by a premature precipitation into telogen. Upon restoration of the homeostatic *status quo ante*, follicular activity restarts and many hairs are shed at the same time, *telogen defluxion*.[4]

Hormonal imbalances upset the normal periodicity of, and the initiation of, spontaneous hair replacement. The exact nature of each hormonal imbalance determines whether or not follicles become active. The alopecia seen in most endocrine dermatoses is due to a failure to initiate anagen and the synchronisation of large numbers of follicles in telogen, when the hair is easily epilated by minor friction. Thus, in rats, oestrogens, testosterones and adrenal steroids delay the initiation of anagen, whereas thyroid hormones have the opposite effect.[4,16] However, except for oestrogens, hormones have little effect on the cycle of growth once it has been initiated. Oestrogens are unique in that they prolong the entire period during which existing hairs grow and they delay shedding of club hairs. Endocrine aberrations affect the physical qualities of the hair in addition to affecting follicular activity.[16]

- Alopecia may not be apparent until 30% of the hair in any given area is lost.
- Endocrinopathy is suggested by bilaterally symmetrical alopecia.
- The alopecia is initially non-pruritic and is often associated with hyperpigmentation of the affected skin.
- Elevated adrenal steroids result in decreased hair fibre diameter whereas testosterone increases fibre diameter.
- Systemic signs such as lethargy, polydipsia, polyuria, alterations in body shape and gynaecomastia may be noted.
- Most endocrinopathies occur in middle-aged animals.
- Consider an underlying endocrinopathy in cases of recurrent pyoderma, particularly if there is minimal inflammation or large, flaccid pustules.

Hypothyroidism

Hypothyroidism is the most common endocrine dermatosis of the dog but has not yet been reliably documented in the cat. Ninety per cent of the cases of canine hypothyroidism are of the acquired, primary type, i.e. due to a loss of productive capacity in the thyroid gland.[2] There are two main causes of primary hypothyroidism, lymphocytic thyroiditis and idiopathic thyroid atrophy.

Lymphocytic thyroiditis is considered to be an autoimmune disorder with antibodies to various components of the thyroid such as thyroglobulin, colloid antigen 2, microsomal and cell surface components, T3 and T4.[23]

Idiopathic thyroid atrophy is characterised by a non-inflammatory loss of thyroid tissue and it has been suggested that the latter condition represents end stage lymphocytic thyroiditis.

Naturally-occurring secondary hypothyroidism (i.e. due to deficiency of thyroid stimulating hormone, TSH) accounts for about 10% of the canine disease and is usually associated with pituitary dwarfism and neoplasia. It has been suggested that a failure in the peripheral conversion of thyroxine (T4) to the metabolically active triiodothyronine (T3) may be involved in the aetiology of some of the canine disease, but this has not yet been documented.[2,10]

Certain breeds are predisposed to hypothyroidism: Golden retrievers, Doberman pinschers, Dachshunds (both miniature and standard) Shetland sheepdogs, Irish setters, Pomeranians, miniature Schnauzers, Cocker spaniels and Airedales. In these predisposed breeds the disease may have a tendency to occur in young adults rather than middle-aged individuals.[9] Females are predisposed.

Clinical signs of hypothyroidism are very variable.[2] The most constant clinical signs are lethargy and cold and exercise intolerance. There may be a gradual slowing of mental activity evidenced by reduced excitability and alertness and loss of interest in walks and in play. Other systemic signs include bradycardia, weak pulse, reduced body temperature, a cool skin, increased body weight, neurological signs (especially head tilt, dragging of front paws and unilateral facial paralysis), and anoestrus and lack of libido.[2,11]

Dogs with hypothyroidism are often disinterested in their surroundings (**451** and **452**). This is unusual in the consulting room and should arouse suspicion. Suspicion may be heightened by a slow heart rate (<100) and a rectal temperature below 101ºF, both unusual in dogs in a consulting room. Haematological changes are non-diagnostic. Hypercholesterolaemia is a common finding.

Skin changes depend upon the length of time the disease has been in existence. Usually, but not invariably, there is a bilaterally symmetrical alopecia which tends to spare the head and the extremities (**453–461**). The hair coat is dry, brittle and dull, and the hairs are easily pulled out. The skin is thickened, cool, non-pitting and puffy. These changes are particularly noticeable on the face and forehead where they impart a tragic, sleepy expression (**462**). Alopecic skin is usually hyperpigmented with a fine sandpaper-like feel.

Another frequent sign is a hairless dorsal surface of the tail. In the giant breeds skin changes are often confined to the legs from the elbow and mid-thigh ventrally. In some individuals the failure to initiate the anagen phase and consequent retention of the old hair may lead to hypertrichosis, an excessively long, thick coat (**463**). Many hypothyroid dogs develop a secondary pyoderma which may be pruritic, causing some diagnostic confusion (**464**). There may be xerosis, particularly if large areas are affected (**465**) and poor wound healing may be noted (**466**).

> **Hypothyroidism is characterised by:**
> - Slow heart rate.
> - Low body temperature.
> - Disinterest in the consulting room.
> - Hypercholesterolaemia.

451

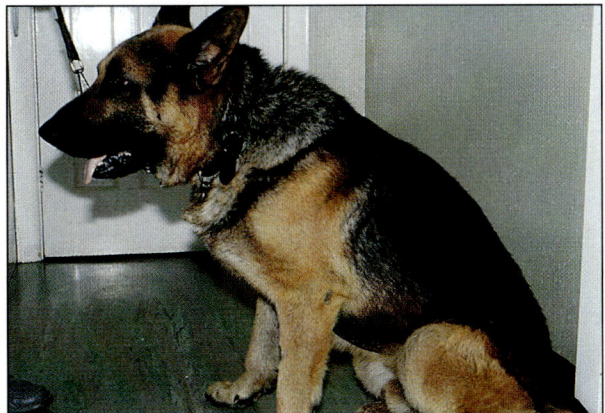

452

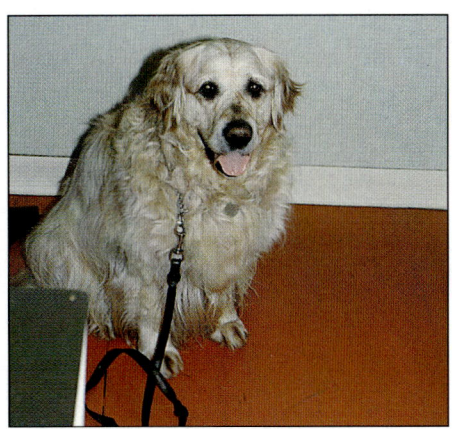

451   Hypothyroidism. Suspicion may be aroused by the lethargic attitude of the dog. This German shepherd dog has no interest in the surroundings.

452   Hypothyroidism. Obesity is another feature of hypothyroidism, although not all animals are as gross as this Labrador retriever.

453

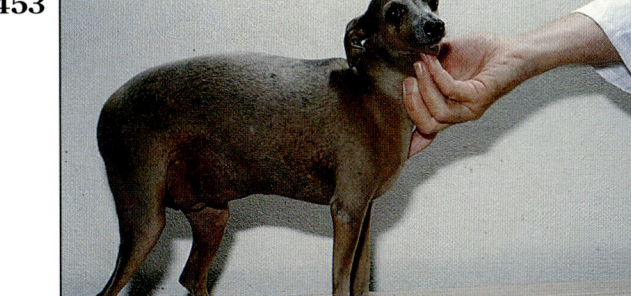

454

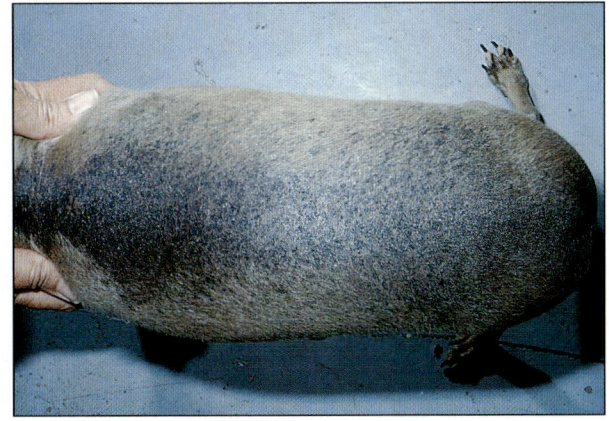

453 and 454   Hypothyroidism. Many cases show a combination of systemic and cutaneous signs. This Italian Greyhound bitch demonstrates obesity, alopecia and macular hyperpigmentation of the skin.

455

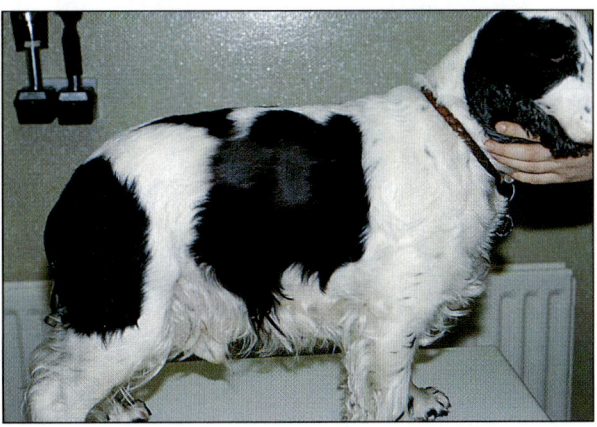

455   Hypothyroidism. Bilaterally symmetrical alopecia is the cardinal sign of any endocrine dermatosis and is not diagnostic for hypothyroidism. It is, however, a feature of many cases. Note the discrete patches of alopecia confined to the sub-lumbar fossa in this Cocker spaniel.

456

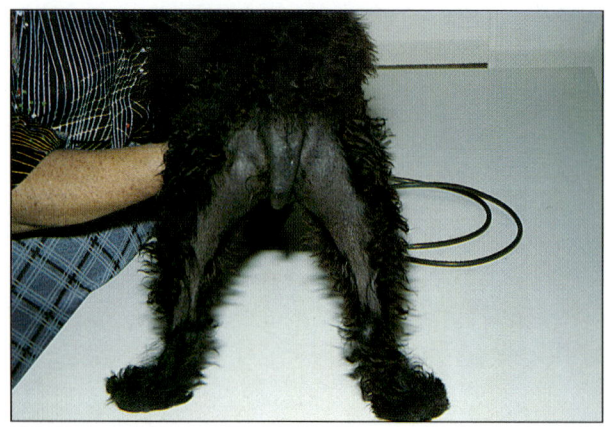

457

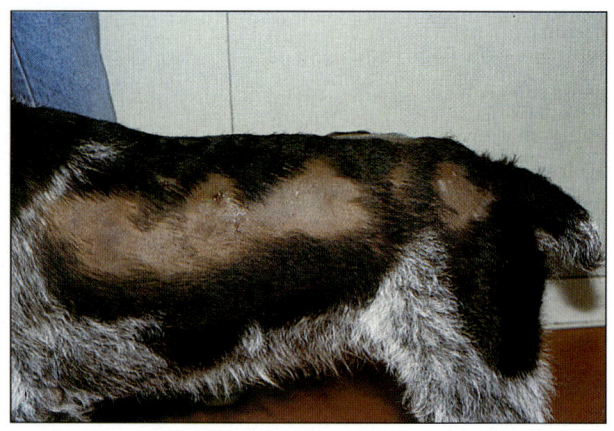

456   Hypothyroidism. Alopecia may begin in areas of the body subject to friction such as the dorsal surface of the tail or, as in this case in a miniature Poodle bitch, the caudal aspect of the thighs.

457   Hypothyroidism. Most cases, although not all, demonstrate hyperpigmentation of the alopecic areas. This was not the case in this German wire-haired pointer.

458

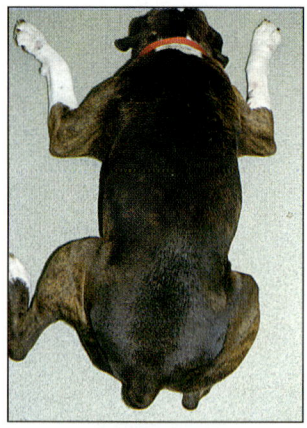

459

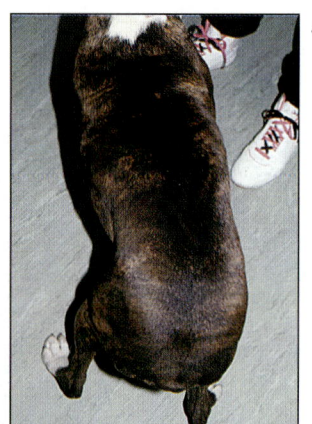

458 and 459   Hypothyroidism. The alopecia may be very extensive, as in this boxer, which is not sedated, where it extends along the entire dorsal trunk. **459** depicts the same dog as in **458** some 6 months after therapy with T4 was initiated. Note regrowth of hair, loss of weight and ability to stand.

460

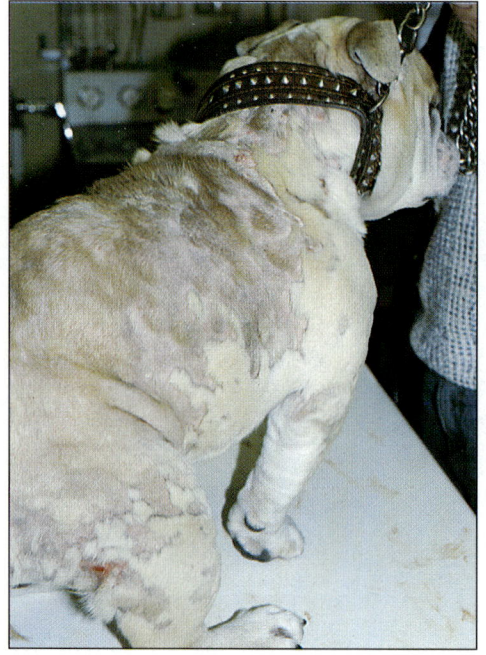

461

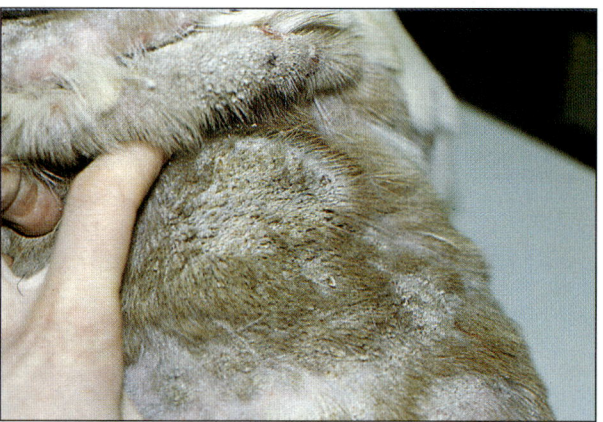

460 and 461   Hypothyroidism. Not all cases demonstrate well-defined areas of hair loss. In this English bulldog there is patchy alopecia, associated with a superficial pyoderma. This secondary infection will confuse the diagnosis because a variable degree of pruritus is present.

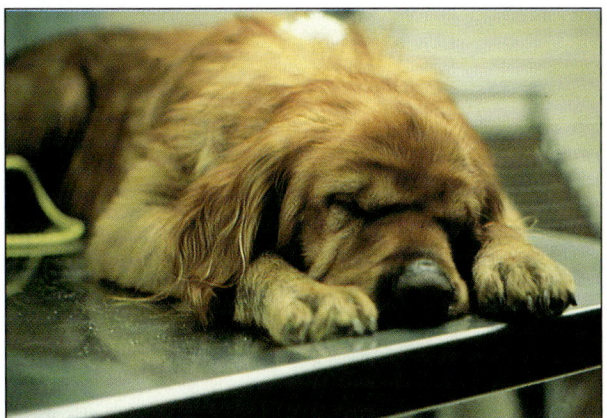

462 Hypothyroidism. Sleepy, 'tragic' expression on the face of a Cocker spaniel dog due to thickening and myxoedema of the skin. (Illustration courtesy of J. A. Yager.)

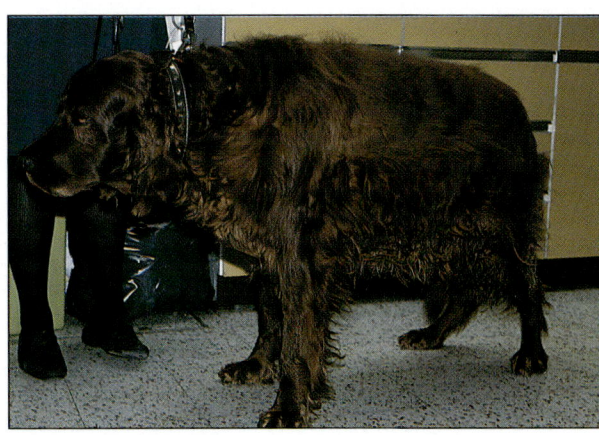

463 Hypothyroidism. Occasionally, a paradoxical retention of hair will occur rather than alopecia. This Irish setter is overweight, lethargic and has hypertrichosis.

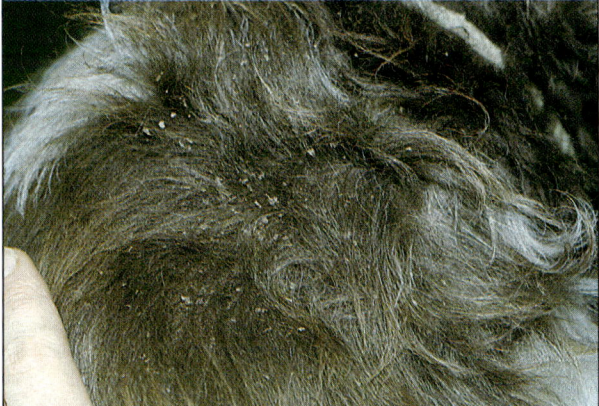

464 Hypothyroidism. Secondary superficial pyoderma and scale is a common feature of hypothyroidism and is nicely demonstrated in this English Springer spaniel.

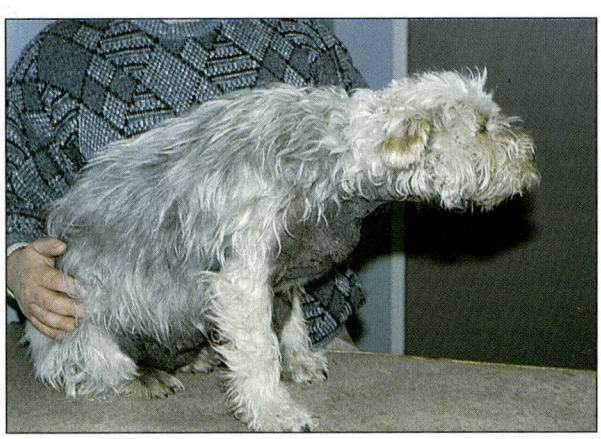

465 Hypothyroidism. In some cases extensive defects in keratinisation produce very severe changes. Extensive ventral alopecia, hyperpigmentation and xerosis in this cross-bred dog caused severe pruritus.

Hypothyroidism is characterised by:
- Very variable systemic signs.
- Bilaterally symmetrical alopecia.

Differential diagnoses include:
- Other endocrinopathies.
- Defects in keratinisation.

Diagnosis can be made by:
- Consideration of the history and clinical signs.
- Demonstration of low T4 and T3 levels, in association with a fasting hypercholesterolaemia.
- Lack of response to administration of TSH or TRH.

466 Hypothyroidism. Poor wound healing may be noted, a consequence of the reduced cutaneous metabolism. In this case there is a proliferative granuloma at the site of a wound on the distal limb.

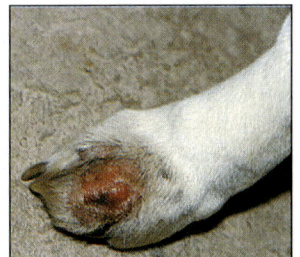

- The dermatohistopathological features of the endocrinopathies are similar to epidermal atrophy, follicular atrophy and hyperkeratosis.[17] Telogen hair follicles predominate. Histopathological findings are rarely diagnostic.

467

468

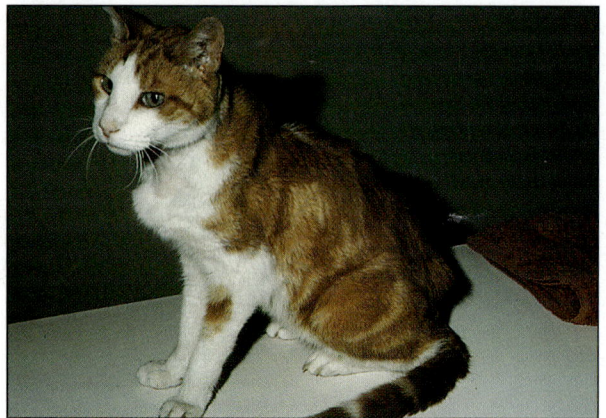

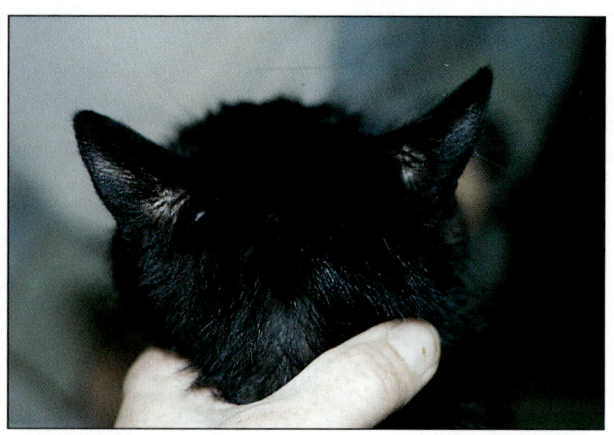

467 **Feline hyperthyroidism.** The elevated metabolic rate may be associated with cutaneous signs such as the emaciation and unkempt coat in this case.

468 **Feline hyperthyroidism.** Bilateral alopecia on the pinnae associated with overgrooming.

Feline hyperthyroidism

Feline hyperthyroidism is now recognised as a significant clinical entity in old cats. It is associated with functional adenoma, or more rarely adenocarcinoma, of the thyroid glands. The condition occurs mainly in cats over ten years of age. The main clinical signs are weight loss despite a normal or increased appetite, hyperactivity, diarrhoea with steatorrhoea, tachycardia and skin changes.[24] The latter consist of an unkempt coat with greasy seborrhoea, patchy alopecia and matting in long-haired animals (**467** and **468**). It is thought that these changes are mainly the result of a reduction in grooming activities.

Feline hyperthyroidism is characterised by:
- An unkempt coat allied to weight loss, despite normal or increased appetite.
- Hyperactivity, tachycardia and diarrhoea.

Differential diagnoses include:
- Other causes of weight loss, e.g. chronic renal failure, alimentary lymphosarcoma, malnutrition.

Diagnosis can be made by:
- Demonstration of elevated serum thyroxine levels.

469

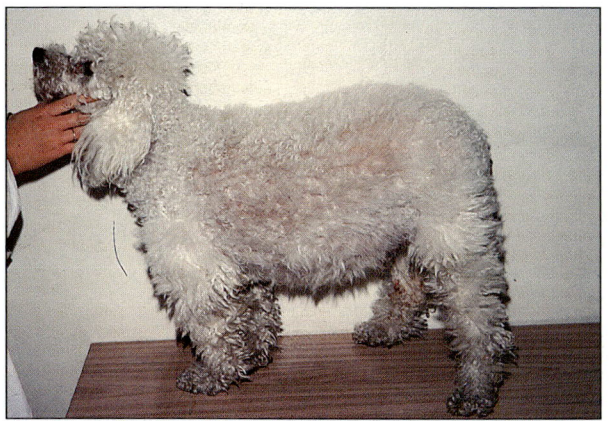

470

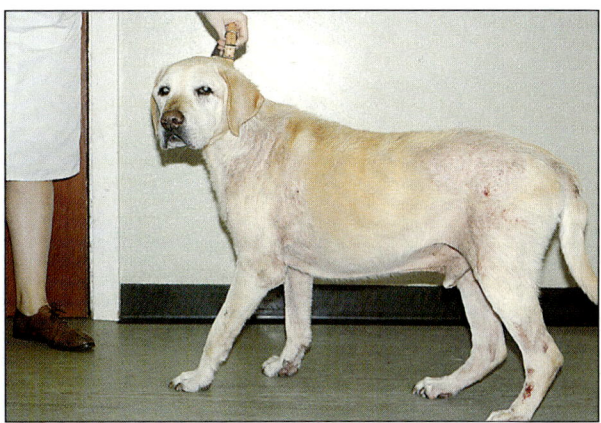

469 Canine hyperadrenocorticism. Miniature Poodle bitch showing characteristic pendulous abdomen and commencing alopecia over the trunk.

470 Canine hyperadrenocorticism. More advanced case in a Labrador retriever. Note the alopecia, pendulous abdomen and flaccid sheath.

Canine hyperadrenocorticism

Hyperadrenocorticism is due to an excess of glucocorticoids. Iatrogenic hyperadrenocorticism may result from excessive or prolonged administration of glucocorticoids and constitutes the most common form of the disorder at the present time. The naturally-occurring form of the disease is associated with two different entities:

1 Pituitary-dependent hyperadrenocorticism (PDH) results from excessive secretion of adrenocorticotrophic hormone (ACTH) by the pituitary gland with consequent bilateral hyperplasia of the adrenal cortex. This form makes up 80% of cases of spontaneous canine hyperadrenocorticism. About 20% of these cases are associated with the presence of a functional pituitary tumour. The remainder are thought to be due to a defect in hypothalamic regulation and the negative feedback system.

2 A functional adrenocortical tumour. Such tumours are usually unilateral, often involving the right gland, and may be benign or malignant. As their secretory activity is autonomous there is atrophy of the non-neoplastic adrenocortical tissue.

There is no sex predisposition for PDH but females are predisposed to adrenocortical tumours.[12] There is a steadily increasing risk with advancing age which levels off at about 7–9 years of age. Dachshunds, Poodles, Boxers, Boston terriers and Silky terriers are predisposed, but not to the same sub-set of the disease. Thus poodles are associated with PDH, dachshunds with adrenal

neoplasia and boxers are predisposed to pituitary tumours.[26] The presenting signs usually include polydipsia, polyuria with a low specific gravity (1.005–1.010), polyphagia, a change in body conformation with decreased muscle mass and a dropped abdomen, hepatomegaly due to a steroid induced hepatopathy, lethargy and alopecia.

Other systemic signs are weakness, anoestrus and virilisation, with clitoral hypertrophy in bitches, testicular atrophy in males, neurological signs due to pituitary neoplasia or metastatic adrenocortical tumours and osteoporosis. Urinary tract and ocular infection may occur. Diabetes mellitus occurs concurrently in up to 15% of cases and is accompanied by elevated blood insulin levels. Although there is often a combination of clinical signs, some animals may present with one sign only. The progression of the disease is also very variable.

Skin changes may include a bilaterally symmetrical alopecia involving the trunk, the dorsum, the chest and the abdomen but sparing the head and extremities[25] (**469–471**). Focal alopecia may be the only clinical sign in some cases (**472** and **473**). The remaining hair is dry, dull, brittle and easily epilated. The skin is thin and hypotonic, so that it mimics dehydrated skin and tends to become permanently wrinkled (**474** and **475**). It bruises easily, shows an increased susceptibility to bacterial infection and heals poorly.

The thinning of the skin renders subcutaneous vessels more visible, especially on the ventral

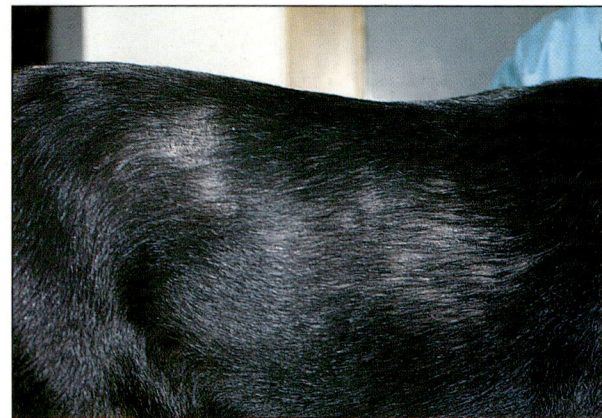

471   Canine hyperadrenocorticism. Extensive alopecia on the lateral trunk in a case of iatrogenic disease in a Labrador retriever.

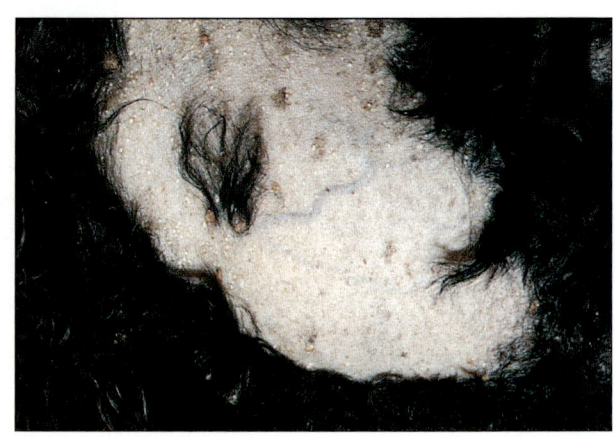

472   Canine hyperadrenocorticism. Focal area of alopecia on the lateral thoracic wall of a miniature Poodle.

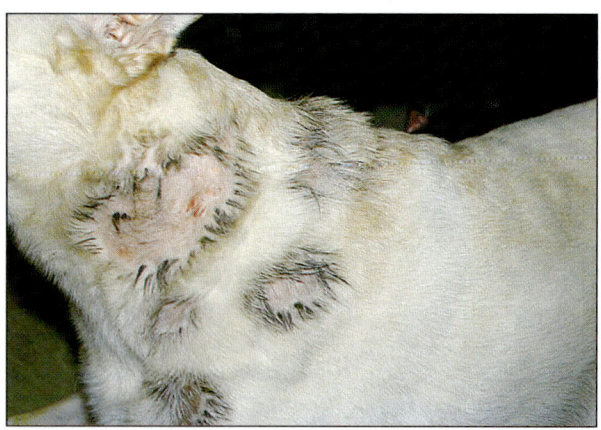

473   Canine hyperadrenocorticism. Multiple, focal, non-inflammatory areas of alopecia associated with pyoderma in a case of iatrogenic disease in a Labrador retriever.

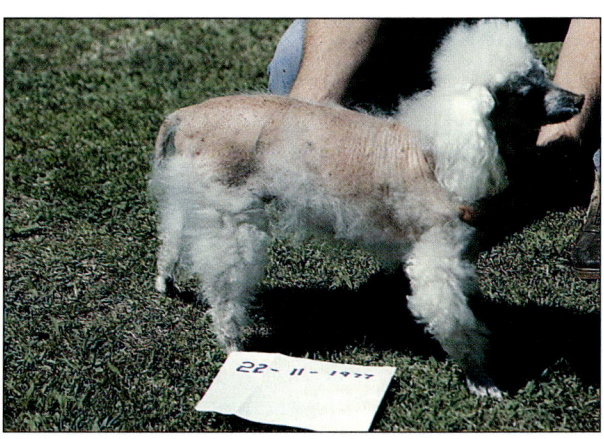

474 and 475   Canine hyperadrenocorticism. Miniature Poodle bitch showing extensive alopecia over the trunk and characteristic wrinkling of the skin due to loss of elasticity resulting from catabolism of skin collagen and elastin. Note also the comedones and follicular cysts in the affected skin.

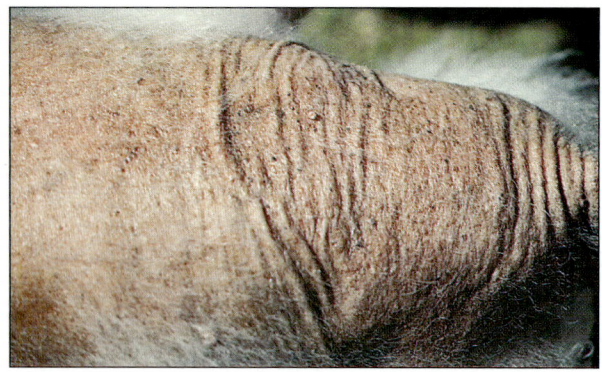

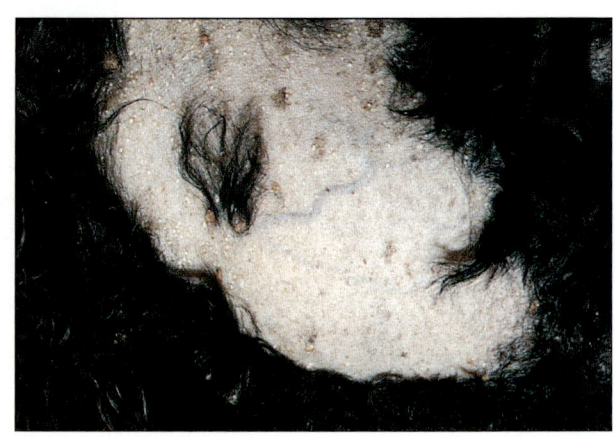

476   Canine hyperadrenocorticism. Bull terrier bitch with grossly distended abdomen. prominent subcutaneous veins and two early lesions of calcinosis cutis.

477

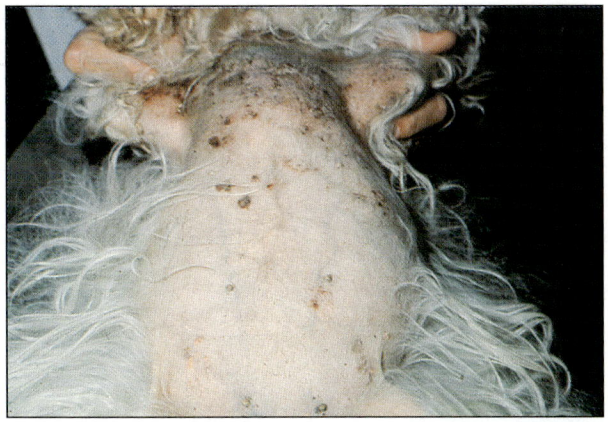

478

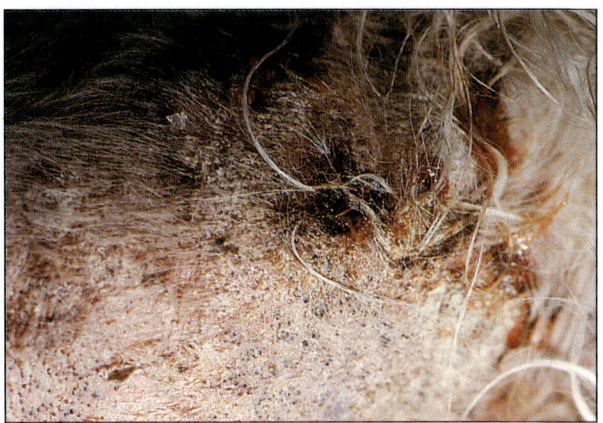

477 and 478   Canine hyperadrenocorticism. Maltese terrier bitch showing how the subcutaneous vessels of the ventral abdomen have become more visible. Note also the grey colouration of the skin of the ventral thorax due to numerous comedones (**478**).

479

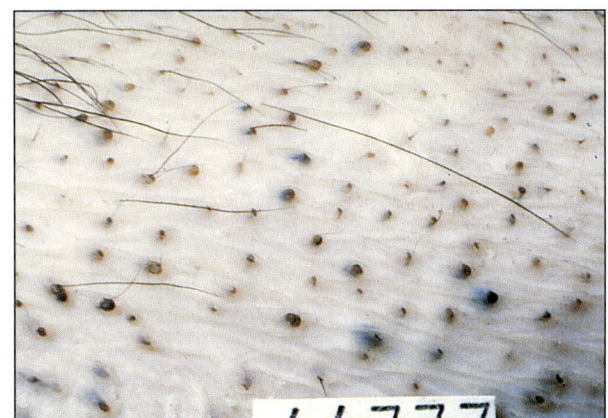

479   Canine hyperadrenocorticism. Comedone formation. (Illustration courtesy J. A. Yager.)

abdomen (**476–478**). Comedones are frequently present around the nipples and the ventral chest and abdomen, where they may be sufficiently numerous as to impart a grey colour to the skin (**479**). Cutaneous phlebectasias have been reported.[18]

Calcinosis cutis (dystrophic mineralisation) occurs in about 40% of cases, predilection sites being the dorsum and the inguinal and axillary regions. It may appear as hard, raised, bluish black or yellow nodules or provoke a severe foreign body reaction which may become secondarily infected and pruritic (**480–482**). The majority of the cutaneous lesions resolve with appropriate therapy.

Laboratory findings include lymphopaenia, eosinopaenia, hypercholesterolaemia, elevated alkaline phosphatase (mainly due to a steroid-induced isoenzyme, probably of hepatic origin) and alanine transaminase, and there may be hyperglycaemia.

In cats the clinical signs of polyuria and polydipsia predominate and there is a strong association with diabetes mellitus.[10,13] Cutaneous signs are similar to those seen in the dog with patchy or symmetrical alopecia and a thin, easily wrinkled skin.

Hyperadrenocorticism has been reported in hamster and in the ferret.[3] In both species the signs were of bilaterally symmetrical alopecia. In the hamsters this was accompanied by hyperpigmented, atrophic skin.

480

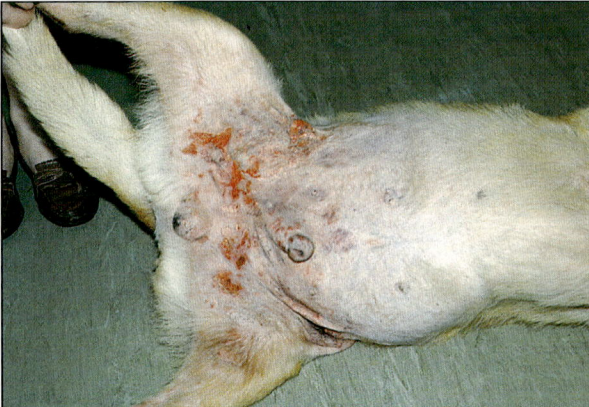

480   Canine hyperadrenocorticism. Early lesions of calcinosis cutis in the groin of a Labrador cross. Calcinosis cutis is considered to be virtually pathognomonic of canine hyperadrenocorticism.

481

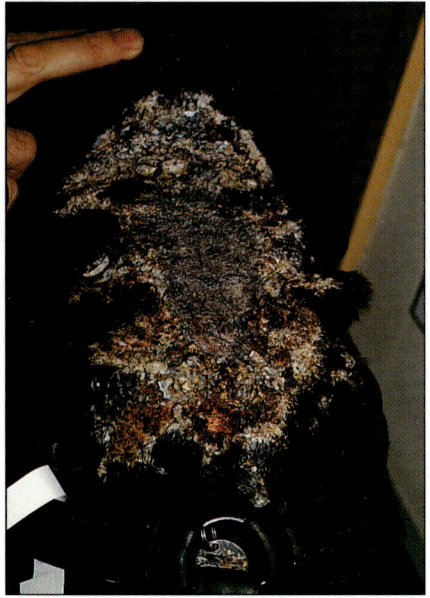

481   Canine hyperadrenocorticism. Huge area of calcinosis cutis on the dorsum of a dog with severe hyperadrenocorticism.

482

482   Canine hyperadrenocorticism. Severe foreign body reaction to calcinosis cutis in the inguinal region of a Maltese terrier bitch.

> **Hyperadrenocorticism is characterised by:**
> - Bilaterally symmetrical alopecia and changes in the hair.
> - Thin, hypotonic skin.
> - Polydipsia, polyuria.
>
> **Differential diagnoses include:**
> - Polydipsia and polyuria.
> - Diabetes insipidus.
> - Renal disease.
> - Symmetrical alopecia.
> - Endocrine alopecias.
>
> **Diagnosis can be made by:**
> - Consideration of the history and clinical signs.
> - Serum biochemistry and haemogram.
> - Adrenal function tests, viz. ACTH response and dexamethasone suppression tests.

Adrenocortical hyperprogestism and hyperandrogenism has been proposed to account for the bilaterally symmetrical alopecia of the trunk and caudal thighs in Pomeranians.[15] These dogs had xylazine response tests similar to those of normal Pomeranians and both groups had elevated xylazine responses compared to control dogs. In addition both affected and normal Pomeranians demonstrated elevated progesterone, 17-hydroxyprogesterone and dehydroepiandrosterone after ACTH administration. A partial deficiency in 21-hydroxylase was proposed to account for these endocrine aberrations.

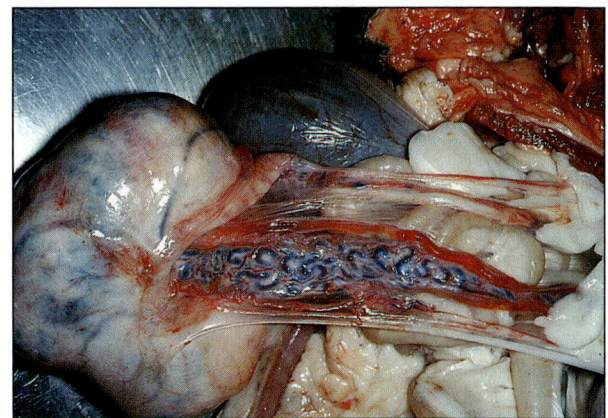

483   Sertoli-cell tumour. Large tumour formation in a retained testis.

Gonadal hormones

That there is a relationship between hair growth and gonadal hormones is indisputable. Problems arise when attempting to classify these relationships. The gonadal steroids all affect cells in a similar manner, by interaction with the genome, each via their own specific receptor. The results of this interaction are typically an increase in the synthesis of various proteins which affect the cell in one manner or another. Different hormones thus have varying effects on the skin and hair cycle.

- **Oestrogens** have been shown to inhibit hair growth in the dog if applied topically or given systemically. They appear to have the power, not only to inhibit initiation of the hair replacement, but also to prolong the actual period of growth of existing hair. Oestrogens decrease sebaceous gland size and function and stimulate epidermal mitosis. Oestrogens increase the melanin content of melanocytes in some species.
- **Progesterone** has no effect on hair growth in the dog but has recently been shown to have an inhibitory effect in the cat. Progesterone has little effect on pigmentation or sebaceous gland function.
- **Androgens** appear to have a stimulatory effect on mitotic activity in the epidermis but have little effect on hair growth, beyond possibly producing a coarser type of hair coat. Androgens cause increased epidermal thickness and appear to have little effect on pigmentation. Androgens increase sebaceous gland size and function. They cause prostatomegaly, may induce adenomatous changes in the perianal glands and cause hyperplasia of the tail gland.

In reality, every hair follicle is exposed to varying concentrations of a number of gonadal hormones and the response is as much a response to the binding of these various hormones as to intrafollicular factors.

Notwithstanding the above, a number of clinical syndromes are recognised.

Sertoli-cell tumour

This tumour of the testis sometimes stimulates marked skin changes. Feminisation may also be seen; a consequence of oestrogen secretion by the neoplastic Sertoli cells. Boxers, Shetland sheepdogs and Weimaraners are predisposed. Most cases develop in dogs that are over six years old. Some animals become anaemic, a consequence of oestrogen suppression of the bone marrow. Although it may occur in scrotal testes, inguinal and abdominally-retained testes are predisposed (**483**). The uninvolved testicle is usually atrophic. Rarely the tumour will become malignant and metastasise. Suspicion of metastasis may be aroused by a lack of response to castration and persistently elevated plasma oestrogen levels — a justification for pre-operative assay of oestrogen.

There are cutaneous changes in addition to alopecia.[6,16] There are hyperpigmented macules and blotchy areas of hyperpigmentation may be apparent. The skin is dry. The hair becomes brittle, epilates easily and is not replaced. The skin may be thinner than usual in the affected areas. Bilaterally symmetrical alopecia occurs in the genital area from which it may extend to the ventral abdomen, the chest, flanks and the neck region (**484** and **485**).

484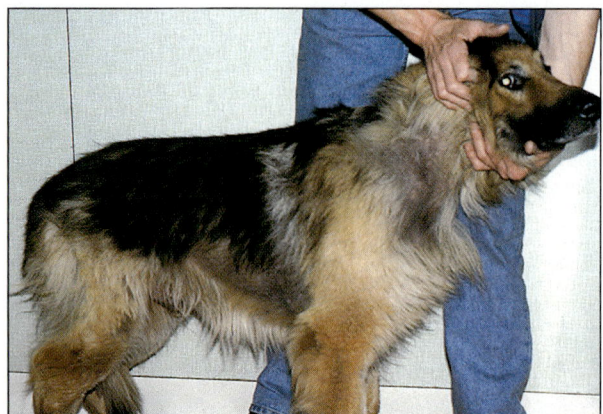

485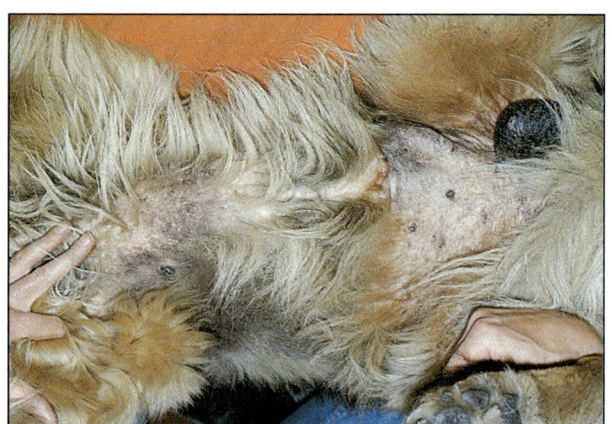

486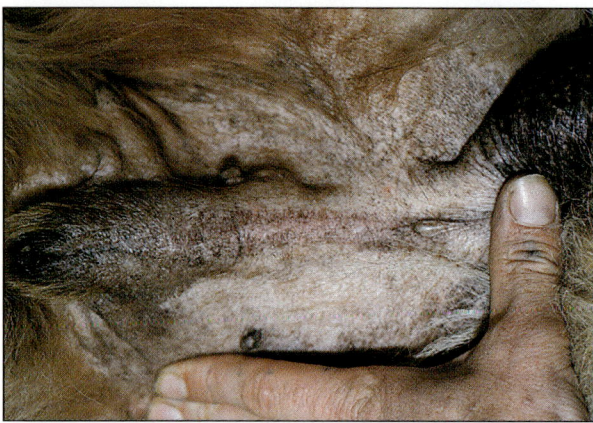

487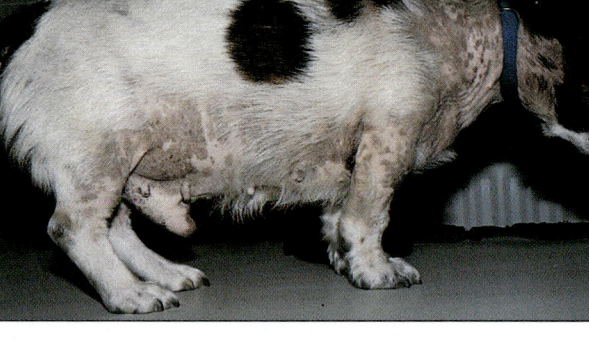

484–486   Sertoli-cell tumour. This German shepherd dog exhibits a number of features suggestive of this disorder. There is hyperpigmented skin associated with alopecia on the neck (**484**), alopecia in the groin (**485**) and there is an erythematous, linear patch along the ventral midline of the sheath (**486**).

487   Sertoli-cell tumour. This Jack Russell terrier exhibits a similar distribution of alopecia. Note the blotchy hyperpigmentation and the ventrally-directed sheath. This dog also had oestrogen-induced bone marrow suppression.

There may be a linear erythematous patch along the ventral midline of the prepuce (**486**). The prepuce becomes hairless and pendulous (**487**). There may be gynaecomastia (**488**), a lack of normal male libido and some affected dogs will become attractive to other male dogs. Cytological examination of cells from the mucosal lining of the prepuce may reveal cornifying cells, similar to those present in the vagina when under the influence of oestrogen. In very chronic cases the hair is lost from the entire body except for the head, the lower limbs and along the dorsum of the trunk and metastasis may be noted (**489–491**).

Sertoli-cell tumour is characterised by:
- Bilaterally-symmetrical alopecia associated with gynaecomastia.
- A palpably-enlarged testis or evidence of cryptorchidism.
- Feminisation.

Differential diagnoses include:
- Other endocrinopathies.

Diagnosis can be made by:
- Consideration of the history and clinical signs.
- Elevated plasma oestrogen levels.
- Response to castration.

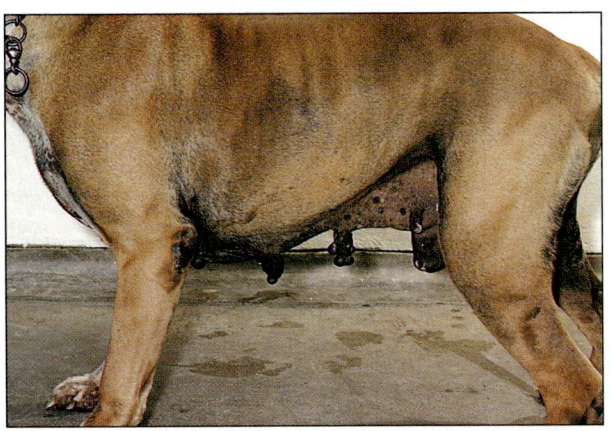

488   **Sertoli-cell tumour.** Boxer dog showing gynaecomastia, pendulous prepuce and early alopecia in the ventral and lateral thorax and the flanks.

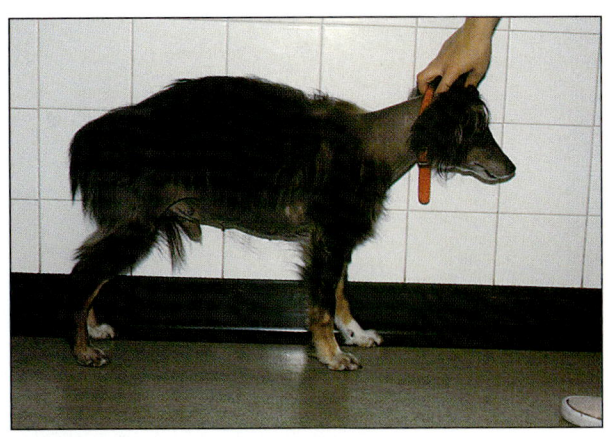

489–491   **Sertoli-cell tumour.** This Shetland sheepdog has signs of advanced changes due to a massive, abdominal, testicle. There were severe adhesions and metastases to other organs. The dog was euthanased during surgery.

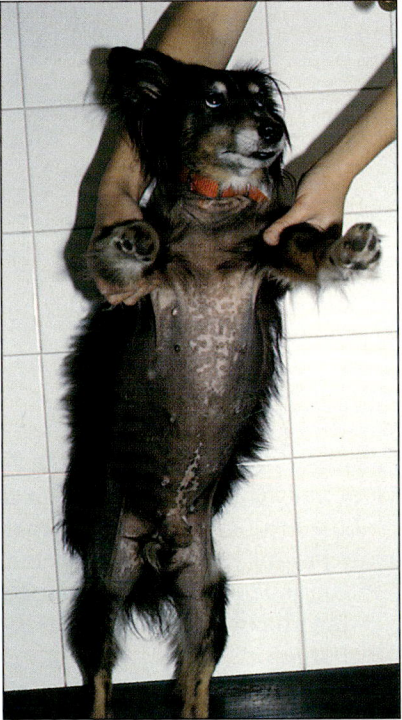

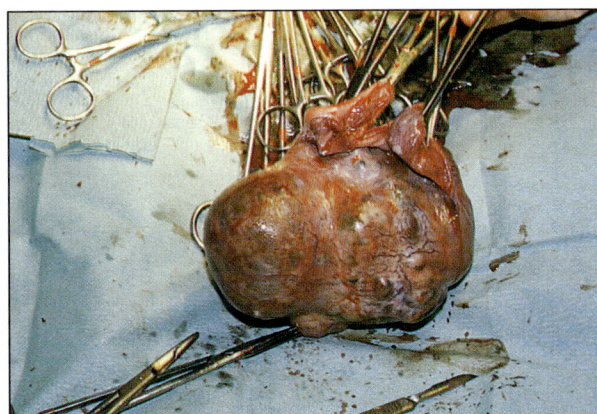

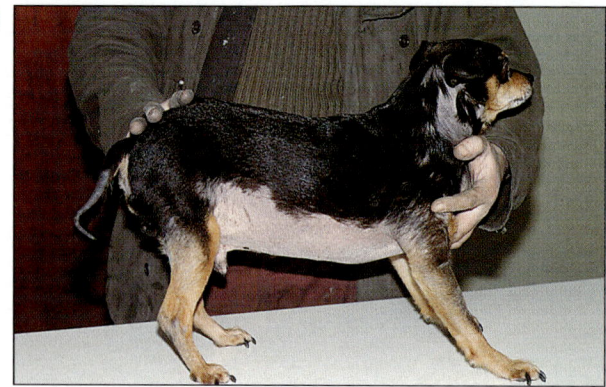

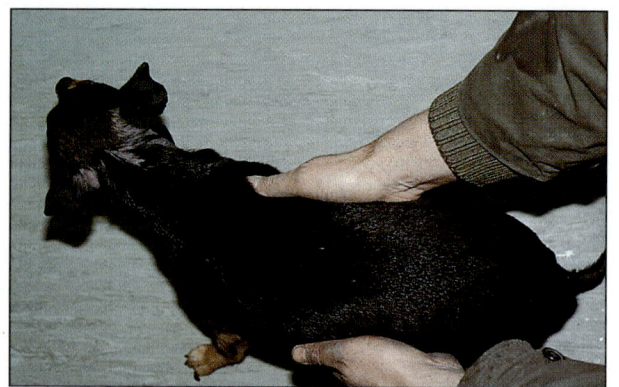

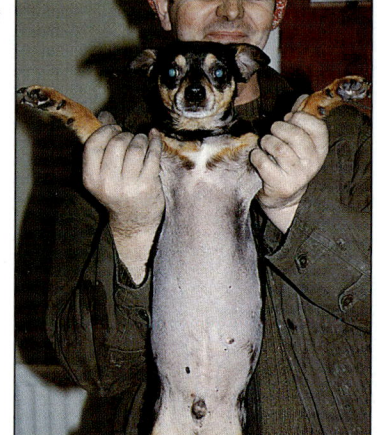

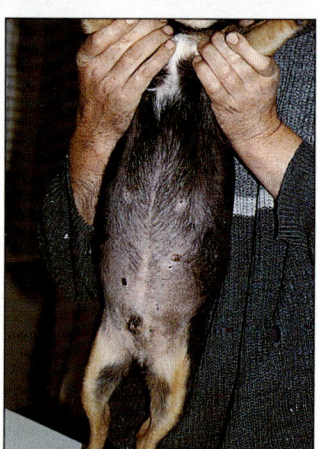

492–495   Male feminising syndrome. Chihuahua with extensive alopecia of the groin, tail, flanks and neck. **495** depicts the same dog after castration. Note the regrowth of hair. No neoplasia was detected in either testis.

Idiopathic male feminisation syndrome

This is a rare, but clear-cut, syndrome in which there is feminisation accompanied by bilaterally symmetrical alopecia and severe seborrhoea. The syndrome bears some resemblance to that seen with Sertoli's cell tumour but in this case the testicles are normal.

Originally the condition was thought to be due either to hypoandrogenism or hyperoestrogenism but studies have shown that affected dogs have normal plasma levels of both androgens and oestrogens and that testis development and spermatogenesis are normal.[8] It has been suggested that the cause is an androgen-blocking factor in the plasma. Presumably in the absence of suffi-

cient androgen reaching the nucleus of the target cell, oestrogen, which is normally present in the male plasma, is free to exert inhibitory effects on the skin and to produce systemic signs of feminisation.

Skin changes commence in the genital and perineal areas and consist of a bilaterally symmetrical alopecia (**492–495**) often accompanied by secondary seborrhoea, lichenification and marked hyperpigmentation. In advanced cases these changes may extend to involve the ventral abdomen and from there the remainder of the body. The seborrhoea is greasy and usually pruritic. Gynaecomastia is a constant finding and bilateral ceruminous external otitis is usually

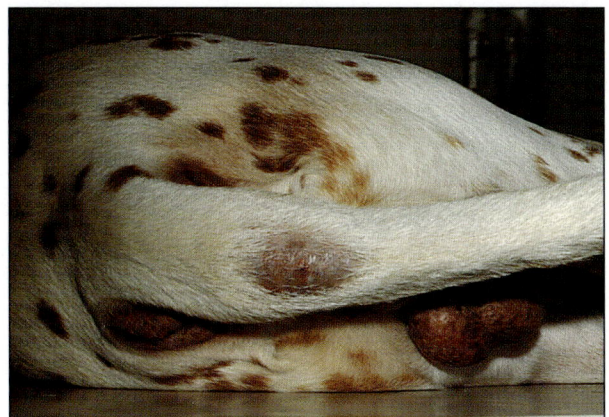

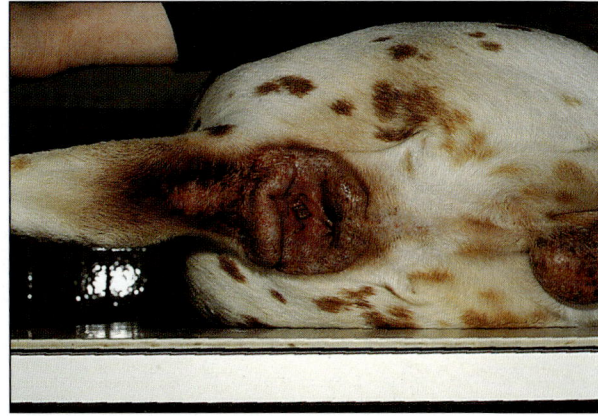

496 and **497   Hyperandrogenism.** The triad of enlarged tail gland, hyperplastic or adenomatous perianal glands and prostatomegaly accompany a testosterone-producing neoplasm. Similar changes may also be found in adult, usually elderly, male dogs with no detectable neoplasia.

present. The prepuce may become hairless and pendulous, the latter due to relaxation of the preputial ligament, and the affected animal may become attractive to other male dogs.

Male feminisation syndrome is characterised by:
- Bilaterally symmetrical alopecia.
- Seborrhoeic skin changes, hyperpigmentation and lichenification.
- Feminisation with gynaecomastia and pendulous prepuce.
- Normal testicles.

Differential diagnoses include:
- Endocrine dermatoses.
- Defects in keratinisation.

Diagnosis can be made by:
- Consideration of the history and clinical signs.
- Response to castration or administration of testosterone.

Hyperandrogenism

This is not uncommon in elderly males (**496** and **497**). The triad of hyperplastic tail gland, perianal gland hyperplasia, or adenomata, and prostatomegaly has been associated with the presence of testicular neoplasia, particularly of the interstitial cells.[21] It may also occur in elderly male dogs with no palpable neoplasia. There are no associated changes in hair coat. Castration is curative.

Castration-responsive dermatosis

This is a rare dermatosis.[14] Keeshonds, Alaskan malamutes, Siberian huskies and Pomeranians may be predisposed. Clinical signs include a dull, dry coat, fading of coat colour and a dry, scaly, hyperpigmented skin. There may be an associated alopecia, particularly of the neck, perineum and ventrum. There is an elevated level of plasma 17 oestradiol in most cases. Castration is curative.

498

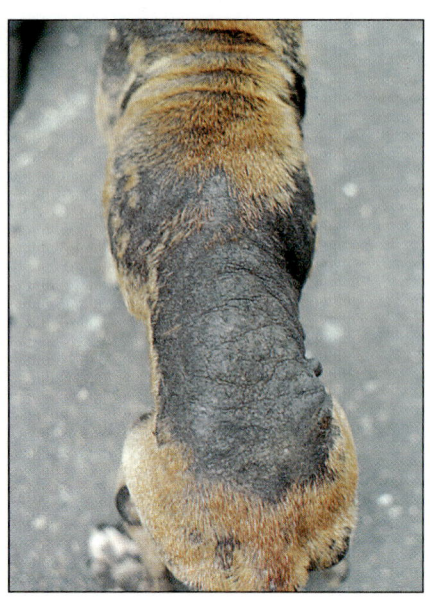

499

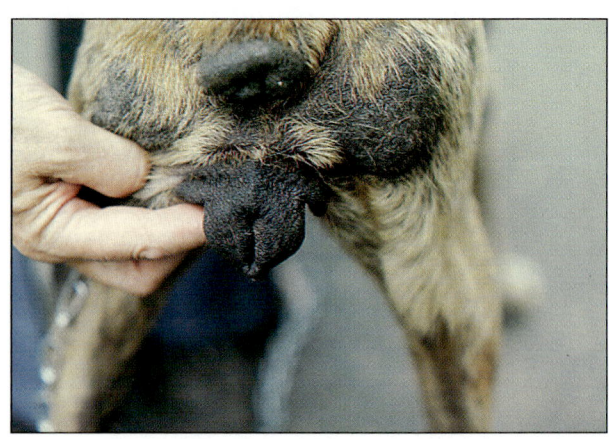

498 and 499   Hyperoestrogenism. Also known as Ovarian imbalance Type I, this condition occurs due to elevated plasma oestrogens. Boxer bitch showing chronic hyperpigmented alopecia and tumefied vulva.

Ovarian imbalance

This is a catch-all term which probably embraces several entities but until hormone levels of the bitch are fully documented the clinician must rely on the clinical signs presented in order to arrive at a diagnosis. Two syndromes are currently recognised.[16]

Hyperoestrogenism

A rare condition occurring in entire bitches (previously known as 'Ovarian imbalance Type I') which is characterised by bilaterally symmetrical alopecia, hyperpigmentation and lichenification of the skin of the perigenital, perineal and axillary regions. The condition is associated with cystic ovaries and, more uncommonly, with functional ovarian tumours, e.g. granulosa cell tumours. Skin changes are most often seen in bitches that are several years old. The skin changes commence with alopecia and hyperpigmentation of the flanks, genital areas and perineum with the axillae becoming involved later (**498–500**).

Lichenification of the skin is a fairly constant finding in advanced cases. Ceruminous otitis externa and pruritic seborrhoeic skin disease are common and comedones are a regular feature. Often the vulva is enlarged and hyperpigmented and there is tumefaction and crusting of the nipples. Irregular oestrous cycles, anoestrus and pseudocyesis are frequently reported.

500

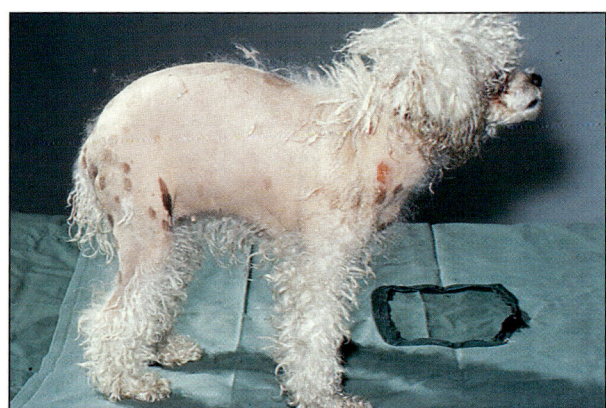

500   Hyperoestrogenism. Alopecia and patchy pigmentary changes in a miniature poodle bitch which were associated with cystic ovaries and cystic endometrial hyperplasia.

Hyperoestrogenism is characterised by:
- Bilaterally symmetrical alopecia.
- Enlargement and tumefaction of the vulva and nipples.

Differential diagnoses include:
- Endocrine dermatoses.
- Defects in keratinisation.
- Hormonal hypersensitivity.

Diagnosis can be made by:
- Consideration of the history and clinical signs.
- Normal thyroid and adrenal function tests.
- Response to ovarohysterectomy.

501

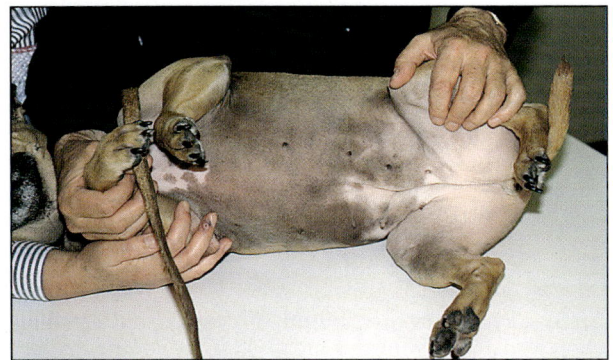

502

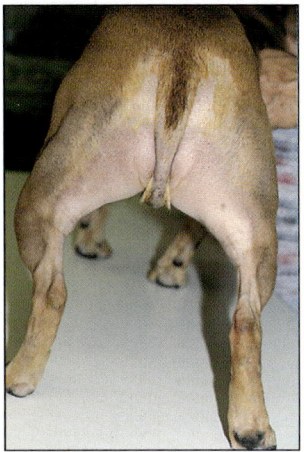

503

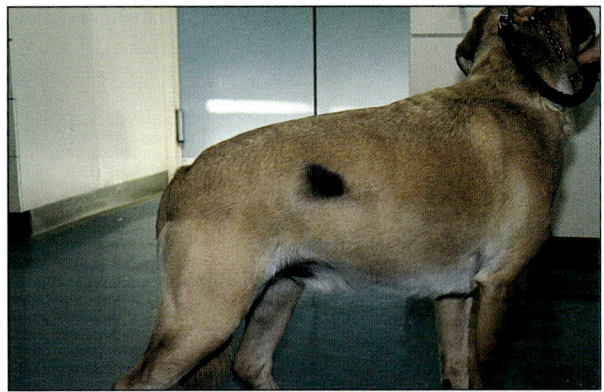

504

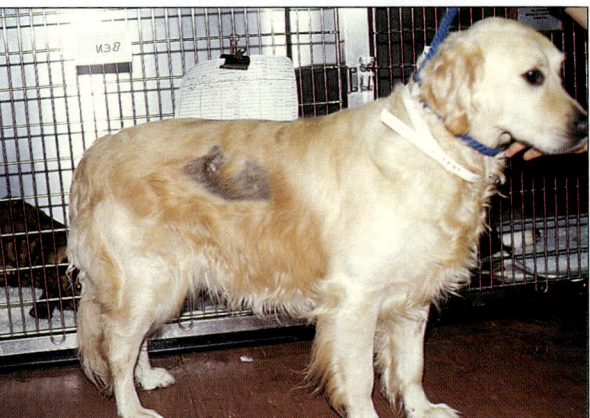

501 and 502 Hypo-oestrogenism. Also known as Ovarian imbalance Type II, this condition is considered to result from either a reduced plasma oestrogen concentrations or to reduced local receptor response to oestrogen. This Staffordshire bull terrier exhibits alopecia of the ventral trunk and caudomedial thighs. There is no accompanying inflammation or hyperpigmentation.

Hypo-oestrogenism

A rare condition (previously called 'Ovarian imbalance Type II') of unknown aetiology. It may be associated with ovarohysterectomy at an early age. There is symmetrical hair loss, especially on the ventral surface of the trunk from where the alopecia may extend to involve the caudal thighs and even the neck and pinnae (**501** and **502**). The skin of the affected area is thin, soft and pliable in most cases with no hyperpigmentation or lichenification. The hair is fine and soft and is easily epilated. The nipples and the vulva may appear infantile.

Hypo-oestrogenism is characterised by:
• Bilaterally symmetrical alopecia.

Differential diagnoses include:
• Hypothyroidism.
• Follicular dysplasia.

Diagnosis can be made by:
• Consideration of the history and clinical signs.
• Normal thyroid and adrenal function tests.
• (Response to administration of oestrogens.)

503 and 504 Idiopathic flank alopecia. These two dogs exhibit the typical features of this condition. There is bilateral alopecia, often in the sub-lumbar fossa. Both dogs had normal TSH and low dose dexamethasone responses. The male Labrador retriever (**503**) had a permanent alopecia whilst the female golden retriever (**504**) exhibited cyclical alopecia, the hair falling out in the late winter and growing in the summer.

Idiopathic flank alopecia

This is a condition of unknown aetiology which occurs in both entire and neutered animals of either sex.[20] There is a bilaterally symmetrical alopecia, sometimes with hyperpigmentation, which commences on the flank, in the sub-lumbar fossa (**503** and **504**). In other animals the alopecia may follow the line of the posterior ribs. The alopecia may wax and wane and may be seasonal in some cases, being most obvious in the late winter and early spring. In other cases the area of alopecia is static for years. Spontaneous regrowth may occur. In every other respect the affected animal appears to be normal.

505

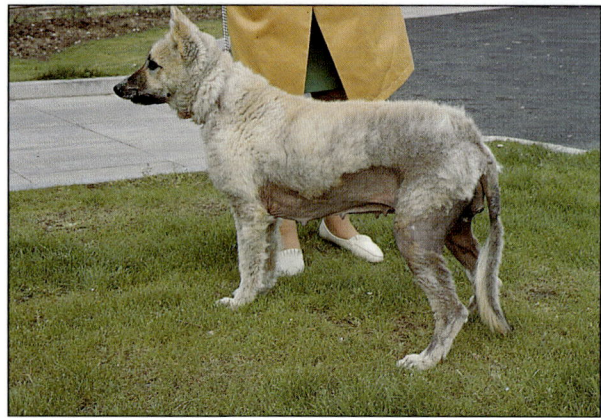

505   Pituitary dwarfism. Four-year-old German shepherd bitch showing small stature, ventral hyperpigmented alopecia and the puppy-like, downy nature of the coat.

506

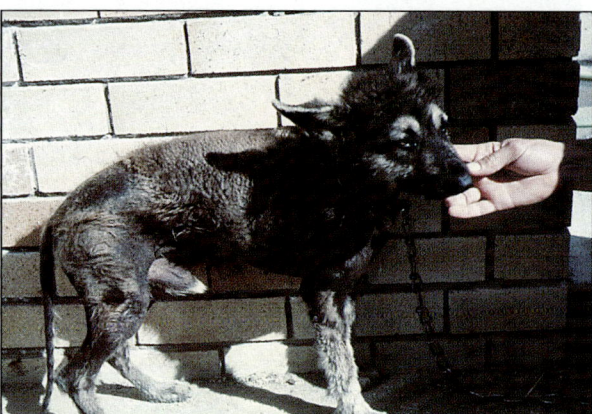

507

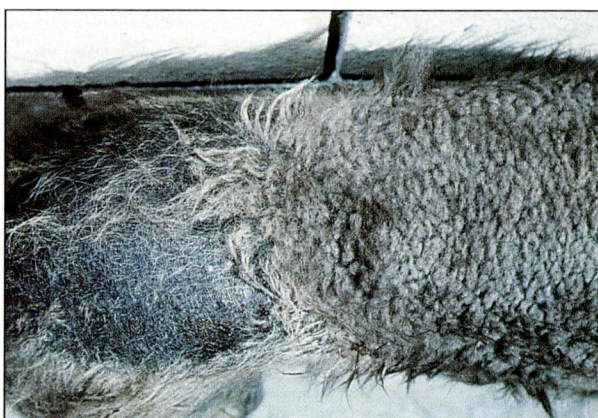

506 and 507   Pituitary dwarfism. Ten-month-old German shepherd dog showing small stature, hyperpigmented alopecia and retained puppy coat. Note the enlarged penis (enlargement of the external genitalia is often noted in this condition). Close-up (**507**) demonstrating puppy-like downy nature of the remaining hair and the hyperpigmented alopecia.

Pituitary dysfunction

Apart from its indirect effect on the skin and hair growth via the medium of other endocrine glands, the pituitary exerts a direct effect through somatropin, the growth hormone. Hypophysectomy accelerates the initiation and spread of spontaneous activity in which the hair cycle is normal but the pelage is infantile (lanugo) in type. Somatropin will restore the pelage to an adult texture but gonadal hormones do not.

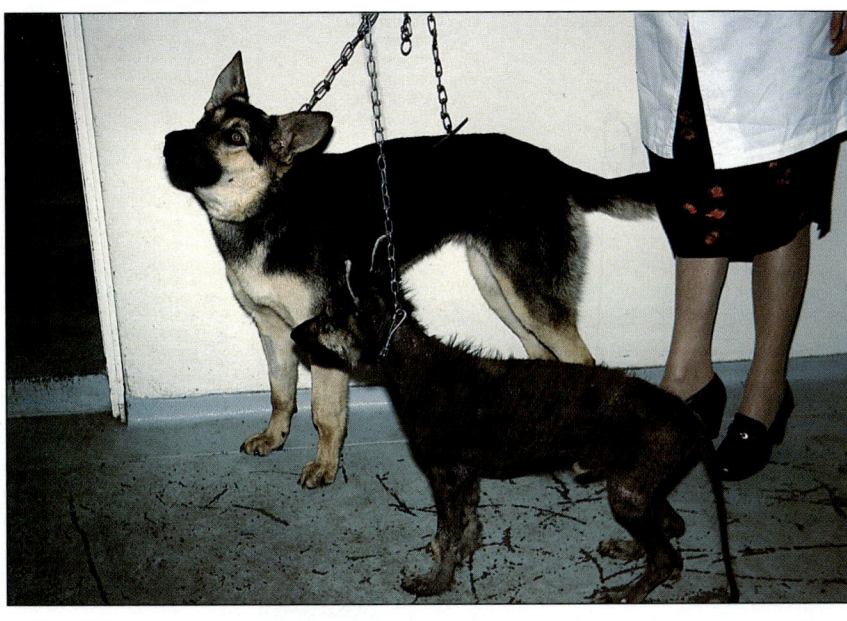

508   Pituitary dwarfism. Another ten-month-old German shepherd dog alongside a normal dog of the same age.

Pituitary dwarfism

An anterior pituitary insufficiency due to cyst formation (Rathke's cleft cyst) in the pituitary gland. The condition is thought to be inherited as a simple autosomal recessive condition in the German shepherd and Karelian bear dog, the breeds most commonly affected. Although affected puppies appear to be normal at birth, after the age of about three months they do not grow normally and are permanent dwarfs.

Primary hairs fail to develop, except for on the lower limbs and the face, and the soft woolly puppy coat of secondary hairs is retained (505–508). These hairs are easily epilated and a bilaterally symmetrical alopecia develops in the friction areas of the lateral aspects of the thighs and around the neck. The skin in the alopecic areas becomes progressively more hyperpigmented, scaly and thin and there may be comedone formation. The external genitalia may be atrophic or hypertrophic depending upon the nature of any gonadal dysfunction.

Pituitary dwarfism is characterised by:
- Dwarfism together with retention of puppy coat.
- Absence of primary hairs and bilaterally symmetrical alopecia.

Differential diagnosis is:
- Congenital hypothyroidism.

Diagnosis can be made by:
- Consideration of the history and clinical signs.
- Negative response to growth hormone stimulation tests.
- Insulin induced severe and prolonged hypoglycaemia.
- Histopathological examination of biopsy material.

509

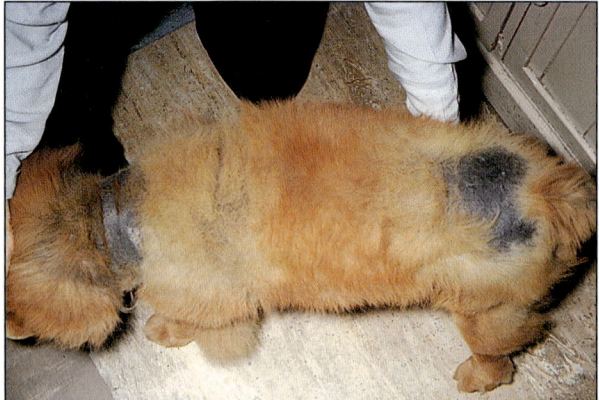

510

511

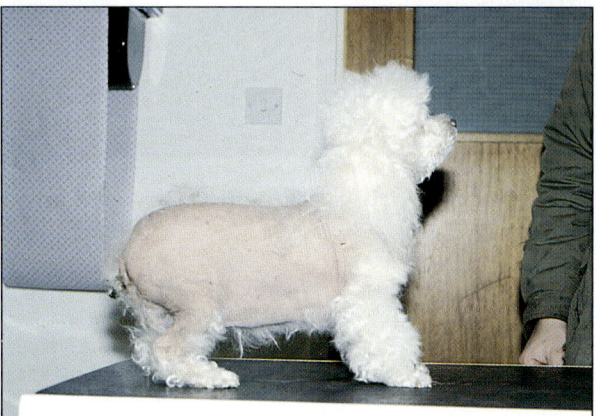

509 and 510   Adult onset growth hormone-responsive dermatosis. Chow chow dog showing alopecia and hyperpigmentation of the skin in the characteristic distribution pattern seen in this condition. Apart from the skin lesions affected dogs are normal.

511   Adult onset growth hormone-responsive dermatosis. This miniature Poodle exhibits the full extent of the alopecia associated with this condition. Note the sparing of the extremities.

Adult onset growth hormone responsive dermatosis

A rare, bilaterally symmetrical alopecia with hyperpigmentation occurring in one- to two-year-old male dogs predominantly of the Chow Chow, miniature Poodle, Pomeranian and Keeshond breeds.[22] The cause of the condition is unknown.[7] The alopecia spares the extremities and the areas usually affected are the trunk, the medial and caudal aspects of the thighs, the neck, pinnae and tail (**509–511**). Here the hair is easily epilated and the skin may be hypotonic and thin. Apart from the skin and coat changes, affected dogs are normal.

Adult onset growth hormone responsive dermatosis is characterised by:
- Bilaterally symmetrical hyperpigmented alopecia without systemic signs.

Differential diagnoses include:
- Other endocrinopathies.

Diagnosis can be made by:
- Consideration of the history and clinical signs.
- Normal thyroid and adrenal function tests, abnormal, blunted response to xylazine stimulation.

512

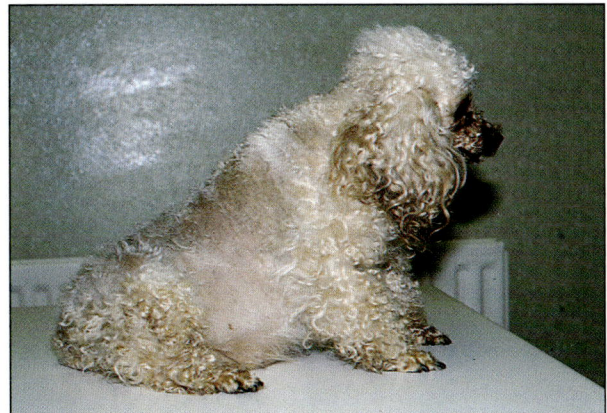

513

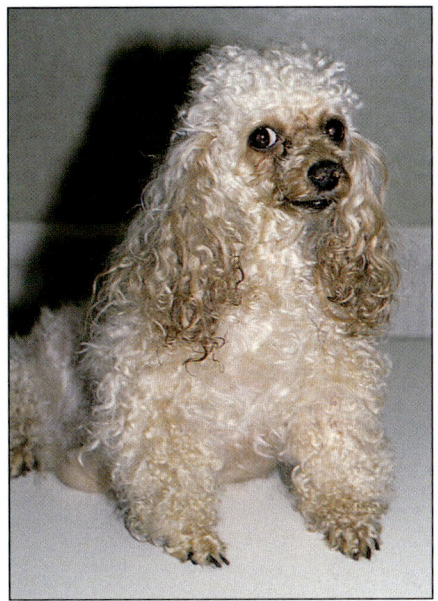

512 and 513   Canine acromegaly. A rare condition. This entire Poodle bitch has hypotrichosis of the trunk, hepatomegaly, abdominal distension, muscular weakness, enlarged interdental spaces and an abnormal stature

Acromegaly

A rare condition associated with hypersecretion of growth hormone in mature animals resulting in overgrowth of connective tissue, bone, muscle and viscera. In the dog the spontaneous condition is confined to entire bitches where it occurs in dioestrus. The iatrogenic condition is more common and typically follows long, continued administration of progestagens.[5] In the cat pituitary neoplasia is the most common cause.[13]

Systemic signs include polydipsia, polyuria, polyphagia, fatigue, inspiratory stridor and frequent panting. There is increased body size, abdominal enlargement and increased interdental spaces (**512** and **513**). Skin changes consist of thickening, the formation of exaggerated folds and myxoedema and occur mainly on the face and the extremities. There is usually hypertrichosis. Histopathological examination of biopsy specimens demonstrates increased collagen and mucin and epidermal and appendageal hyperplasia.

Acromegaly is characterised by:
- Inspiratory stridor.
- Increased body size, polydipsia, polyuria.
- Exaggerated skin folds.

Diagnosis can be made by:
- Consideration of the history and clinical signs.
- Histopathological examination of biopsy samples.
- Plasma growth hormone levels cannot be suppressed by intravenous injection of 1g glucose/kg.

References

1. Al-Bagdadi, F. A., Titkemeyer, C. W. and Lovell, J. E. (1977). Hair follicle cycle and shedding in male beagle dogs. *American Journal of Veterinary Research*, **38**: 611–616.

2. Chastain, C. B. (1982). Canine hypothyroidism. *Journal of the American Veterinary Medical Association*, **181**: 349–353.

3. Collins, R. R. (1987). Dermatologic disorders of common small nondomestic animals. In: Nesbitt, G. H. (Ed.). *Contemporary Issues in Small Animal Practice, No. 8 Dermatology*. Churchill Livingstone, New York.

4. Dawber, R. P. R., Ebling, F. J. G. and Wojnarowska, F. T. (1992). Disorders of hair. In: Champion, R. H., Burton, J. L. and Ebling, F. J. G. (Eds.), *Textbook of Dermatology*, Volume 4, pp. 2533–2638. Blackwell Scientific Publications, Oxford.

5. Eigenmann, J. E. and Venker-Haagen, A. J. (1981). Progestagen-induced and spontaneous canine acromegaly due to reversible growth hormone overproduction: clinical picture and pathogenesis. *Journal of the American Animal Hospital Association*, **17**: 813–822.

6. Lipowitz, A. J., Schwartz, A., Wilson, G. P. and Ebert, J. W. (1973). Testicular neoplasms and concomitant clinical changes in the dog. *Journal of the American Veterinary Medical Association*, **163**: 1364–1368.

7. Lothrop, C. D. (1988). Pathophysiology of canine growth hormone-responsive alopecia. *Compendium on Continuing Education*, **10**: 1346–1349.

8. Mattheeuws, D. and Comhaire, F. (1975). Oestradiol and testosterone in male dogs with alopecia and feminization without testicular neoplasia. *British Veterinary Journal*, **131**: 65–68.

9. Milne, K. L. and Hayes, H. M. (1981). Epidemiologic features of canine hypothyroidism. *Cornell Veterinarian*, **71**: 3–14.

10. Nelson, R. W., Feldman, E. C. and Smith, M. C. (1988). Hyperadrenocorticism in cats: Seven cases (1978–1987). *Journal of the American Veterinary Medical Association*, **193**: 245–250.

11. Panciera, D. L. (1990). Canine hypothyroidism. Part 1. Clinical findings and control of thyroid hormone secretion and metabolism. *Compendium on Continuing Education*, **12**: 689–701.

12. Peterson, M. E. (1986). Canine hyperadrenocorticism. In: Kirk. R. W. (Ed.) *Current Veterinary Therapy IX*, pp. 963–972. W. B. Saunders, Philadelphia.

13. Peterson, M. E. (1988). Endocrine disorders in cats: four emerging diseases. *Compendium on Continuing Education*, **10**: 1353–1360.

14. Rosser, E J. (1989). Castration responsive dermatosis in the dog. In: von Tscharner, C. and Halliwell, R. E. W. (Eds.) *Advances in Veterinary Dermatology*, pp. 34–42. Baillière Tindall, London.

15. Schmeitzel, L. P. and Lothrop, C. D. (1990a). Hormonal abnormalities in Pomeranians with normal coat and in Pomeranians with growth hormone-responsive dermatosis. *Journal of the American Veterinary Medical Association*, **197**: 1333–1341.

16. Schmeitzel, L. P. and Lothrop, C. D. (1990b). Sex hormones and skin disease. *Veterinary Medicine Report*, **2**: 28–41.

17. Scott, D. W. (1982). Histopathologic findings in endocrine skin disorders of the dog. *Journal of the American Animal Hospital Association,* **18**: 173–183.

18. Scott, D. W. (1985). Cutaneous phlebectasias in cushingoid dogs. *Journal of the American Animal Hospital Association,* **21**: 351–354.

19. Scott, D. W. (1989). Biology of hair growth. In: von Tscharner, C. and Halliwell, R. E. W. (Eds.) *Advances in Veterinary Dermatology*, pp. 3–33. Baillière Tindall, London.

20. Scott, D. W. (1990). Seasonal flank alopecia in ovaro-hysterectomized bitches. *Cornell Veterinarian*, **80**: 187–195.

21. Scott, D. W. and Reimers, T. J. (1986). Tail gland and peri-anal gland hyperplasia associated with testicular neoplasia and hypertestosteronemia in a dog. *Canine Practice*, **13**: 15–17.

22. Scott, D. W. and Walton, D. K. (1986). Hyposomatotropism in the mature dog: a discussion of 22 cases. *Journal of the American Animal Hospital Association,* **22**: 467–473.

23. Thacker, E. L., Refsal, K. R. and Bull, R. W. (1992). Prevalence of autoantibodies to thyroglobin, thyroxine, or tri-iodothyronine and relationship of autoantibodies and serum concentrations of iodothyronines in dogs. *American Journal of Veterinary Research*, **53**: 449–453.

24. Thoday, K. L. and Mooney, C. T. (1992). Historical, clinical and laboratory features of 126 hyperthyroid cats. *Veterinary Record*, **131**: 257–264.

25. White, S. D., Ceragioli, K. L., Bullock, L. P., Mason, G. D. and Stewart, L. J. (1989). Cutaneous markers of canine hyperadrenocorticism. *Compendium on Continuing Education*, **11**: 446–464.

26. Willeberg, P. and Priester, W. A. (1982). Epidemiological aspects of clinical hyperadrenocorticism in dogs (canine Cushing's syndrome). *Journal of the American Animal Hospital Association*, **18**: 717–724.

Chapter 11:

Nutritional dermatoses

Nutritional dermatoses due to absolute dietary deficiencies are rare in animals fed commercially-produced food.[7,10] However, because these diets are well-balanced it is possible for an unwitting owner to over-supplement the diet and this may result in a relative deficiency of one component being induced. Thus, dietary calcium competes for absorption with dietary zinc and therefore over-supplementation with calcium may result in a relative deficiency of zinc.

Most nutritional dermatoses are ill-defined and have only been produced experimentally but the clinical signs are similar with scale, erythema, a dry, lustreless and easily epilated coat and a greasy skin, often accompanied by secondary bacterial infection.[7] These changes reflect alterations in the process of keratinisation, the fundamental metabolic activity of the skin and the adnexae.

Although many components of the diet have some function in one or more aspects of cutaneous homeostasis, the essential fatty acids, vitamin A and zinc are the most important from the clinician's point of view. In addition, a number of other dietary components such as biotin, the retinoids, niacinamide and vitamin E, have been investigated for their potential in the control of skin disease both in dogs and cats.

Protein/calorie deficiency

Long-term protein/calorie deficiency is unlikely to be encountered in clinical practice but may be seen in animals maintained for prolonged periods on very low-protein diets or with long-standing illness such as chronic renal failure (**514** and **515**). There is hyperkeratosis, epidermal hyperpigmentation and the normal coat is gradually replaced by a thin, poor, lustreless coat.[1,5,10]

514
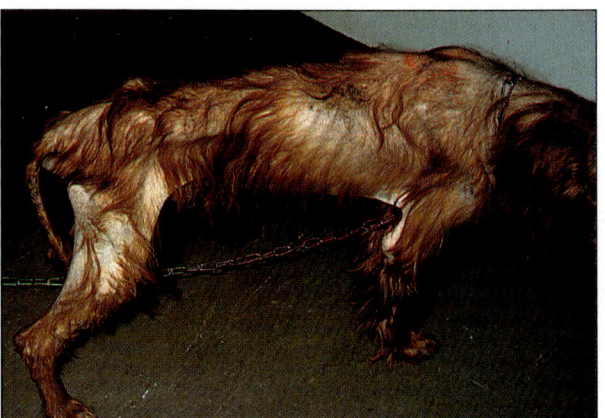

515
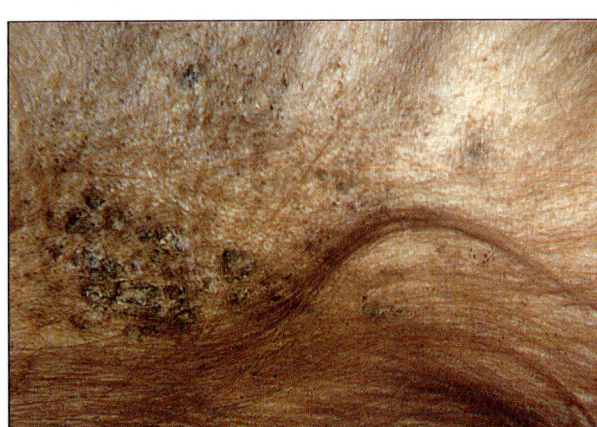

514 and 515 Dermatosis associated with malnutrition. Irish setter which had suffered from intermittent anorexia for nearly two years when presented. Note the symmetrical and extensive hair loss, the emaciation and the crusted skin lesions.

516

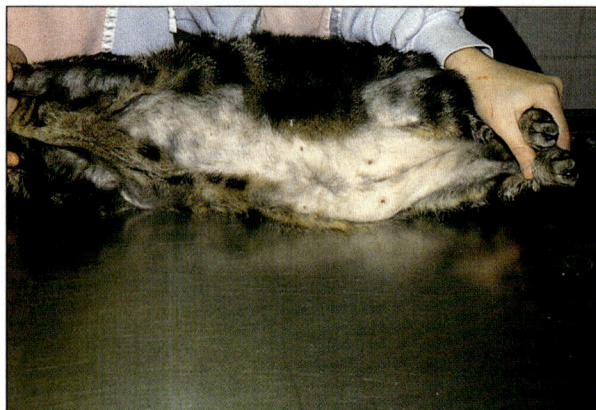

516 Telogen defluxion in a cat with chronic renal failure. Note the symmetrical loss of hair on the ventral body surfaces.

517

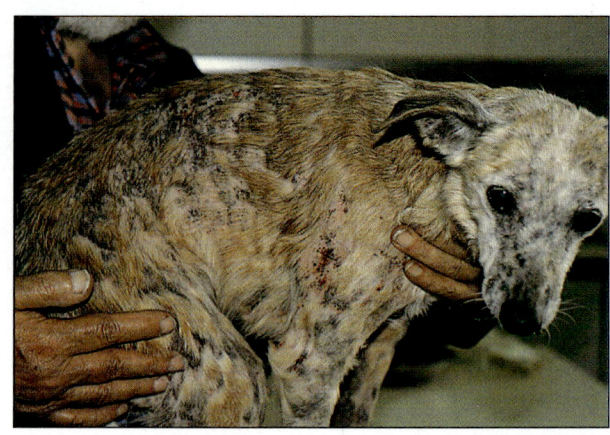

517 Anagen defluxion. A dog with generalised patchy alopecia. The animal suffered from acute nephritis some 6 weeks prior to the photograph. The severe systemic disease resulted in anagen arrest and accounts for the patchy loss of hair.

518

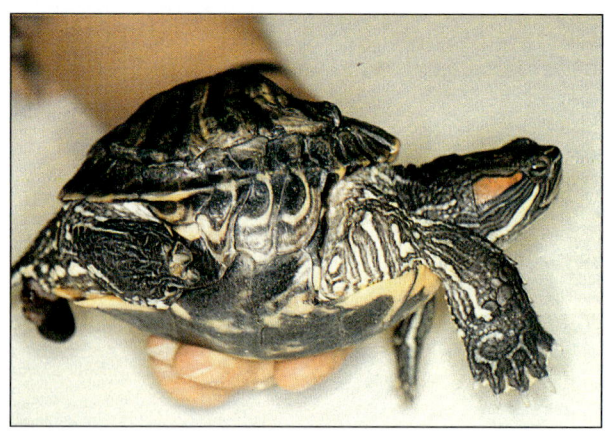

518 Soft shell in young chelonia is a result of high growth rates and insufficient dietary calcium. The soft shell may be pulled out of shape by the contracture of limb muscles which insert on the underside of the shell. (Illustration courtesy M. P. C. Lawton.)

Eventually alopecia may result through the gradual cessation of growth in the hair follicles, telogen defluxion (**516**). Sudden cessation of anagen may occur in severe systemic disease, resulting in localised areas of weakness in the hair shaft. As the regrowing shaft emerges from the protection of the follicle it breaks, resulting in an uneven, rough, dry pelage, anagen defluxion (**517**).

High protein levels may be a cause of disease in reptiles, particularly gout.[9] Although hind-limb paralysis is a major sign there may be subcutaneous deposits of uric acid, visible as small white nodules. The combination of high protein and low calcium and phosphorus which occurs in vegetables and fruit may cause shell problems in young chelonia. The high protein encourages a rapid growth rate, outstripping available calcium and phosphorus. This results in nutritional secondary osteodystrophy and the production of soft shell (**518**). Deformation may occur as limb muscles exert forces on the shell via their attachments.

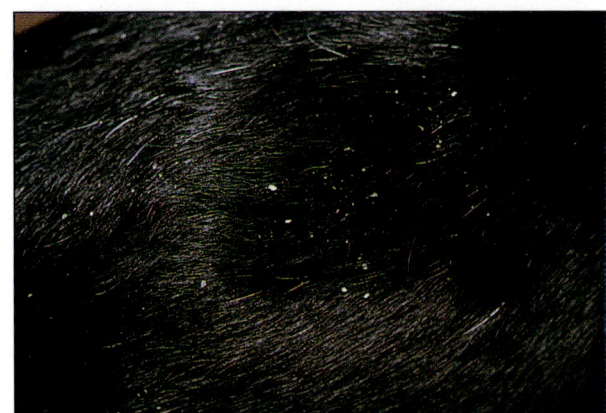

519

519 **Essential fatty acid** may result from the feeding of complete diets which have been subjected to prolonged storage. A fine scale is the earliest sign.

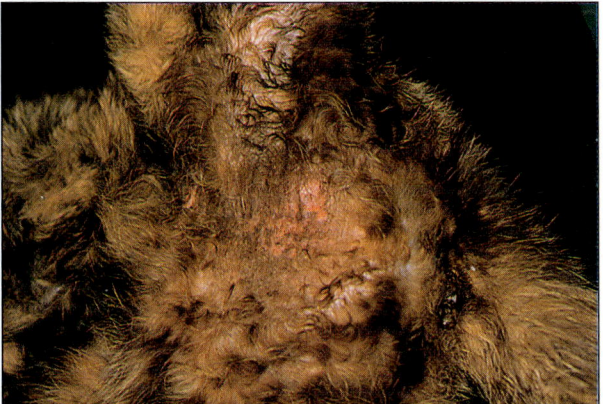

520

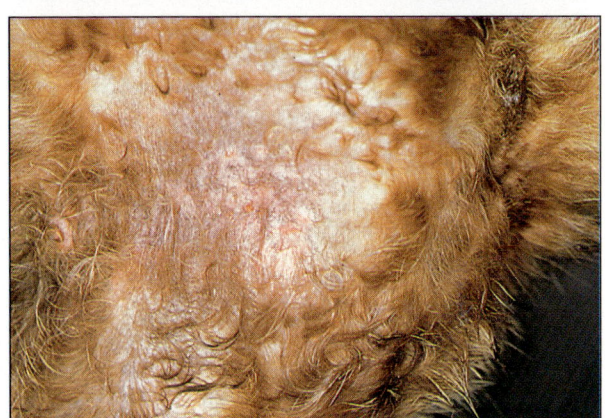

521

520 and 521 **Pansteatitis.** This cat exhibits the clinical signs of a nodular dermatosis accompanied by alopecia and discharging sinus formation. The cat was fed canned tuna. (Illustrations courtesy D. H. Scarff.)

Essential fatty acid deficiency

Commercially-prepared, canned diets are adequately supplemented, but the fat content of the dried-type is low compared to canned and moist diets and the level of linoleic acid may fall below adequate if the food is stored for too long, particularly in a warm, damp environment. Cutaneous signs compatible with essential fatty acid deficiency may accompany chronic internal disease such as malabsorption and liver disorders.

The early signs of essential fatty acid deficiency are a dull coat accompanied by a fine scale[6] (**519**). Prolonged deficiency results in alopecia, a greasy skin particularly on the pinnae and feet, exfoliative dermatitis and secondary pyotraumatic dermatitis.[1]

The metabolism of fatty acids results in the production of lipid peroxides and free radicals which are potentially toxic. Post δ-6 desaturase fatty acids, vitamin E and ascorbic acid all have antioxidant and free-radical scavenging capacity. Imbalances of the relationship between any of these substances, particularly a relative deficiency in vitamin E, may result in disease.

Thus, pansteatitis in cats results from inflammation of the subcutaneous fat deposits which become softened and contain firm, painful nodules. There is usually pyrexia, lethargy and inappetance and there may be draining tracts (**520** and **521**). Typically associated with diets containing oily fish, it may also be seen in animals on commercially- prepared food. Naturally-occurring vitamin E deficiency has not been recorded in dogs.

522

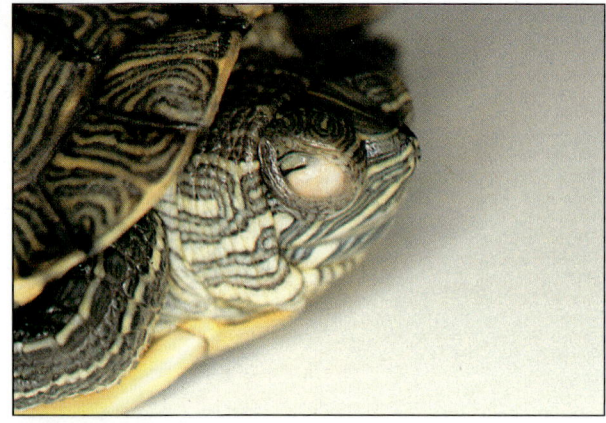

522   **Blephroedema** (swollen eyelids) and caseous material over the cornea in a red-eared terrapin due to vitamin A deficiency. (Illustration courtesy M. P. C. Lawton.)

523

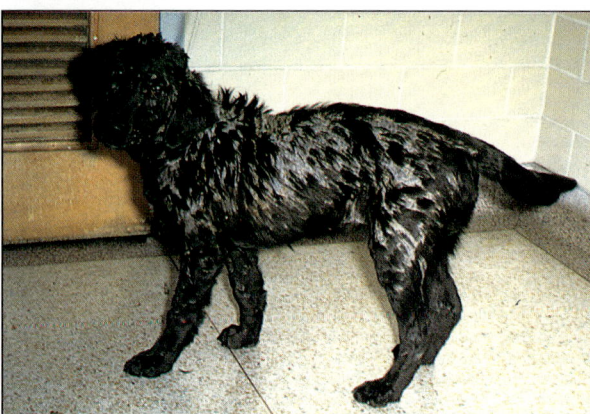

524

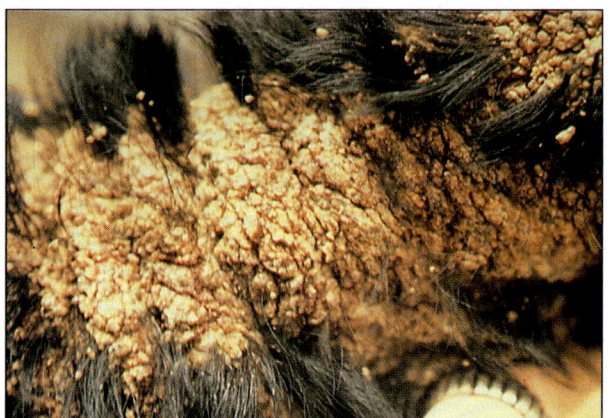

523 and 524   Vitamin A responsive dermatosis. Cross-bred retriever bitch showing extensive patches of hair loss and seborrhoeic dermatitis. **524** illustrates the crusted nature of the lesion. (Illustrations courtesy J. A. Yager.)

Vitamin A deficiency

Vitamin A deficiency is rare but is most likely to occur during growth, pregnancy or lactation, in animals on fat-restricted diets or those with poor fat absorption. Deficiency of vitamin A occurs most frequently in cats as their daily requirement is quite high and they are unable to synthesise the vitamin from carotene present in the diet. The hair coat becomes dry, lustreless, harsh and brittle, there is loss of hair and the skin is dry and erythematous. There is hyperkeratosis of the epidermis, follicles and the sebaceous glands and there may be a papular eruption, a consequence of blocked, hyperkeratotic sebaceous gland ducts. There is increased susceptibility to bacterial infection.[1,10]

Vitamin A deficiency is seen more frequently in exotic species, particularly red-eared terrapins (*Trachemys scripta elegans*), and the acute form presents as an ocular disorder with swollen eyelids and corneal oedema[9] (**522**). More chronic deficiency may result in hyperkeratosis of the skin as in mammals.

Vitamin A–responsive dermatosis

This is a rare condition almost entirely confined to Cocker spaniels.[3] There is no evidence that affected animals have deficient diets. Signs are of a severe and more or less generalised defect in keratinisation. There may be a greasy coat, loss of hair, mild to moderate pruritus and secondary pyoderma. The condition is characterised by focal areas of follicular plugging with plaque-like accumulations of keratin (**523** and **524**). Histopathological examination of these areas reveals a markedly disproportionate follicular hyperkeratosis. The lesions slowly resolve with doses of 10,000 IU vitamin A daily. Since this is in excess of the dietary requirement, care must be taken to eliminate other causes of the dermatosis before treatment is initiated.

525

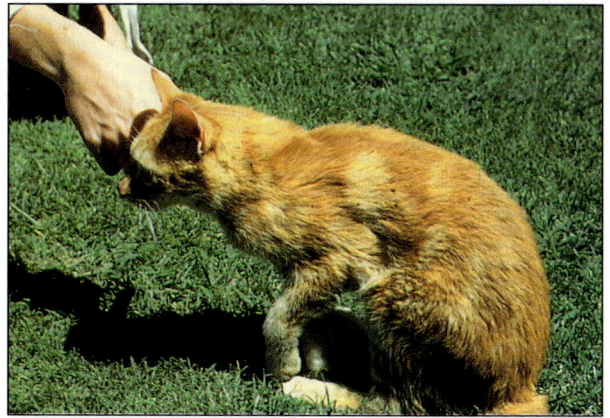

526

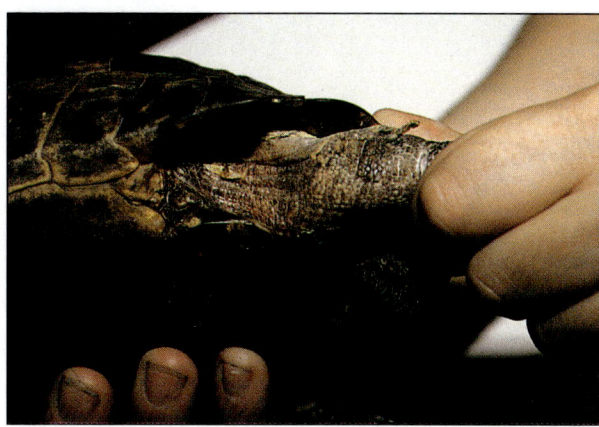

525   Hypervitaminosis A. Cat with marked cervical spondylitis leading to the assumption of 'marsupial posture'. Note the rough, unkempt coat resulting from the cat's inability to groom itself due to neck rigidity.

526   Erosive dermatosis on the forelimb of a tortoise due to iatrogenic hypervitaminosis A. (Illustration courtesy M. P. C. Lawton.)

Hypervitaminosis A

This may occur in cats addicted to foodstuffs rich in vitamin A, typically liver or cod-liver oil.[1] Extensive confluent bony exostoses form mainly on the cervicothoracic vertebrae which eventually prevent the cat from bending its neck. As a result the coat becomes unkempt, rough and staring due to the cat's inability to groom itself (**525**). Iatrogenic hypervitaminosis A may result in an erosive dermatosis in chelonia (**526**).

B vitamin deficiency

Individual deficiency of B group vitamins is reported to be very rare in dogs and cats in clinical practice. Deficiencies of the B vitamins are usually considered together as the clinical syndromes are similar, consisting of alopecia, anorexia and weight loss combined with a dry, flaking seborrhoea.[10] Single deficiencies of riboflavin, niacin and biotin may produce variations on this common theme. Deficiency of water-soluble vitamins may occur in conditions associated with water loss such as enteritis or where prolonged antibacterial therapy has reduced the synthesising ability of enteric flora.

Occasionally, animals on bizarre diets may exhibit signs of single B vitamin deficiency.[1] This is because dietary components may inactivate specific vitamins. For example avidin in raw egg-white will bind biotin and the niacin in corn is bound and unavailable. Riboflavin deficiency causes seborrhoea-like dermatitis especially around the eyes, the lips and the ventral body surfaces in dogs and alopecia of the head in cats.[10] Niacin deficiency causes canine pellagra, a condition characterised by a dry, harsh and staring coat, diarrhoea, oral ulceration and loss of condition.

A black tongue is considered to be pathognomonic of the condition, which used to be seen quite frequently in Scottish sheepdogs which were fed almost exclusively on maize. Biotin deficiency in dogs is associated with crusted lesions on the face, neck, body and legs coupled with anorexia, emaciation, diarrhoea and lethargy.[2] A characteristic feature is the spectacled appearance produced by periorbital alopecia.

527

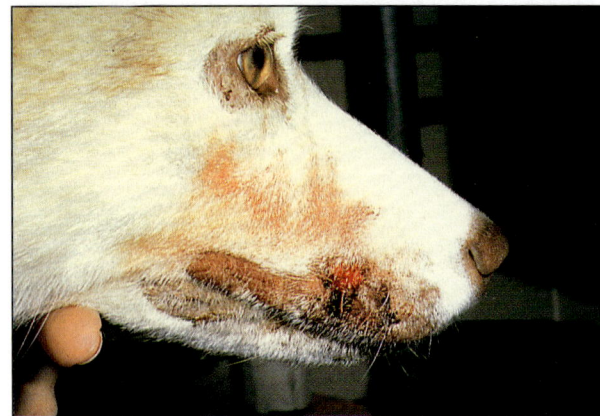

527   Zinc-responsive dermatosis Type I. Siberian husky showing dermatitis around eyes and mouth. (Illustration courtesy J. A. Yager.)

528

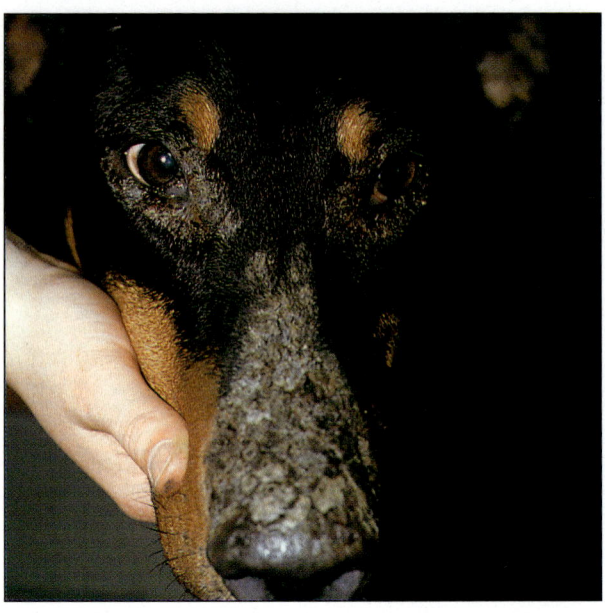

528   Zinc-responsive dermatosis in a Doberman pinscher. Note the symmetrical distribution of the facial lesions.

529

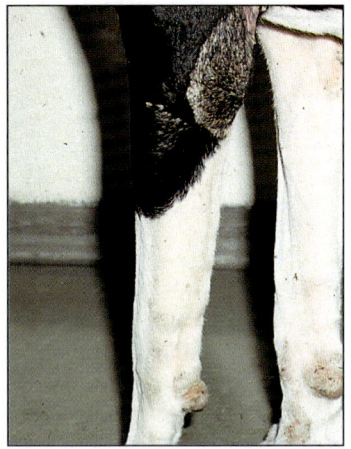

529   Zinc-responsive dermatosis. Focal areas of hyperkeratosis may occur on the trunk or limbs, particularly over pressure points. (Illustration courtesy A. H. M. Van Den Broek.)

Zinc deficiency

Most commonly, signs of zinc deficiency are due to interaction with other dietary components rather than absolute deficiency. Thus the absorption of zinc from the gut is inhibited by iron, copper and calcium which compete with zinc for absorption[11], whilst intestinal phytate and inorganic phosphate bind zinc and thus hinder absorption.[1]

In cases of absolute zinc deficiency, or a metabolic inability to utilise zinc, there may be systemic as well as cutaneous signs. In less severe cases, associated with relative dietary deficiency or interaction, the cutaneous signs predominate. These appear over the pressure points and adjacent to the mucosae, in a more or less symmetrical manner; around the mouth and periorbitally, peripinnal, perineal and on the limbs[7,11] (**527** and **528**). Areas of crusting are typically well demarcated with an erythematous border and may be mistaken for pyoderma (**529**). The coat is dull, harsh and occasional areas of achromotrichia may be noted. Lymphadenopathy is a common feature, particularly in younger animals.

530

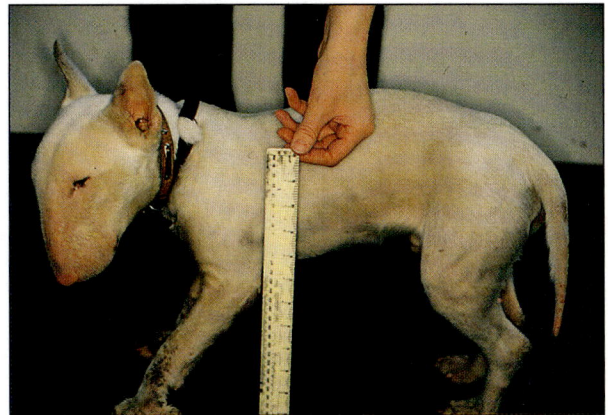

531

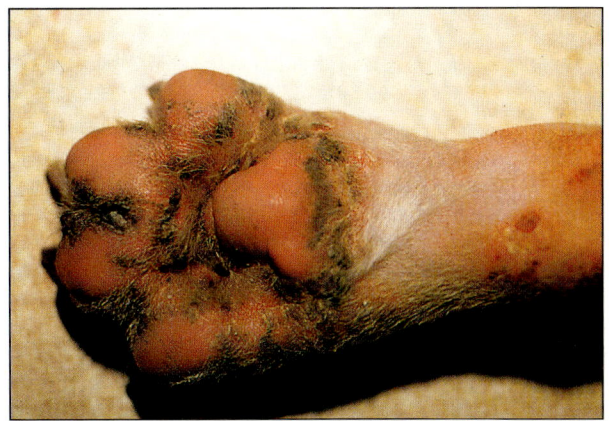

532

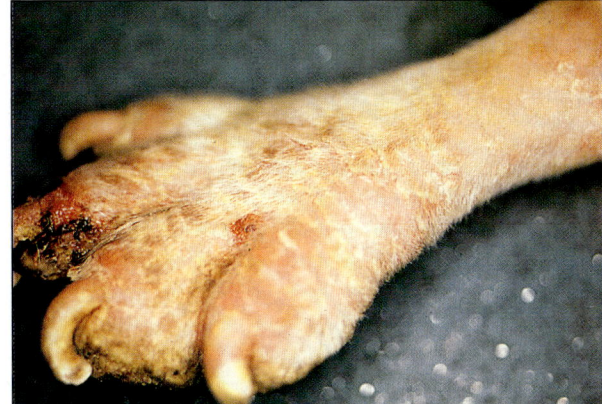

530–532 Lethal acrodermatitis in English Bull terriers. These illustrations depict a typical case. Note the emaciation and stunted growth (**530**), poor conformation and pododermatitis (**531** and **532**). (Illustrations courtesy of N. A. McEwan.)

Two groups of animals appear to be at risk from zinc-responsive dermatosis.[7] The distinction between groups is not absolute and the cutaneous lesions are similar.

In the first group ('Syndrome 1') certain individuals of many breeds of dog, but of Siberian huskies and Alaskan malamutes in particular, appear unable to absorb sufficient zinc from the intestine, even when fed a nutritionally-balanced diet. The condition may be precipitated by stress.

The second type of zinc-responsive dermatosis ('Syndrome 2') may occur in any breed of dog. Typically it is seen in rapidly-growing animals fed zinc-deficient diets or diets in which nutritional antagonism occurs, particularly diets over supplemented with calcium or high in phytate.

A recessive, lethal, acrodermatitis associated with an inability to utilise zinc has been reported in English bull terriers.[4] Clinical signs included growth retardation, conjunctivitis and keratitis, emaciation, pododermatitis and immunoincompetence (**530–532**).

References

1. Buffington, C. A. (1987). Nutrition and the skin. *Proceedings of the 11th Annual Kal Kan Symposium for the Treatment of Small Animal Diseases.* pp. 11–16.

2. Fromageot, D. and Zaghroun, P. (1990). The potential role of biotin on canine dermatology. *Recueil de Medicine Veterinaire,* **166**: 87–94.

3. Ihrke, P. J. and Goldschmidt, M. H. (1983). Vitamin A-responsive dermatosis in the dog. *Journal of the American Animal Hospital Association,* **182**: 687–690.

4. Jezyk, P. F., Haskins, M. E., MacKay-Smith, W. E. and Patterson, D. F. (1986). Lethal acrodermatitis in bull terriers. *Journal of the American Veterinary Medical Association,* **188**: 833–839.

5. Lewis, L. D. (1981). Cutaneous manifestations of nutritional imbalances. *Proceedings of the 48th Annual Meeting of The American Animal Hospital Association.* pp. 263–272.

6. MacDonald, M. L., Anderson, B. C., Rogers, Q. R., Buffington, C. A. and Morris, J. G. (1984). Essential fatty acid requirements of cats: Pathology of essential fatty acid deficiency. *American Journal of Veterinary Research,* **45**: 1310–1317.

7. Miller, W. H. (1989). Nutritional considerations in small animal dermatology. *Veterinary Clinics of North America: Small Animal Practice,* **19**: 497–511.

8. Scott, D. W and Sheffey, B. E. (1987). Dermatosis in dogs caused by vitamin E deficiency. *Companion Animal Practice,* **1**: 42–46.

9. Scott, P. W. (1992). Nutritional diseases. In: Beynon, P. H., Lawton, M. P. C. and Cooper, J. E. (Eds.) *Manual of Exotic Pets,* pp. 138–152, British Small Animal Veterinary Association, Cheltenham.

10. Sousa, C. A. (1987). Nutritional Dermatoses. In: Nesbitt, G. H. (Ed.) *Contemporary Issues in Small Animal Practice Volume 8 Dermatology,* pp. 189–208, Churchill Livingstone, New York.

11. Van Den Broek, A. H. M., and Thoday, K. L. (1986). Skin disease in dogs associated with zinc deficiency: A report of 5 cases. *Journal of Small Animal Practice,* **27**: 313–323.

Chapter 12:

Chemical factors

Natural secretions/excretions

Natural secretions, such as tears, may cause excoriation, hair loss and depigmentation of the skin. Tears often cause a brown discolouration of the coat beneath the medial canthus of the eye in white-coated animals with chronic epiphora (**533**). The underlying cause is often blocked tear ducts, notably in the long-haired (Persian) cat, the miniature poodle and the Maltese terrier. Saliva produces a similar discolouration of the hair coat, and this effect is often a reliable sign that the area is pruritic (**534–536**). Long-term exposure to excretions such as nasal or ocular discharges may

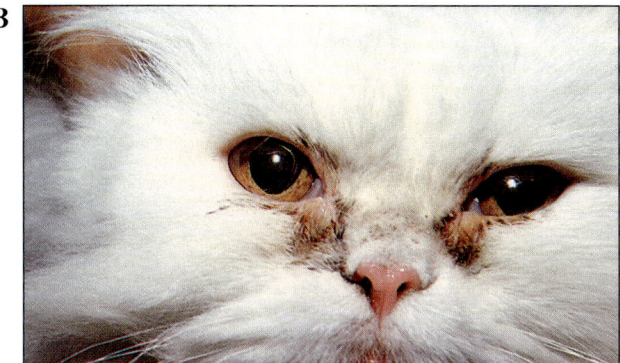

533 Chronic epiphora in a white longhaired cat, showing brown staining of hair coat.

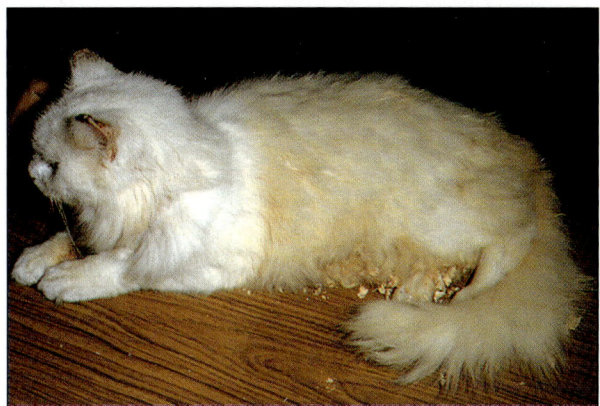

534 Saliva staining of the coat in a white long-haired cat. Note also the bilateral solar dermatitis.

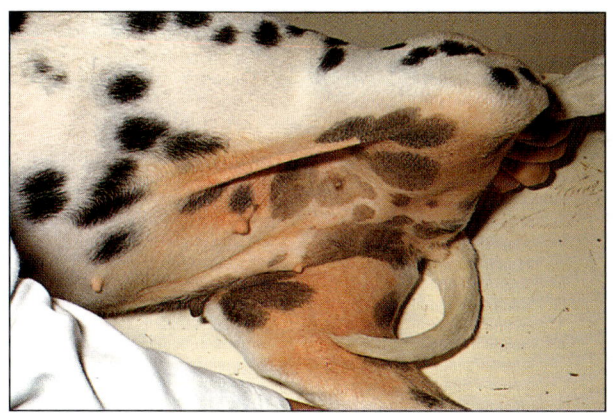

535 Saliva staining of the coat in a Dalmatian bitch associated with pruritus in the groin.

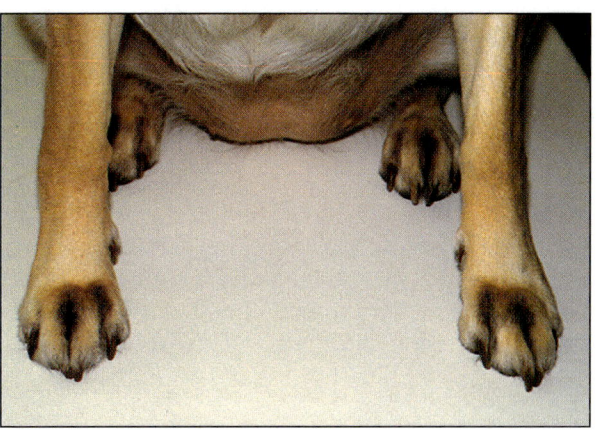

536 Saliva staining on the feet of a Labrador retriever with atopy.

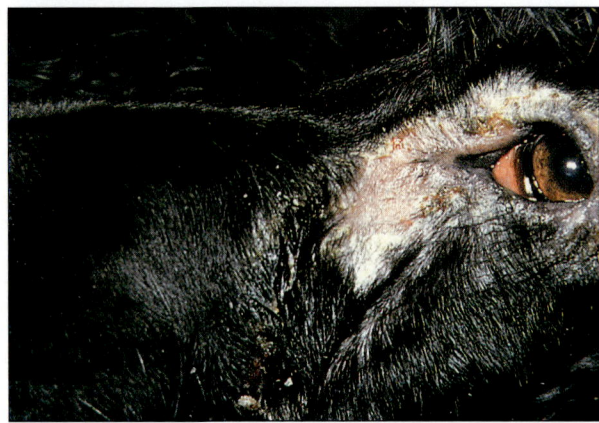

537 **Hair loss and depigmentation of the skin** resulting from chronic ocular discharge in a Cocker spaniel.

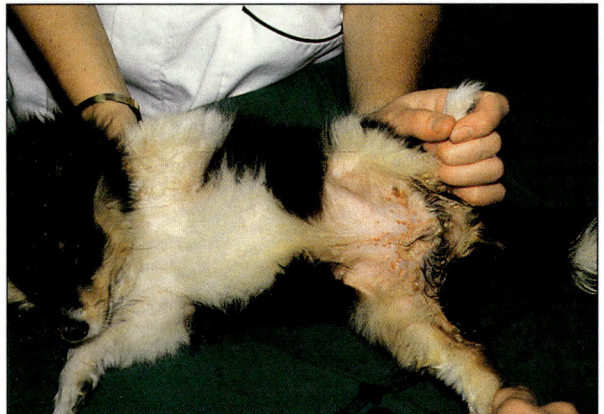
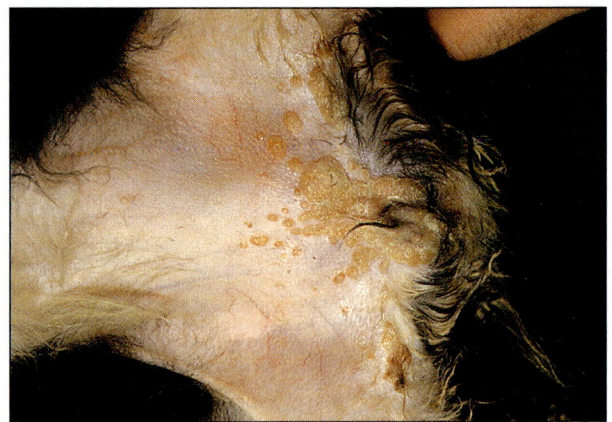

538 and 539 **Crusting papules and secondary superficial pyoderma** in the groin of a Shetland sheepdog pup with urinary incontinence secondary to ectopic ureter.

lead not only to discolouration of the hair but to local alopecia and inflammation (**537**). Chronic exposure to urine will result in inflammation, alopecia, secondary infection and erosions in the perivulval region and the groin (**538 and 539**).

Primary irritant contact dermatitis

Irritant material coming into contact with the skin of any animal can cause a primary contact dermatitis. From a clinical point of view it is not easy to distinguish allergic contact dermatitis from primary irritant dermatitis; indeed, it may not be necessary to do so. The mechanism of irritation and the manner in which epidermal cells are affected will vary from substance to substance. On a microscopic level the changes in the epidermis

540

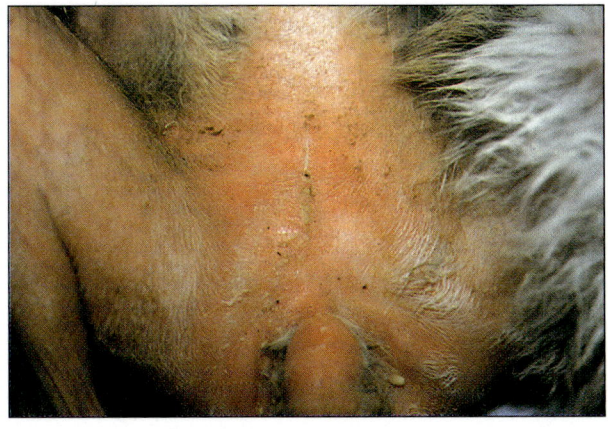

541

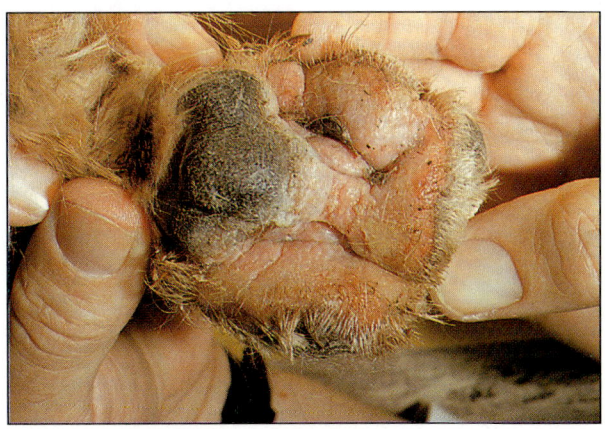

540 **Primary irritant dermatitis.** Extensive erythema and alopecia in the groins and along the medial thighs of a rabbit due to continued use of a topical iodine wash.

541 **Pododermatitis** due to use of over-strong disinfectant on the floor of a dog kennel.

542

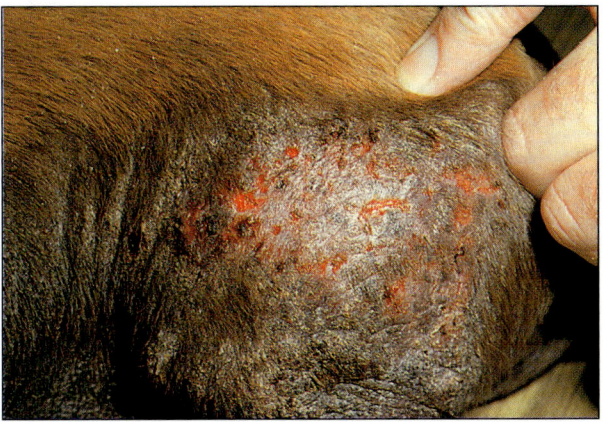

543

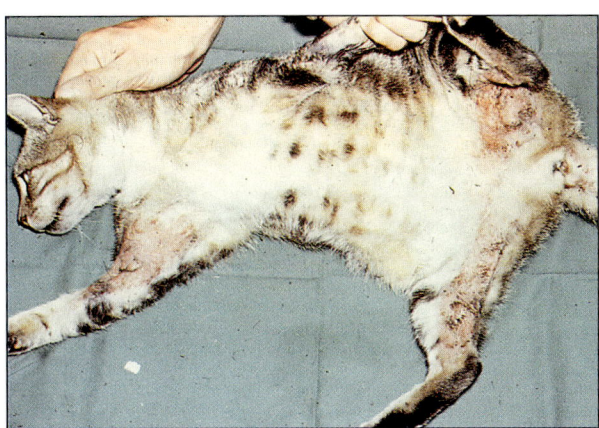

542 **Primary irritant contact dermatitis.** Chronic scrotal dermatitis resulting from bathing the dog in a medicated shampoo.

543 **Primary irritant contact dermatitis.** Characteristic distribution of lesions in a cat.

and the response of the epidermis to different irritants will vary accordingly; irritant contact dermatitis is a heterogeneous disorder with variable clinical manifestations. Such irritants include quite a number of therapeutic agents and chemical dermatitis often results from over-enthusiastic topical therapy. Agents such as iodine, insecticides, topical fungicides and even grooming aids initiate a reaction or aggravate an already inflamed integument (**540**). Insufficient dilution of disinfectant used on kennel floors is a not uncommon cause of pododermatitis (**541**). Bathing of male dogs in medicated shampoos can cause a chronic refractory scrotal dermatitis (**542**). Flea collars may evoke a severe dermatitis initially around the neck, which may spread to neighbouring areas. Exposure to garage and building materials may also be a source of inflammation, particularly of the interdigital regions (**543**).

544

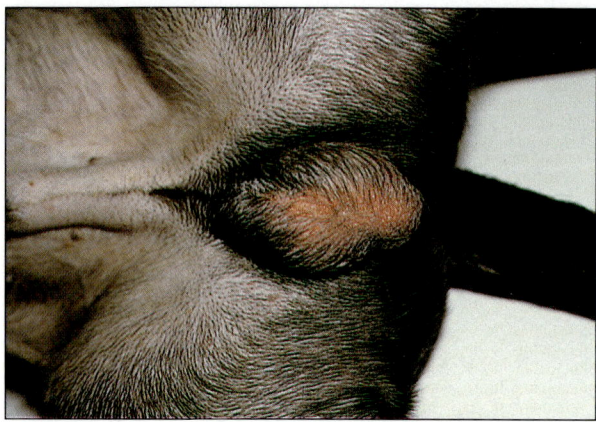

545

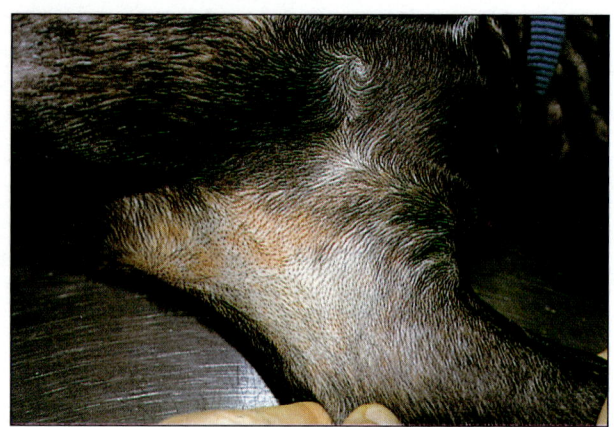

544 and 545   Primary irritant dermatitis. Erythematous lesions on the scrotum and in the axilla of a dog which came into contact with a common household floor cleaner.

546

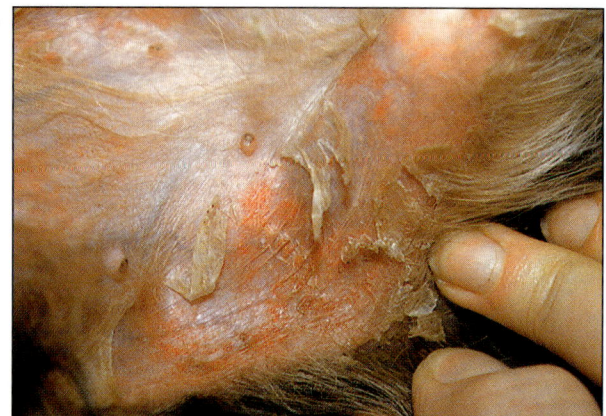

546   Primary irritant contact dermatitis. Multiple erosions on the skin of a show dog as a consequence of using an irritant oil during grooming in preparation for a show.

In cases where there is chronic exposure to a mildly irritant substance such as shampoo, the clinical signs may be limited to the production of scale. In more acute cases the signs of damage will vary from erythema to erosions or ulcerations of the epidermis, depending on irritant potential and duration of contact (**544–546**).

Irritant contact dermatitis is characterised by:
- Variable lesions.
- Variable distribution of lesions.
- Usually an acute history.

The differential diagnoses include:
- Allergic contact dermatitis.

Diagnosis is made by:
- Consideration of the history and clinical signs.
- Demonstration of access to an irritant.
- Resolution after restricting access.

Chapter 13:

Physical factors

Solar radiation

Actinic damage to the skin occurs from repeated sunburn following exposure to solar ultraviolet waves in the range 290 and 320nm (3000 Angstrom band), classified as ultraviolet B.[1] The condition occurs most commonly in unpigmented skin of white and partially white dogs and cats especially in sparsely haired or hairless areas.

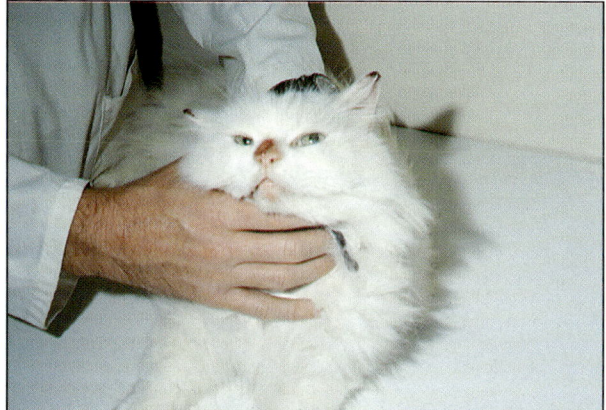

547 **Feline actinic dermatitis**. White cat showing actinic damage to both ear tips, the planum nasale and the chin.

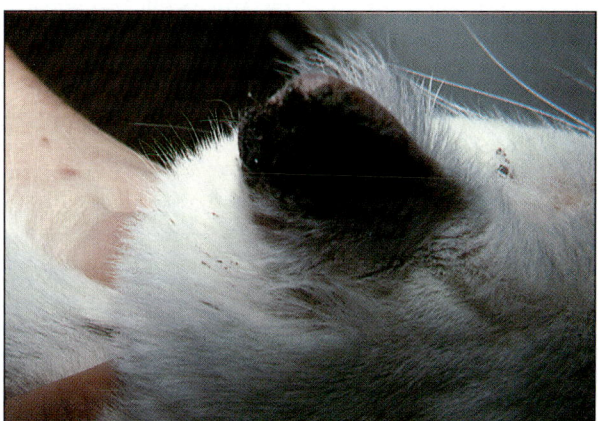

548 **Feline actinic dermatitis.** Precancerous lesion on margin of pinna showing extensive dark crusting of solar keratosis.

Feline actinic dermatitis

The main sites affected are the pinnae and the planum nasale. Occasionally the eyelids and lips also may be involved. The initial lesions on the pinnae consist of erythema, scaling and hair loss, particularly at the distal margins of the pinna. With continuing exposure to the sun the condition progresses; there is peeling of the skin and the formation of black or brown crusting lesions, solar kera-

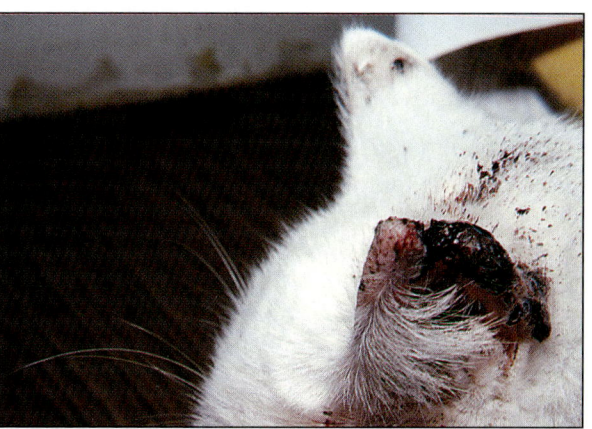

549 **Feline actinic dermatitis.** White cat showing early squamous cell carcinoma of right ear and actinic dermatitis of left ear. Note thickening and dark crusts of solar keratosis of ear margin.

550

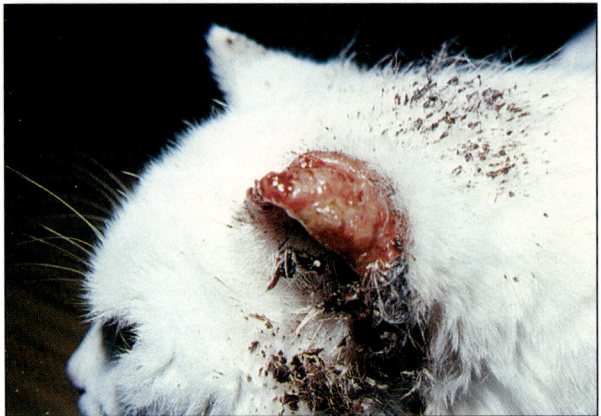

550   Feline actinic dermatitis. Same cat showing progressive development of the carcinoma two months later.

551

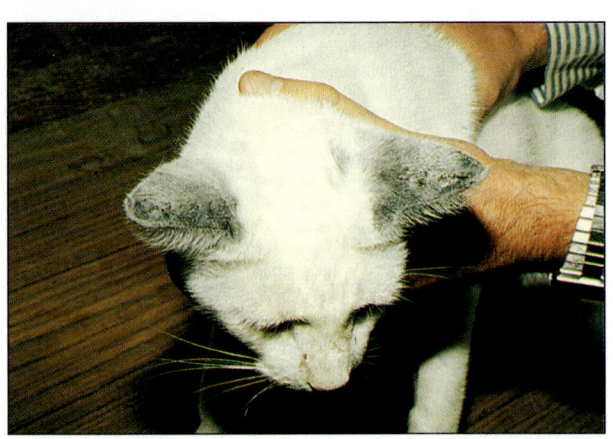

551   Feline actinic dermatitis. Some measure of protection from actinic damage is afforded by tattooing of the unpigmented pinnae. However note the evidence of continuing dermatitis on both ears.

552

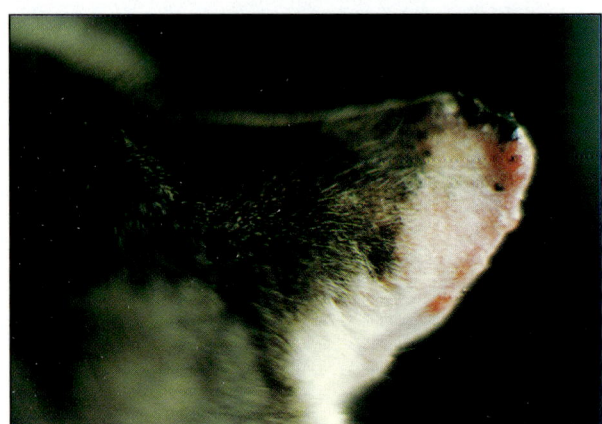

552   Feline actinic dermatitis. Pinna showing hair loss, erythema, scaling, the black crusts of solar keratoses and upward tilting of tip.

553

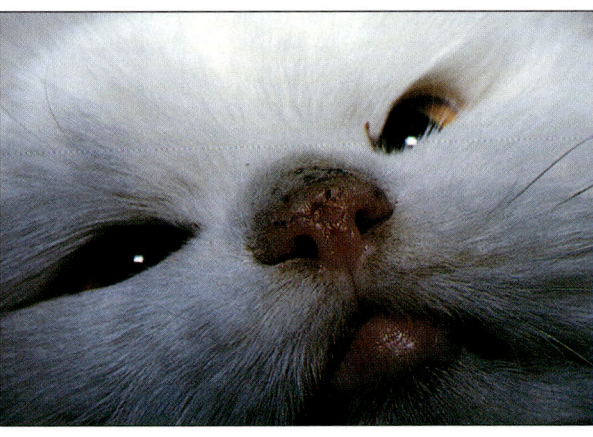

553   Feline actinic dermatitis. Early erosive lesion on the unpigmented planum nasale of a white cat. Note dark crusts of solar keratosis extending on to the bridge of the nose and erythema and swelling of the sparsely haired, unpigmented chin.

toses (**547–551**). Neoplastic transformation may occur and squamous cell carcinoma commonly develops on the affected ears in many cats over six years of age. Self-inflicted trauma may cause additional inflammation. A common feature of the chronic condition is an upward curling of the tip of the pinna (**552**). On the planum nasale the initial lesion is a solar keratosis (**553**), which develops as a small dark crust usually on the dorsal surfaces of the planum, at the junction between normal skin and the planum nasale. A shallow erosion forms on the planum and in many cases this progresses to become an ulcerating squamous cell carcinoma (**554–556**).

554

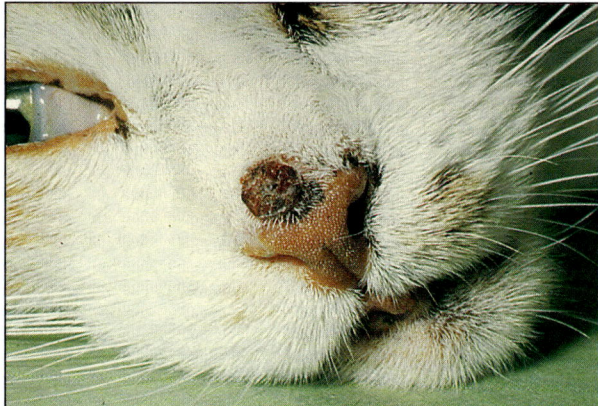

554   Feline actinic dermatitis. A later stage showing extension of the lesion with hair loss and development of several solar keratoses on the bridge of the nose.

555

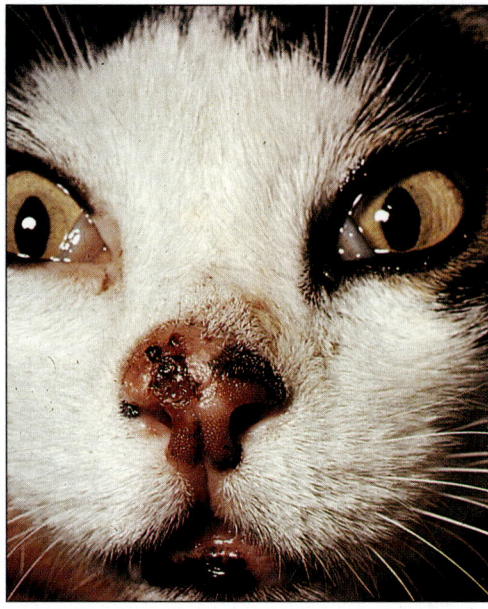

555   Feline actinic dermatitis. A large well circumscribed, crusted solar keratosis which is undergoing malignant change. Note further small keratoses in right nostril.

556

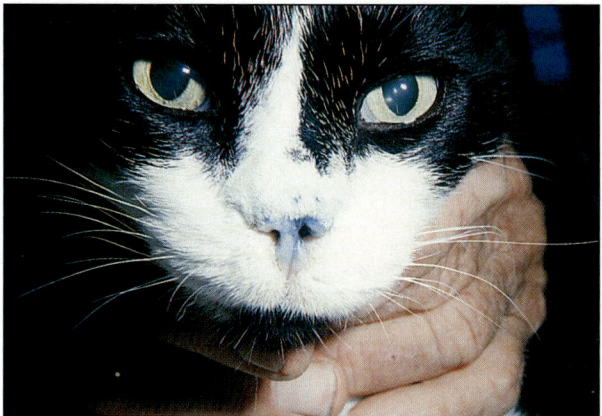

556   Feline actinic dermatitis. Showing planum nasale that has been tattooed following successful X-irradiation of a squamous cell carcinoma. Note the loss of substance in the right nostril caused by erosion by the tumour.

557

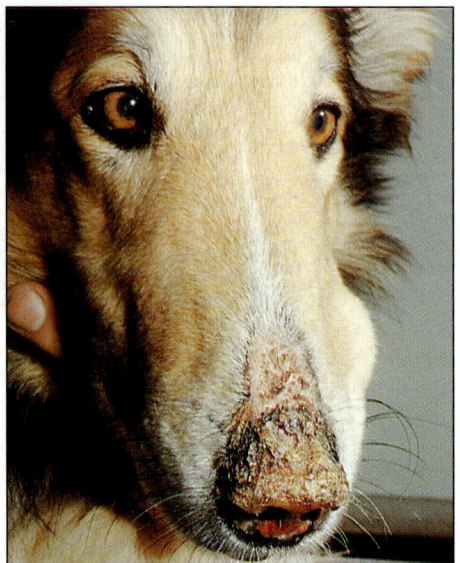

558

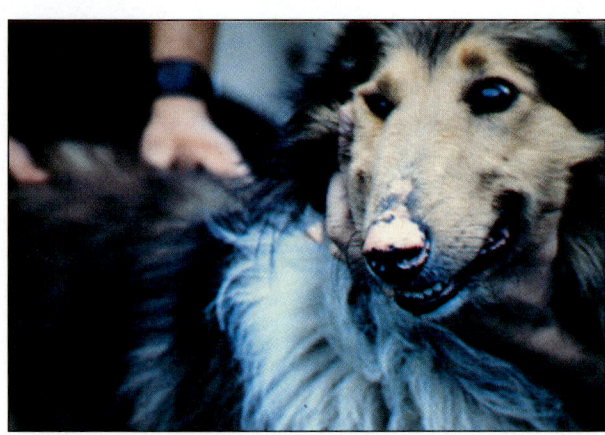

558   Canine actinic dermatitis. Depigmentation of the affected area following resolution and healing. Again note similar change in the floor of the nostrils.

557   Canine actinic dermatitis. 'Collie nose'. Erythema, crusting, erosion and depigmentation of the planum and antero-dorsal aspect of the bridge of the nose. Note the ulceration of the floor of thc nostrils.

559

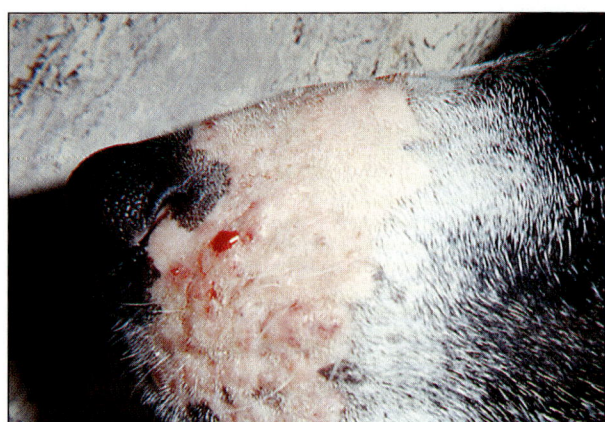

559   Canine actinic dermatitis. Actinic damage to the white nose of a Bull terrier and secondary bacterial infection.

Canine actinic dermatitis

In the dog, lesions occur on the dorsal surfaces of the face. The most common site for neoplastic transformation is an unpigmented area at the junction of normal skin and the planum nasale. Other areas of the face may be affected such as unpigmented areas of the planum, the nares, eyelids and lips, particularly in long-nosed breeds. Actinic dermatoses may also occur on the trunk. Predisposed areas are the unpigmented, sparsely-haired skin in the flank and ventral abdomen of white or partially white dogs, particularly Dalmatians and white Bull terriers.

In the past the condition occurring on the nose has been termed 'collie nose' but there is now some controversy as to whether this exists as a clinical entity (**557–559**). Similar lesions are seen in some autoimmune diseases, such as discoid lupus erythematosus, pemphigus foliaceus and

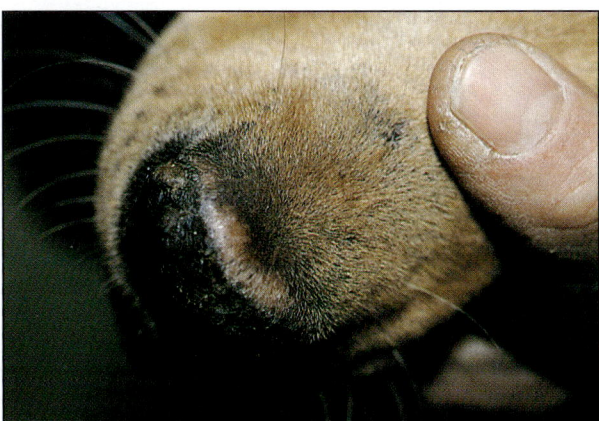

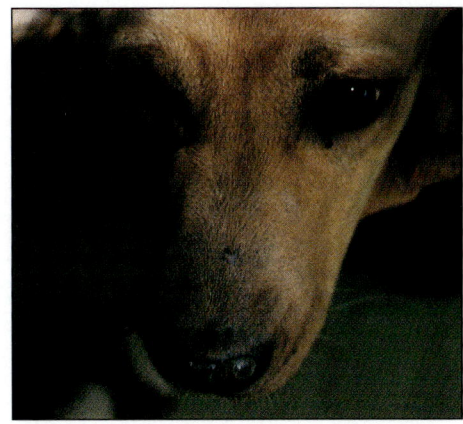

560 and 561 Canine actinic dermatitis. Actinic damage to a 14-month-old Labrador retriever. Second figure shows the same dog photographed during the winter months. Note the virtually complete resolution of the lesion.

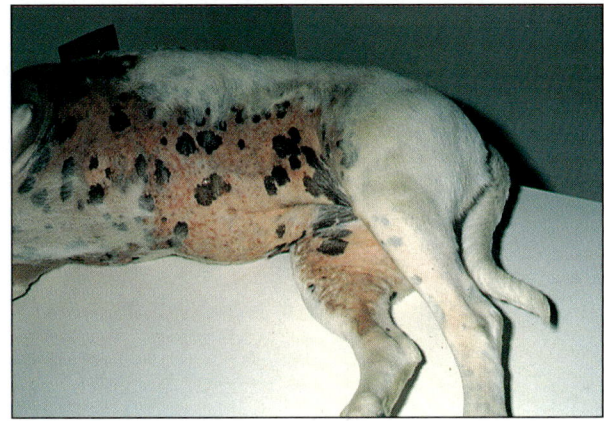

562 Canine actinic dermatitis. Characteristic distribution of 'sunburn' lesions in a white Bull terrier bitch. This was the dog's habitual sunbathing posture. Note the involvement of the medial aspect of the sparsely-haired right thigh. The medial surface of the left thigh unexposed to the sun's rays was unaffected.

erythematosus, nasal pyoderma, dermatomyositis and *Microsporum gypseum* infection. The autoimmune conditions tend to be aggravated by exposure to sunlight and this adds to the confusion as to aetiology. In the early stages there is erythema with loss of hair followed by exudation, crusting and eventually ulceration, especially in the floor of the nostrils. The lesions enlarge and progress with each successive summer, especially in sunny climates (**560** and **561**). If treated with glucocorticoids and protected from sunlight the lesions heal by regeneration of a hairless, unpigmented, thin, fragile epithelium.

Truncal lesions typically occur on dogs which habitually spend long periods lying on one side sunbathing. Unpigmented areas become chronically sunburned with erythema, scaling and thickening of the skin (**562** and **563**). Pigmented areas are

563

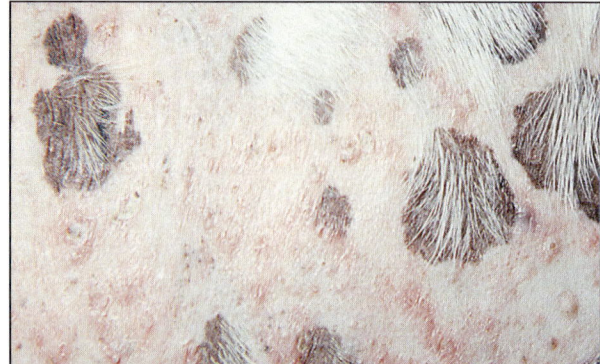

564

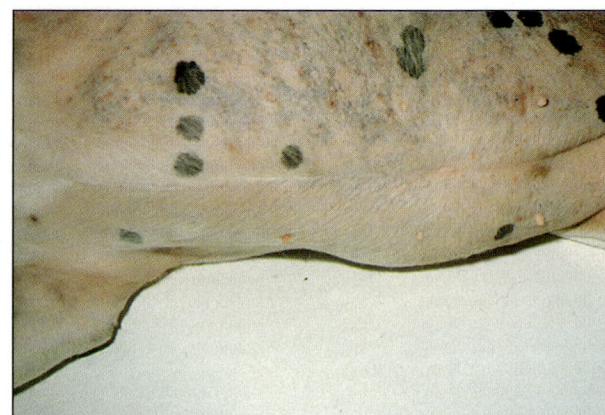

563 Canine actinic dermatitis. Close-up of affected area showing erythema, papules, nodules, crusting and peeling of the skin. Note the lack of involvement of the pigmented areas.

564 Canine actinic dermatitis. White Bull terrier bitch showing grey appearance of the left side of the ventral abdomen produced by the formation of numerous comedones. Note that the underlying right side and the medial surface of the right elbow remain normal.

565

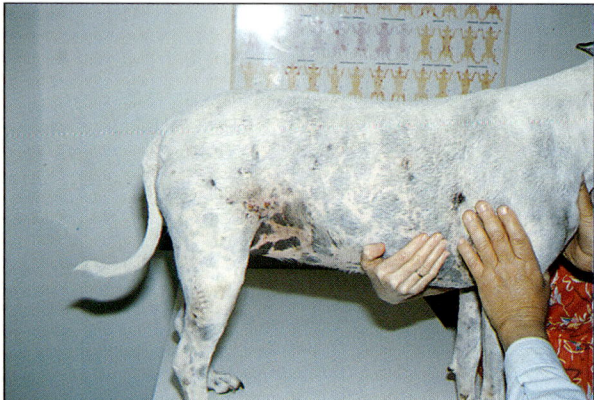

565 Canine actinic dermatitis. Partially white Bull terrier bitch showing early squamous cell carcinoma formation in the predilection site in the sparsely-haired, unpigmented flank area.

Actinic dermatoses are characterised by:
- Chronic exposure to strong sunlight.
- Lesions initially confined to unpigmented and white, sparsely-haired areas.
- Frequent development of squamous cell carcinoma.

Differential diagnoses include:
Cat:
- Insect bite dermatitis.
- Rabbit flea infestation.
- Mosquito bite allergy.
- Pemphigus foliaceus/erythematosus.
- Notoedric mange.
- Dietary intolerance.

Dog:
- Nasal pyoderma.
- Discoid lupus erythematosus.
- Pemphigus foliaceus/erythematosus.
- Dermatophytosis.
- Dermatomyositis.
- Demodicosis.

Diagnosis can be made by:
- Consideration of the history and clinical signs.
- Spontaneous recovery when exposure to sunlight prohibited.
- Histopathological examination of biopsy samples.

unaffected and a distinct demarcation is palpable between thickened and normal skin at the unpigmented: pigmented margin. As exposure to sunlight continues, numerous comedones may appear imparting a grey colour to the area (**564**); there may be erosions and ulceration. Solar keratoses may form and eventually squamous cell carcinoma develops (**565**). Pyoderma may occur in affected areas.

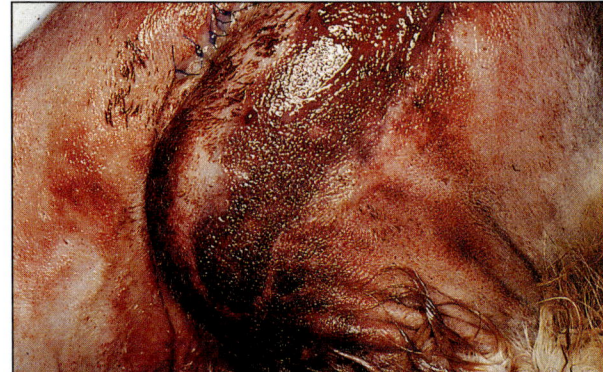

566 **Burn.** Partial thickness thermal burn in a cat associated with the use of diathermy during perineal urethrostomy.

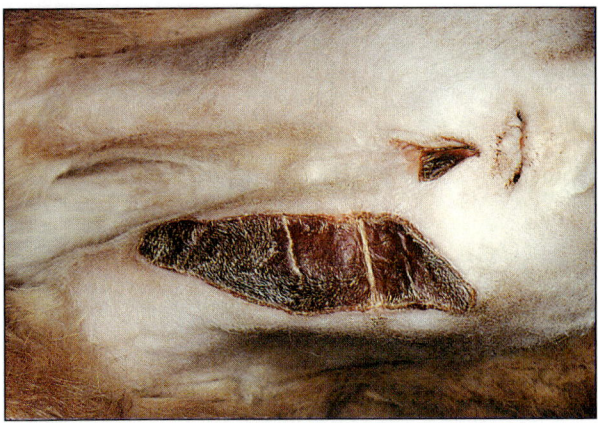

567 **Burn.** Dark, leather-like nature of the slough of necrotic skin occurring ten days after the injury.

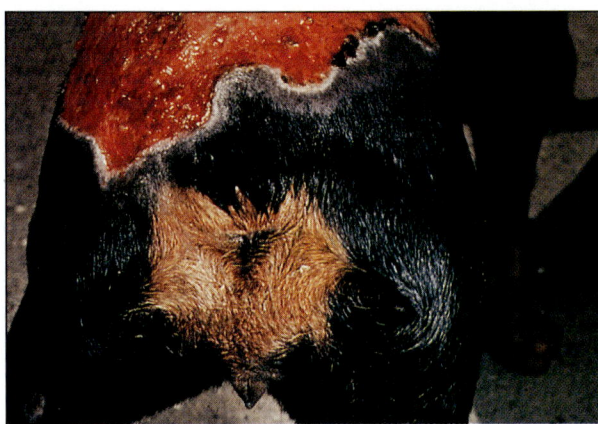

568 **Burn.** Full thickness thermal burn on the back of a rottweiler following sloughing. Note the pale line of commencing epithelialisation around the margin of the lesion.

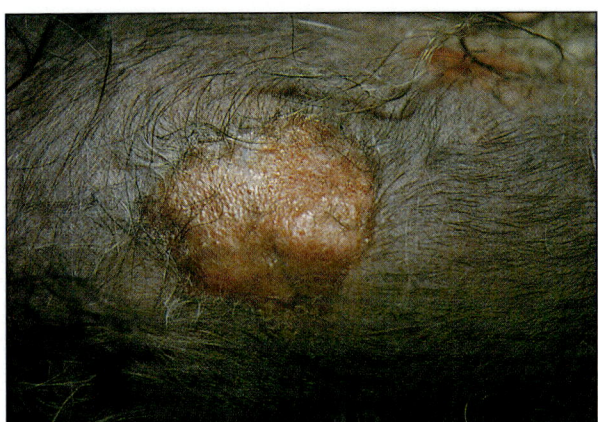

569 **Burn.** Scalds often result in erosions, as in this case in which the dog fell into a hot bath.

Burns

Burns may result from X-irradiation, microwave radiation and thermal or chemical insult to the skin.[3,4] They are now classified as either partial or full thickness lesions rather than first, second and third degree burns. Partial thickness burns do not completely destroy the skin so that healing and re-epithelialisation can occur more rapidly, from the ostia of hair follicles for example (**566**). In full thickness burns, all skin components are destroyed, the affected area sloughs and re-epithelialisation depends upon the migration of epithelial cells from the margins plus contraction of the lesion (**567** and **568**).

Thermal burns may result from the use of over-hot heating pads during surgery, hair driers and diathermy apparatus, from fire and scalds from boiling water or hot cooking oil (**569** and **570**). The initial lesions may be hidden from the owner's obser-

570

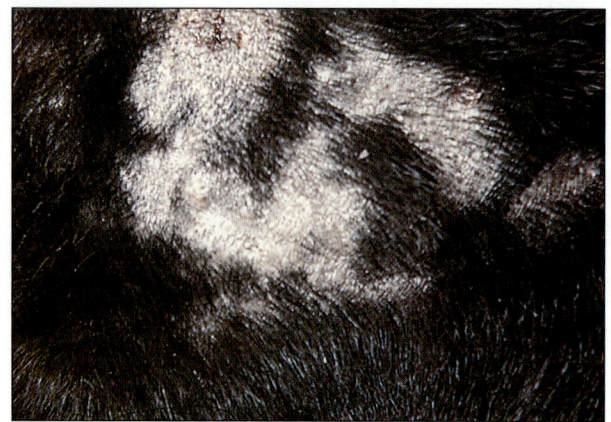

570   Burn. Scald wound on the shoulder of a
Rottweiler that is healing. Note the scale and alopecia.

571

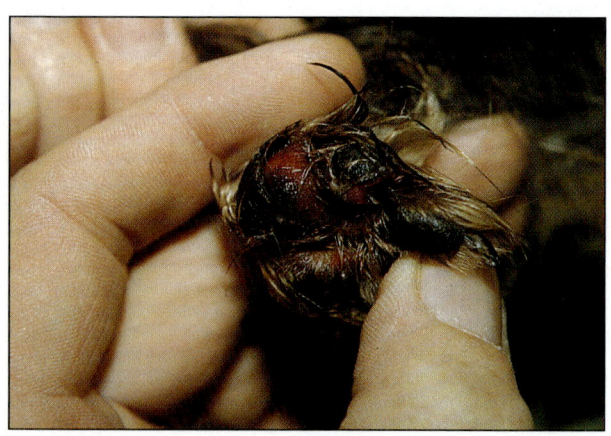

571   Burn. Some delay may occur between the scald
and signs of damage becoming apparent. This Yorkshire
terrier started to shed its nails a few days after immer-
sion in a hot bath (see **569**).

572

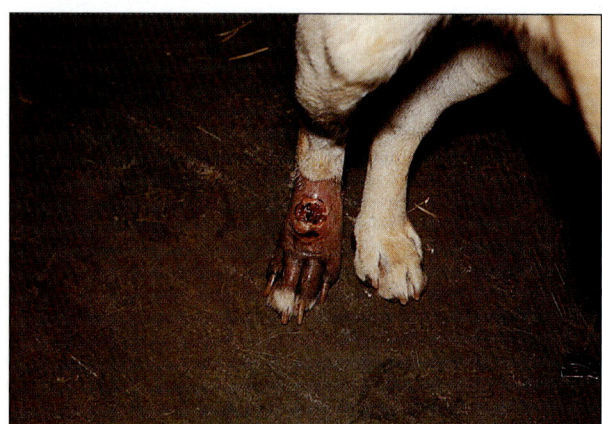

572   Burn. Partial thickness X-irradiation burn on
the hind leg of a Labrador retriever given X-ray therapy
for a fibrosarcoma in the metatarsal region.

vation by the hair coat and this is especially true of
scalds. Sloughing of the nails may follow immer-
sion in scalding water (**571**). Chemical burns
result from contact with caustic or acid materials.
X-irradiation burns result from X-ray therapy for
neoplasia (**572**).

Burns are characterised by:
- Sudden onset.
- Varying degrees of destruction of skin with
  sloughing.
- Slow healing by epithelialisation and con-
  traction.

Differential diagnoses include:
- Road accident trauma especially degloving
  injuries.
- Allergic contact dermatitis.
- Drug eruptions especially toxic epidermal
  necrolysis.

Diagnosis can be made by:
- Consideration of the history and clinical.
  signs.

573

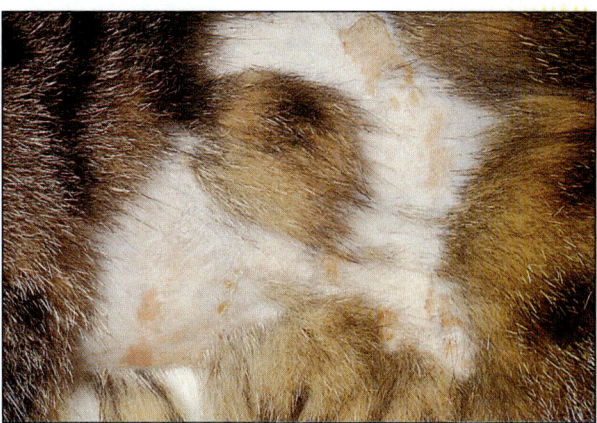

573   Traumatic dermatitis. Severe laceration following road accident.

574

574   Traumatic dermatitis. Lesion produced in a young cat by tearing out of the hair probably in a fight or road accident. Note the quite extensive superficial areas of inflammation, now covered by a thin crust of dried exudate associated with the forcible epilation of the hair.

575

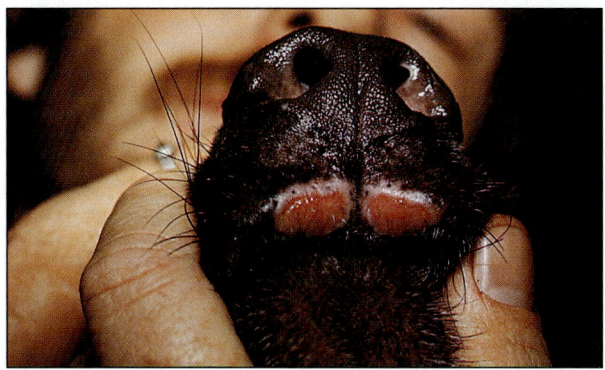

575   Traumatic dermatitis. Traumatic dermatitis. Erosive lesions produced by persistent licking on the upper lip of a Labrador retriever.

576

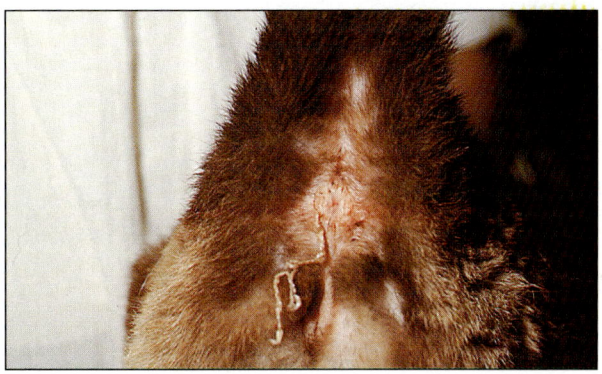

576   Traumatic dermatitis. Impaction and secondary infection of the anal sacs is quite common in the dog but rare in the cat. The irritation produced may lead to self trauma to the skin around the tail, lateral aspect of the upper thighs and the dorsal pelvic area. Anal sac impaction in a cat.

Traumatic dermatitis

Traumatic dermatoses, usually localised, may result from a variety of insults to the skin. Bruises, abrasions and cuts may follow blows, abrasions, lacerations, pressure, biting and continued licking (**573** and **574**). An animal's response to irritation from otitis externa or impacted anal sacs may result in severe trauma to the adjacent skin; pyotraumatic dermatitis may result (**575** and **576**). A characteristic lesion is produced by the malicious application of an elastic band around an extremity; the band gradually sinks into the

depths of the skin by pressure necrosis becoming buried from view by extensive crust formation and the coat (**577**). If placed around a limb or the tail the condition may result in necrosis of the part distal to the band.

Managemental influences such as clipping and tying bows in the hair may also result in dermatoses. 'Clipper burn' occurs in dogs and cats that are close clipped for cosmetic or other reasons. In poodles the predilection sites are the face, the feet and around the tail. The condition occurs within 12

577

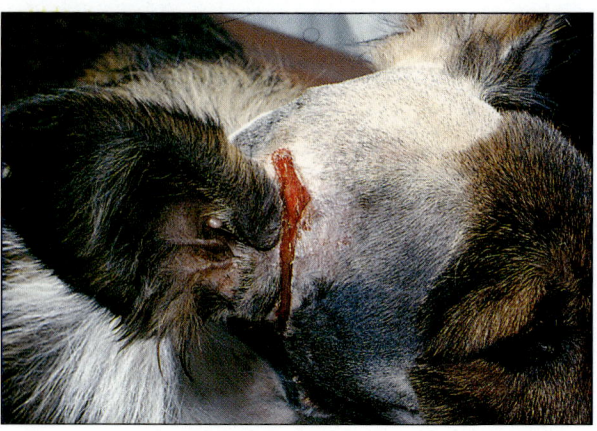

577 Characteristic lesion produced by malicious application of elastic band around the ear of a dog.

578

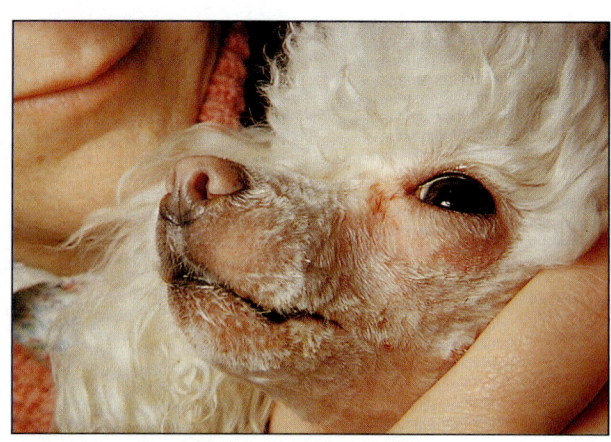

578 Traumatic dermatitis. 'Clipper burn' on the face of a Miniature Poodle.

579

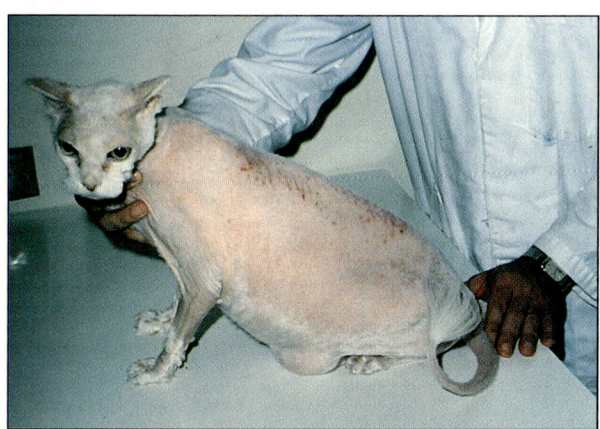

579 Traumatic dermatitis. 'Clipper damage' to a long-haired cat that was clipped to search for ticks in a case of tick paralysis.

580

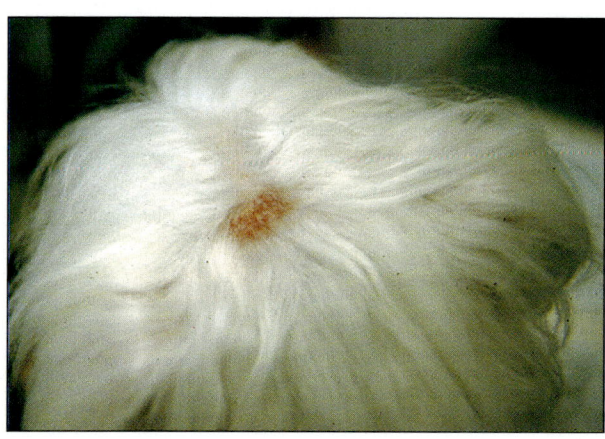

580 Traction alopecia resulting from overtight application of ribbons or bows in pre-show preparation. (Illustration courtesy C. E. Griffen.)

hours of clipping and is sudden in onset. The animal becomes distressed with face rubbing, 'tobogganing', yelping and rushing about the room with tail clamped down. There is erythema initially followed by acute dermatitis due to self trauma (**578** and **579**). Traction alopecia has been reported: overtight application of elastic bands and ribbons to the gathered bunches of hair resulted in permanently scarred hair follicles[5] (**580**).

Callus formation occurs especially in large,

short-coated breeds of dogs such as Great Danes, Boxers and Mastiffs (**581–584**). Pressure produces hyperkeratosis of the skin over subcutaneous bony prominences overlying the elbows, hocks and tuber ischii. The lesions consist of well defined, oval or round areas of very thickened, pigmented or unpigmented skin with a wrinkled surface which may become fissured. Secondary pyoderma, often deep, is common. In some cases the pressure can embed fragments of hair expressed

581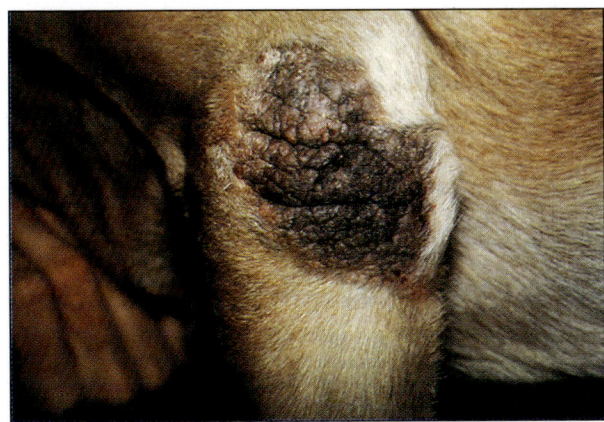

582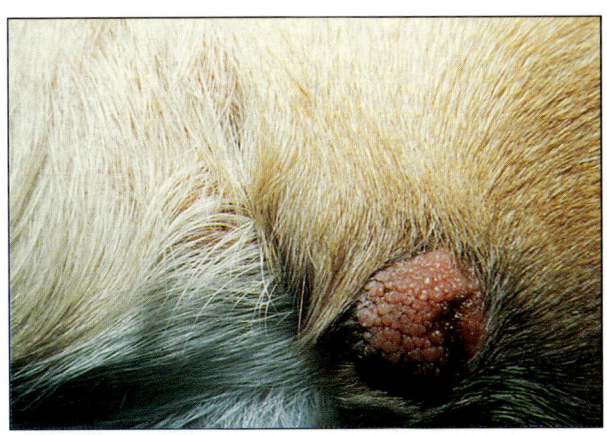

581 and 582   Traumatic dermatitis. Pigmented and unpigmented callus formation on the elbows of two dogs.

583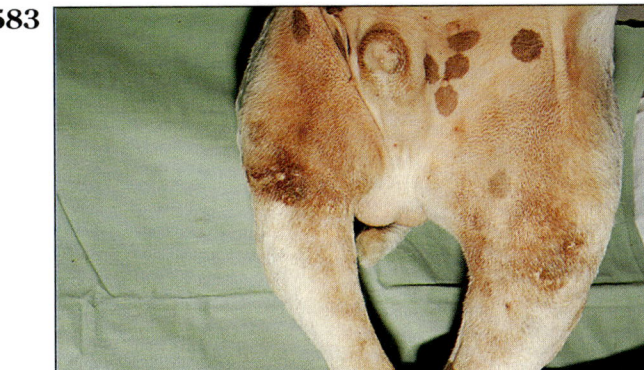

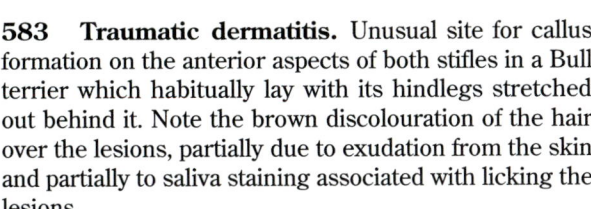

584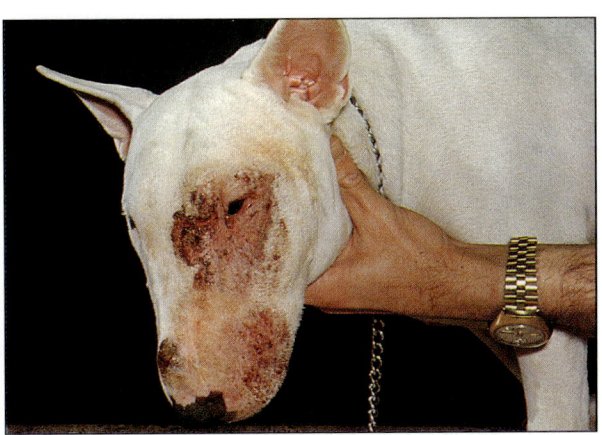

583   Traumatic dermatitis. Unusual site for callus formation on the anterior aspects of both stifles in a Bull terrier which habitually lay with its hindlegs stretched out behind it. Note the brown discolouration of the hair over the lesions, partially due to exudation from the skin and partially to saliva staining associated with licking the lesions.

584   Traumatic dermatitis. Callus formation again in an unusual site on the nose of a Bull terrier bitch which was an avid rooter in the soil, from which she also contracted the *Trichophyton mentagrophytes* infection causing the severe inflammatory lesion on the face.

from the follicles into the dermis setting up a foreign body reaction (**585**). Devitalised and depigmented hairs may be squeezed out in pus from the lesions.

Analagous conditions may be encountered in small mammals. Chronic response to poor environmental conditions results in sore hocks, particularly in rabbits and guinea-pigs (**586 and 587**). Damp bedding, inadequate bedding and hard flooring are thought to contribute to the onset of

these lesions. The plantar aspects of the hocks becomes thickened and erythematous, often complicated by secondary infection. Chronic pododermatitis in some breeds of dog, notably bulldogs, Bull terriers and Boxers, may result, at least in part, from physical factors such as conformation and weight. Although attending to obvious factors such as obesity, bedding, secondary infection and nutrition may help, many of these cases are refractory to treatment.

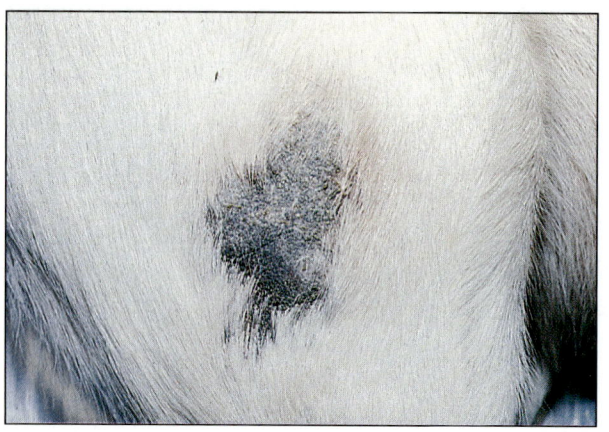

585   Traumatic dermatitis. Callus formation in which embedding of fragments of hair has occurred with subsequent foreign body reaction.

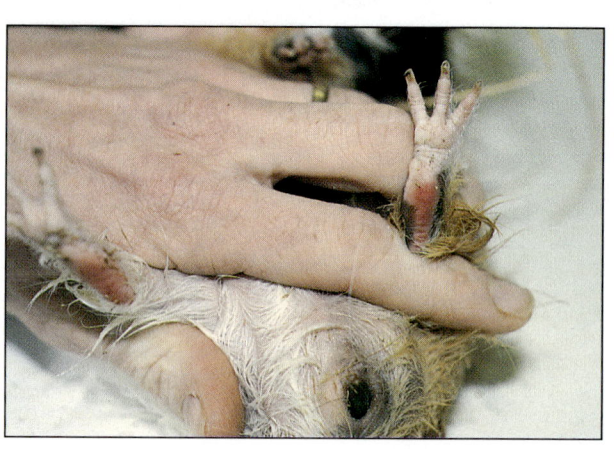

586   Traumatic dermatitis. Sore hocks in a guinea-pig as a result of poor husbandry.

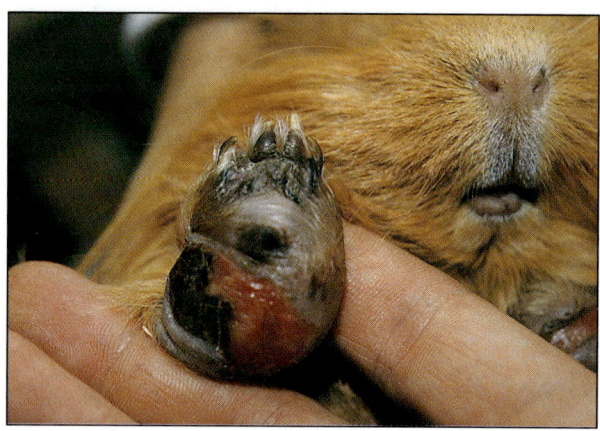

587   Traumatic pododermatitis. Grossly enlarged foot of a guinea pig as a result of secondary infection and poor management.

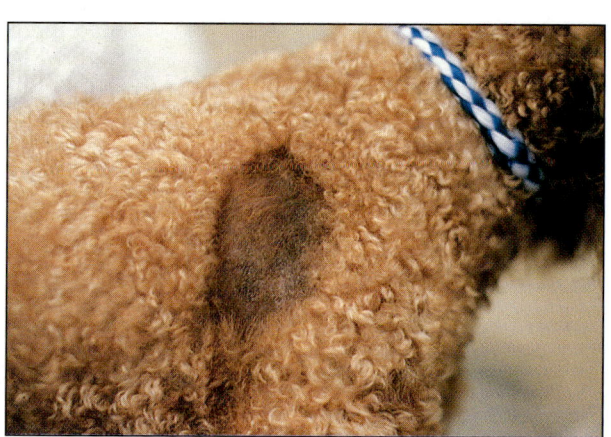

588   Injection reactions may result in permanent alopecia as in this Poodle. (Illustration courtesy C. E. Griffen.)

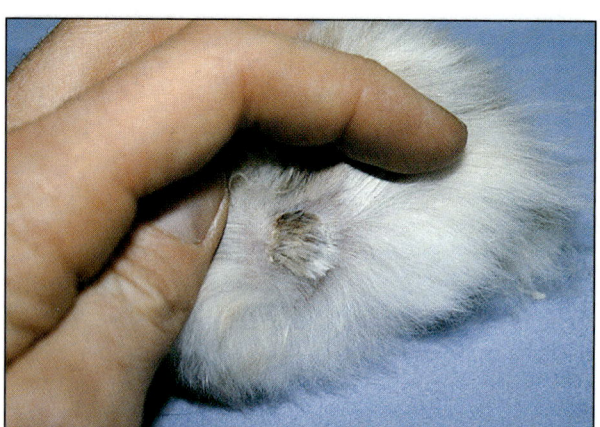

589   Hamster with a focal, crusted, necrotic reaction at the site of subcutaneous injection.

590 **591**

592 **593**

590–593 Injection reactions. Cutaneous atrophy following subcutaneous injection of a depot glucocorticoid into the mid-shoulder region in a corgi dog (**590** and **591**) and into the dorsum of a Miniature Poodle (**592**). Ulceration at the site of perivascular injection of sodium thiopentone in 10% solution (**593**).

Reactions to injections may result in focal reactions at the site and in dogs, notably miniature and toy poodles, focal alopecia may follow rabies vacination (**588**). In very small mammals such as mice focal necrosis may follow subcutaneous injection of many compounds, presumably a result of compromised vascular supply (**589**). Similar reactions may follow the subcutaneous injection of progestagens or depot glucocorticoids (**590– 592**). Focal panniculitis is a rare sequel to subcutaneous injections.[2] A well-circumscribed, solitary nodule is present at the site of injection. Perivascular necrosis and slough following extravascular injection of 5 or 10% sodium thiopentone is an occasional result of anaesthetic administration (**593**).

References

1. Gange, R. W. and Lim, H. W. (1991). Photobiology and Pathophysiology of cutaneous responses to electromagnetic radiation. In: Soter, N. A and Baden, H. P. (Eds.) *Pathophysiology of Dermatologic Diseases,* pp. 395–423. 2nd edn. McGraw Hill, New York.

2. Hendrick, M. J and Dunagan, C. A. (1991). Focal necrotizing granulomatous panniculitis associated with subcutaneous injection of rabies vaccine in cats and dogs: 10 cases (1988–1989).*Journal of the American Animal Hospital Association,* **198**: 304–305.

3. McKeever, P. J. (1980). Thermal injuries. In: Kirk, R. W. (Ed.) *Current Veterinary Therapy VII*, pp. 191–194. W. B Saunders, Philadelphia.

4. Reedy, L. R. and Clubb, F. J. (1991). Microwave burns in a toy poodle: a case report. *Journal of the American Animal Hospital Association,* **27**: 497–500.

5. Rosenkrantz, W. S., Griffen, C. A. and Walder, E. J. (1989). Traction alopecia in the canine: Four case reports. *California Veterinarian*, May/June, 7–12.

Chapter 14:

Neoplastic dermatoses

Introduction

The skin and subcutis constitute the most common sites of neoplasia in the dog (about 30%) and the second most common in the cat (about 20%). Dogs suffer from many more types of skin tumour than do cats. Furthermore, in the dog roughly 50% of the cutaneous neoplasms are benign in nature, whereas in the cat there are three times as many malignant as benign neoplasms. Neoplasia is uncommon in immature dogs but when it occurs it tends to be malignant, with mast cell tumours predominating in one study.[10] Skin tumours are the most frequently and easily recognised neoplastic disorders in domestic animals, so diagnosis is likely to be made early and treatment should be effective. Unfortunately, the harmless appearance of some tumours and their slowly progressive, painless, nature may lead to delay in presentation. This delay may adversely affect therapy.

Clinically, it is impossible to distinguish between benign and malignant neoplasms and surgical excision, where practical, is the preferred course of action. Although palpation may suggest a well-defined, mobile nodule these features do not imply a benign nature and it is advisable to regard any tumour as being potentially malignant.

Aspiration cytology (Chapter 3) may yield useful information on constituent cell-type[2] but, in general, does not provide a sufficient sample size to allow decisions on malignancy to be made. However, cytological examination of suspect neoplasms prior to surgery may be very useful as a guide to the surgical management of the lesion.[2] Thus, identification of mast cells in an aspiration smear is an indication for a 2cm margin of excision.[8] After excision, samples should be submitted for histopathological examination.

> - The most common cutaneous neoplasms in dogs are lipomas, mast cell tumours, sebaceous gland hyperplasia and adenomas and papillomas. Canine cutaneous neoplasia has a 50% chance of being benign.
> - The most common cutaneous neoplasms in cats are basal cell tumours, mast cell tumours, squamous cell carcinomas and fibrosarcomas. The majority of feline cutaneous neoplasms should be regarded as malignant.

219

594

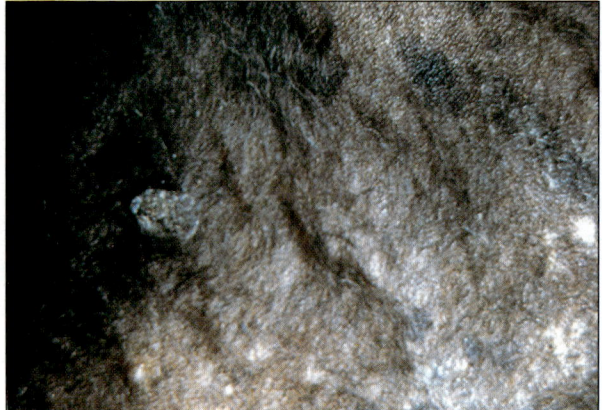

594   Papilloma. These neoplasms may become very large and friable. Pigmentation is variable. Haemorrhage may be a problem with papillomas on the face which become traumatised by the animal. The illustration shows a pigmented papilloma on a dog.

595

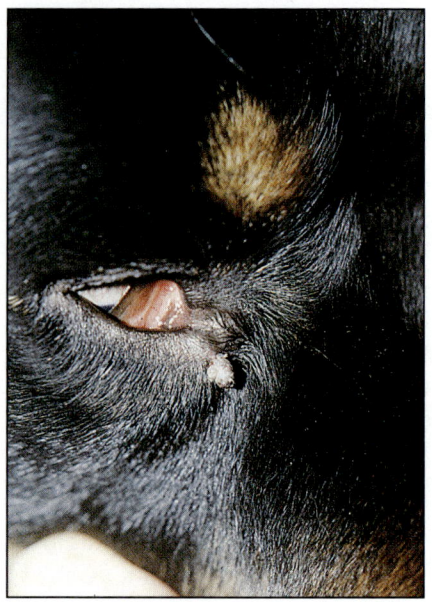

595   Papilloma. A solitary lesion immediately below the right eye of a Rottweiler.

596

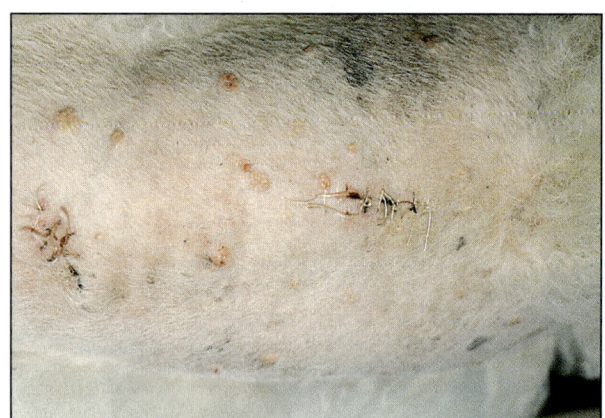

596   Papilloma. Some animals, such as this elderly Bichon frise, exhibit multiple papillomas. Excision of every one is tedious and owners may elect excision of only the largest.

Tumours of epithelial origin

Papilloma

Papillomas are benign tumours arising from the squamous cells of the epidermis. Viral-induced papillomatosis occurs in young dogs, particularly on structures within the oropharynx (see Chapter 6). Papillomas, which are not thought to be virally-induced, occur as cauliflower-like, sessile or pedunculated tumours on the surface of the skin of older dogs (**594**). They are found most commonly on the head (**595**), feet and genitalia.[3] Some animals suffer from large numbers of these papillomas and owners may elect surgery only for large, friable and haemorrhagic lesions (**596**). Oral papillomatosis does not occur in the cat and solitary papillomas are uncommon in this species, although papillomatous growths may occur in the external ear canal (**597** and **598**).

597

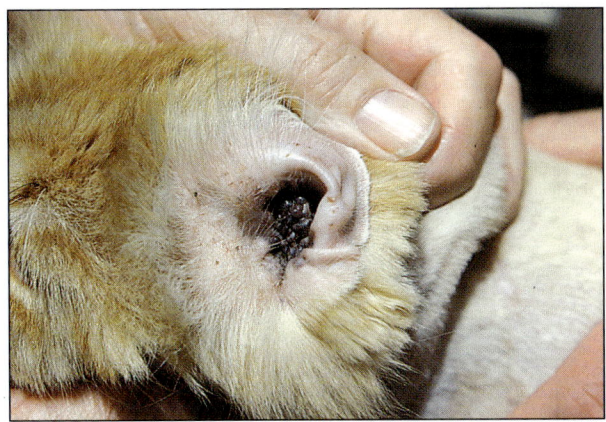

598

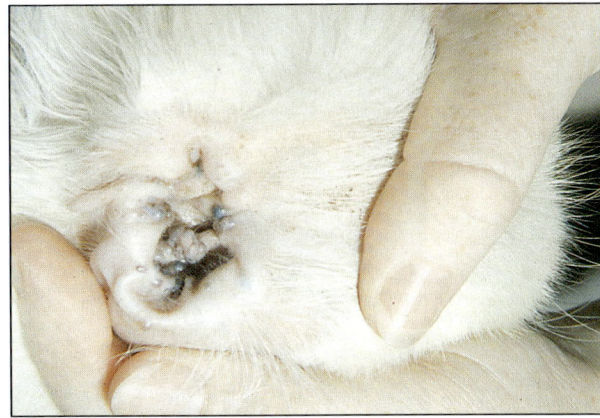

597 and 598   Papilloma. Pigmented and unpigmented, inflammatory papillomatous growths in the external ear canals of two cats. In both cases the condition was bilateral.

599

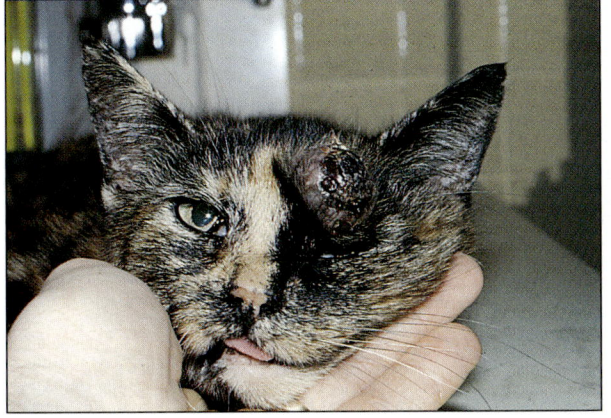

600

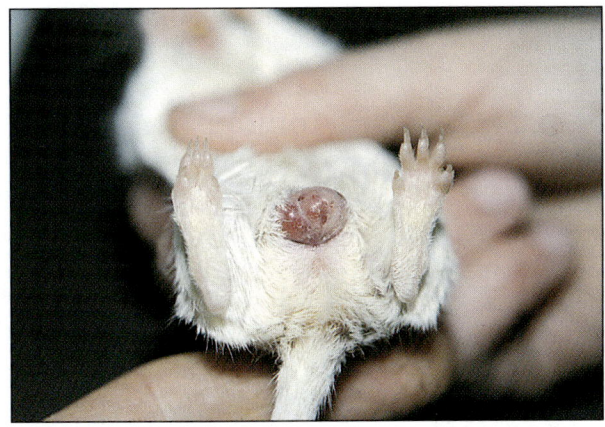

599   Basal cell tumour. Ulcerated nodule on the head of a cat.

600   Basal cell tumour adjacent to the vulva of a gerbil.

Basal cell tumour

Basal cell tumours arise from the basal cells of the epidermis and are common in cats, rather less so in dogs. Basal cell tumours are more common in elderly animals and there is no sex predisposition. Poodles, cocker spaniels and cross-breeds appear to be particularly susceptible.[3] There is no breed predisposition in cats. The majority of these neoplasms are benign, growing slowly and, although sometimes infiltrating neighbouring tissues, rarely if ever metastasising. Tumours are usually solitary, occurring most commonly on the head and neck as firm, discrete masses up to 2·5cm in diameter, which may be ulcerated (**599 and 600**).[12,13,15] They are usually freely movable over the underlying tissues.[3] Pigmentation is variable. About 60% of feline basal cell tumours are cystic.

601

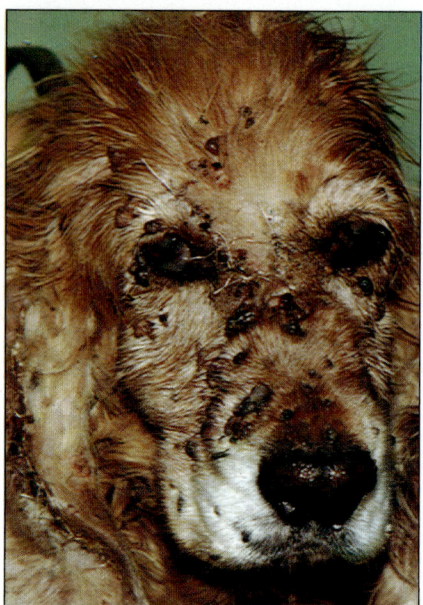

601   Sebaceous gland adenoma.
Multiple tumours on the face of an aged
Cocker spaniel.

602

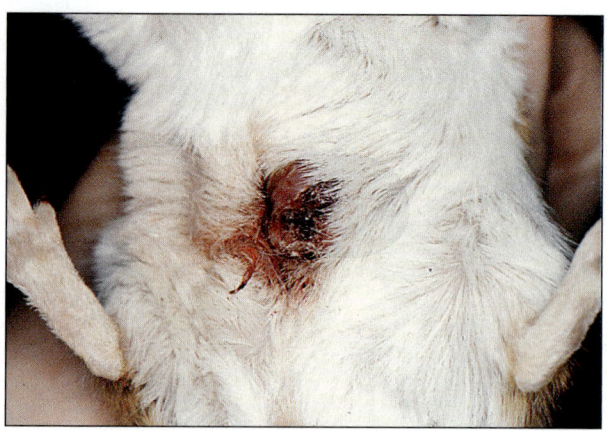

**602   Adenoma of the ventral scent gland of a ger-
bil**. This gland is a common site for neoplastic change in
this species. (Illustration courtesy of M. P. C. Lawton.)

Sebaceous gland tumour

Sebaceous gland tumours can be classified histologically into four types. In one study[3], sebaceous
hyperplasia was the most common, sebaceous
epithelioma next most common, followed by sebaceous adenoma and, the most rare, sebaceous adenocarcinoma. As a group they are very common in
older dogs. Hyperplasia of the sebaceous gland
was more common in miniature Schnauzers,
Cocker spaniels, Poodles and Beagles, and epithelioma of the sebaceous gland was more common
in Shih tzus, Lhasa apsos, malamutes, Siberian
huskies and Irish setters. No breed predisposition
was noted for adenoma or adenocarcinoma of the
sebaceous gland.[16] These tumours are rare in cats,
only sebaceous adenoma being noted in one
study.[12] Tumours may be single or multiple and
may occur anywhere on the body. They show a
predilection for the limbs and head[3], particularly
the eyelids (**601**). They measure up to 2.5 cm in
diameter and are discrete, hairless, firm, dome-
shaped or pedunculated tumours, usually multilobulated and yellowish in colour. When squeezed,
greasy sebaceous material can often be expressed.
Adenomas and adenocarcinomas are frequently
ulcerated.[3] The latter are larger, firm, poorly-

defined tumours that tend to expand and infiltrate
surrounding tissue but rarely metastasise.[16]

The ventral scent gland situated on the ventral thoracic wall of gerbils is derived from sebaceous glands and
is a common site for adenomatous changes, presenting as a reddened nodule (**602**).[5]

Trichoepitheliomas and pilomatricomas

These tumours are derived from the structures of
the hair follicle. Trichoepitheliomas differentiate
towards the hair follicle sheath, or the follicle
sheath and hair matrix, while pilomatricomas (also
called calcifying epitheliomas) are related solely to
the hair matrix. There is no breed predisposition
for trichoepitheliomas, but Kerry blue terriers are
predisposed to pilomatricomas.[3] Both types of
tumour are relatively common in dogs over five years
old[3], but rare in cats. They are usually solitary, firm and
well circumscribed, ranging in size from 2 to 10cm
in diameter. The overlying skin is thin and hairless
and may be ulcerated. They grow slowly, are usually
non-invasive, and do not metastasise.

603

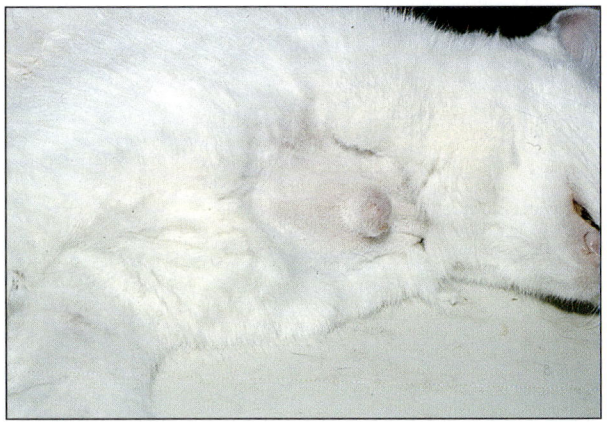

603   Adenoma of the epitrichial (sweat) gland. These are solitary and nodular. This illustration shows a discrete nodule on the ventral neck of a cat.

604

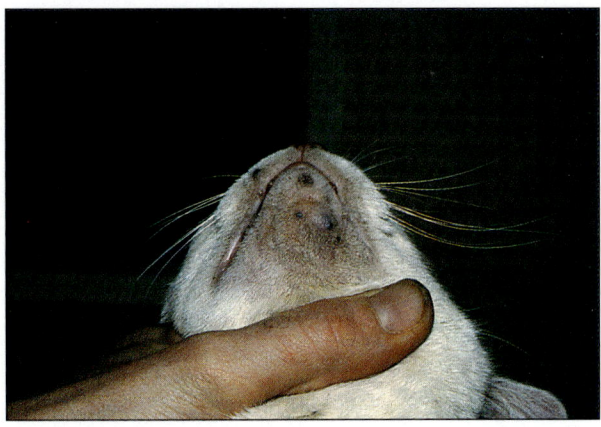

604   Adenoma of the epitrichial (sweat) gland. An unusual case of multiple adenomata on the chin of a cat.

Sweat gland tumours

Tumours which arise from epitrichial sweat glands are relatively uncommon compared to tumours of the sebaceous glands in dogs, whereas in cats they are of roughly equal frequency.[12] Tumours of atrichial sweat glands of the canine foot pad are extremely rare.[3] Tumours of epitrichial sweat glands usually occur in dogs and cats over eight years old.[3] Labrador retrievers were found to be predisposed in one study.[10] Predisposition in male dogs has been reported, although not consistently.

Tumours may be classified as adenomas or adenocarcinomas, the latter being by far the most common.[10] There are no clinical features unique to either type. They may occur anywhere on the body although the head and neck are common sites.[3] They are usually solid and solitary (**603**) although occasionally animals will exhibit multiple lesions (**604**). Although lymphatic invasion is not uncommon, metastasis appears to be rare.[10] Recurrence after surgical removal may be noted.

605

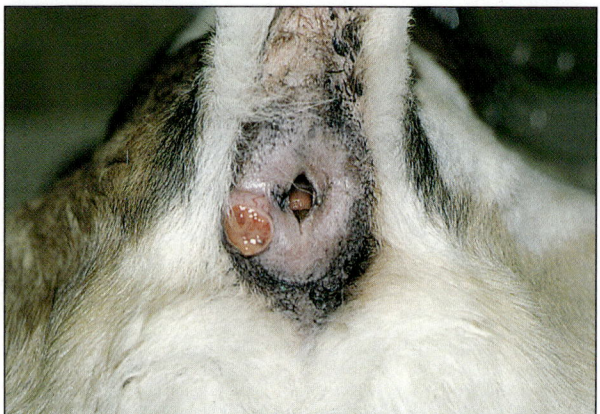

606

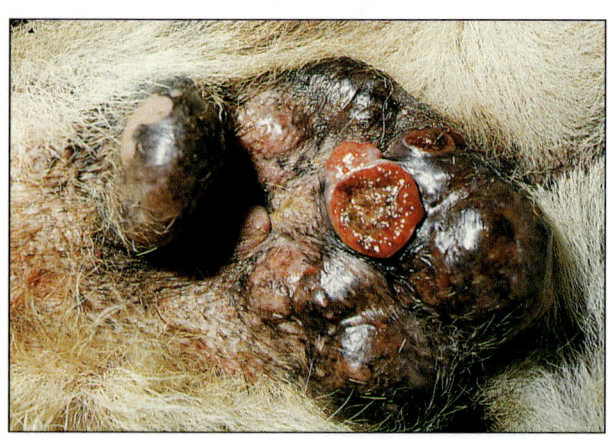

605   Circumanal (perianal) gland tumour. A solitary ulcerated nodule. Note the hyperplasia of the glandular tissue around the anal ring.

606   Large, ulcerating tumours on the anal ring. Lesions such as this are often a cause of dyschezia and haemorrhage.

607

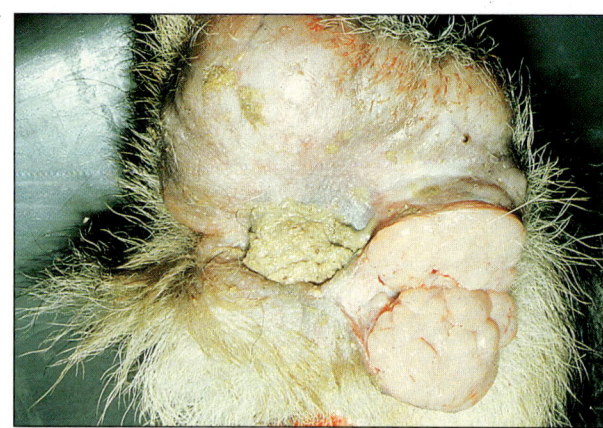

607   Circumanal (perianal) gland tumour. Large tumours involving ventral tail. One tumour has been sectioned to show the encapsulated, multinodular nature of a benign adenoma.

Circumanal (perianal) gland tumours

These tumours (also called hepatoid gland tumours because of their histological resemblance to liver cells) occur only in the dog as the cells of origin are not present in cats. Hepatoid tissue is predominantly found in the perianal region but may be found, in smaller amounts, in the prepuce, on the dorsal lumbosacral region and on the hind limbs[3]. There is a sex predisposition for both adenomatous and adenocarcinomatous changes in these glands, with intact males being predisposed to adenocarcinoma. Cocker spaniels, English bulldogs and Samoyeds are predisposed to adenoma, whilst Samoyeds, arctic breeds in general and German shepherd dogs are predisposed to adenocarcinoma.[18] Dogs over 35 kg are also predisposed. Tumours may be single (**605**) or multiple (**606** and **607**) and occur most commonly around the anus, although they may appear on the tail, the prepuce and the perineum, wherever there is hepatoid tissue.[3,15] In the early stages tumours are firm, round or ovoid but as they get larger they tend to become multinodular and less well defined. They appear to be pruritic and may sustain self trauma as a consequence, with haemorrhage, inflammation and infection. Ulceration is frequent. Most tumours are benign. Adenocarcinomas tend to grow more rapidly, are larger and more often, and more extensively, ulcerated. They may be locally invasive, spread into the pelvic cavity or metastasise to the regional lymph nodes.

608

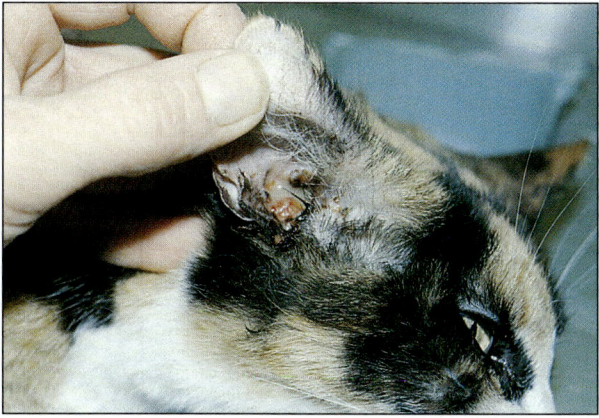

609

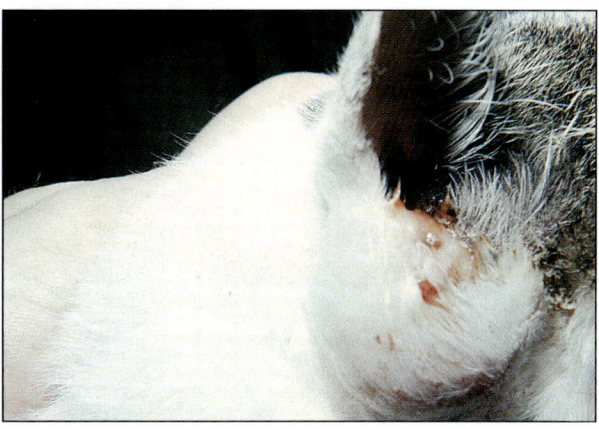

608   Ceruminous gland tumour. This cat presented with an acute, unilateral otic discharge due to the presence of the tumour which obstructed the external ear canal.

609   Ceruminous gland tumour. This adenocarcinoma formed a large mass at the base of the ear of a cat after it had perforated the otic cartilage.

610

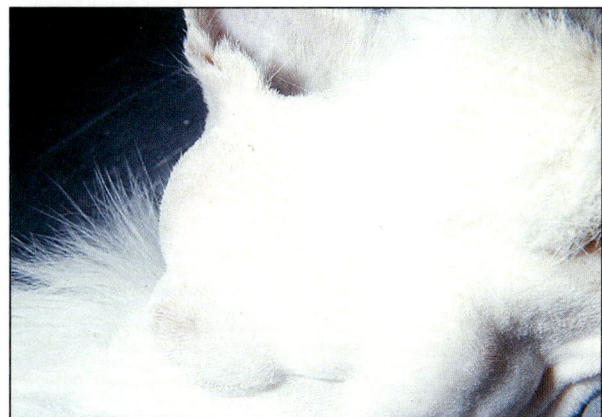

610   Ceruminous gland tumour. Metastasis to the local lymph nodes from an adenocarcinoma which was hidden within the external ear canal of a cat.

Ceruminous gland tumours of the external ear canal

Ceruminous gland tumours arise from the ceruminous glands of the horizontal ear canal. They frequently present with unilateral otic discharge (**608**). Polyps, of pharyngeal or auditory canal origin, may present similarly. Polyps are benign and sometimes bilateral. Ceruminous gland tumours are uncommon, being seen most frequently in old cats. It has been estimated that 50% are malignant.[12] Tumours may be small and pedunculated but may penetrate the cartilage of the ear canal and form a large mass at the base of the ear. Malignant tumours invade the parotid gland and metastasise to regional lymph nodes (**609** and **610**).

611

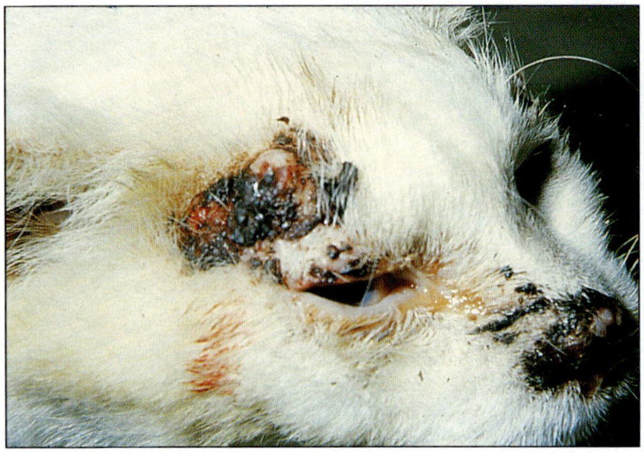

612

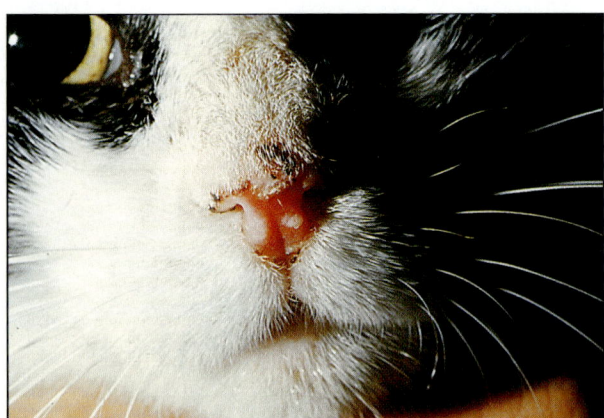

611   Squamous cell carcinoma. Large preneoplastic, dark, crusted solar keratoses on the skin above the eye and on planum nasale of a white cat.

613

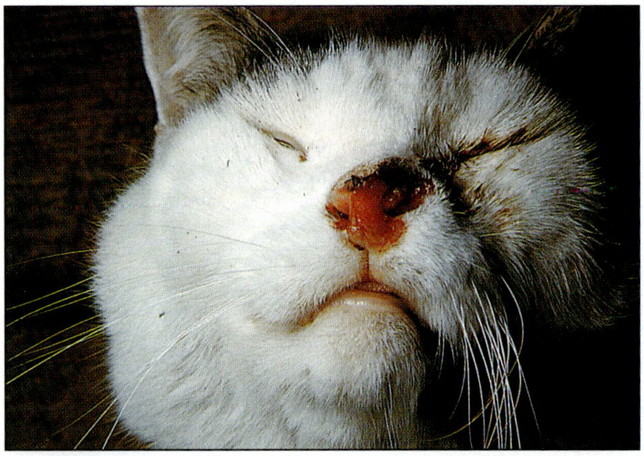

614

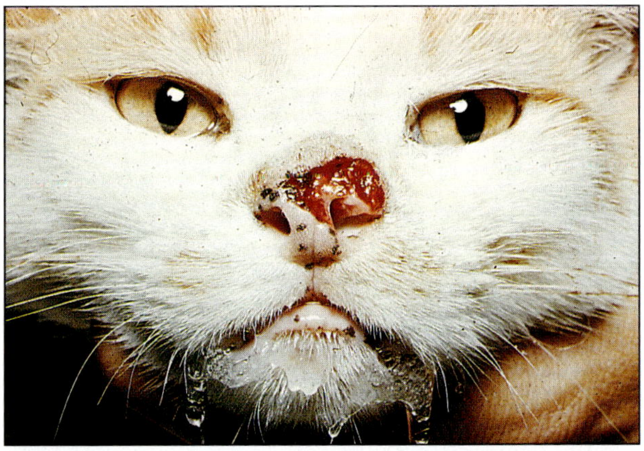

615

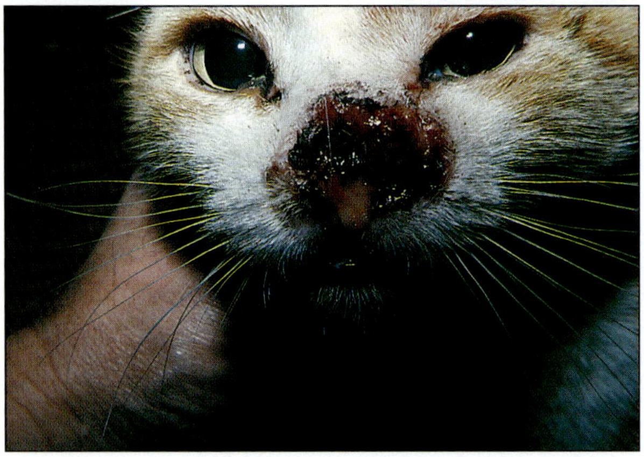

616

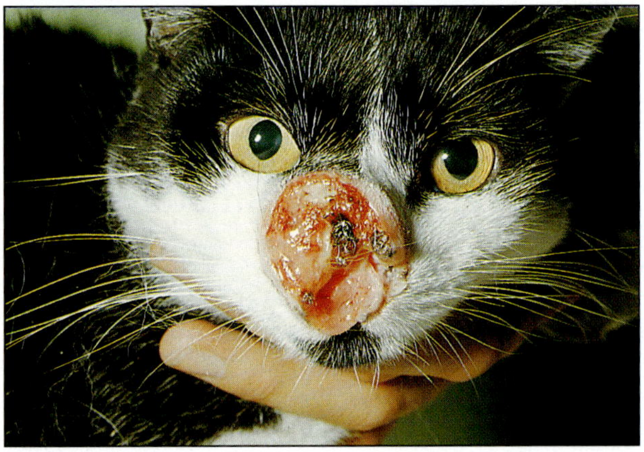

612–616   Squamous cell carcinoma. Stages in the development of the erosive form of the tumour usually associated with chronic exposure to ultra violet radiation.

617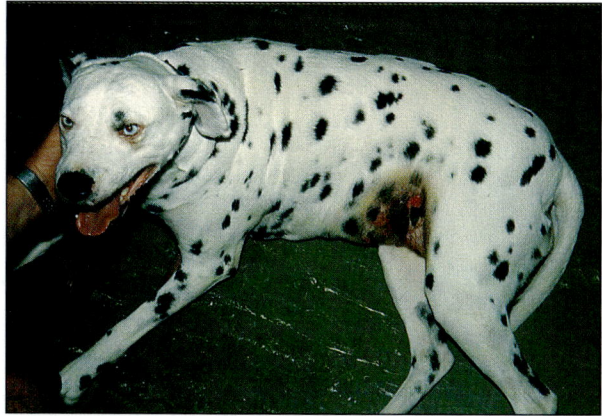

618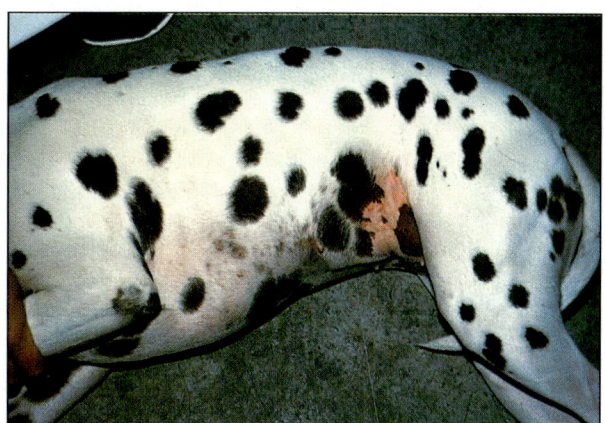

617–619 Squamous cell carcinoma. The flank is a characteristic site for development of solar radiation-induced tumours in Dalmatians and white Bull terriers. Illustrations depict two Dalmatian bitches with lesions in the flank and a close up of one of the tumours.

619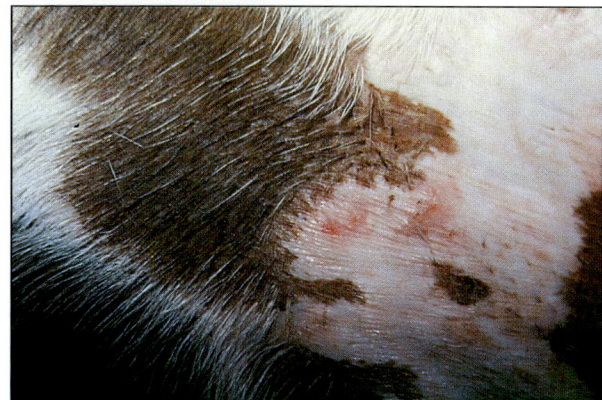

Squamous cell carcinomas

Squamous cell carcinomas are the most malignant epithelial tumours of the skin of the dog.[3] They are common and are derived from squamous epithelium and occur in both the dog and the cat. Animals that lack melanin pigment, such as white-haired cats and dogs, which are exposed to excessive amounts of solar radiation are especially susceptible to tumour development particularly in sparsely-haired areas (see Chapter 13).[11,12] Neoplastic transformation may follow the development of solar keratoses (**611–616**).[3] In cats the predilection sites are the pinnae, the planum nasale and the eyelids.[13] In the dog, particularly the Dalmatian and the white Bull terrier, the sparsely-haired area of the flank and ventral abdomen constitute the prime sites (**617–620**). Tumours arising in the flank are often refractory to treatment, recurring even after wide margins of excision are employed. Predilection sites in normally-pigmented breeds include the scrotum, limbs, digits, nose and lips. Tumours are usually solitary and may be productive or erosive. The

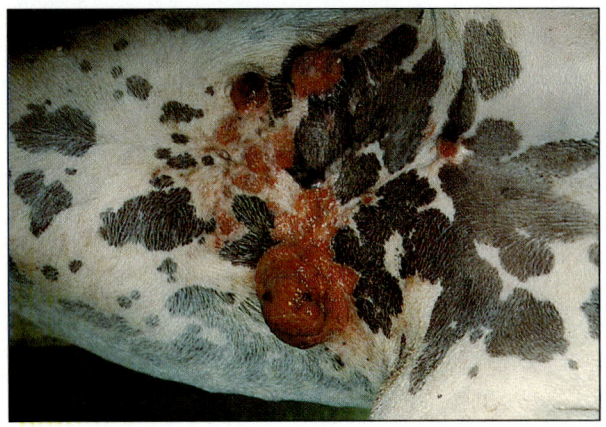 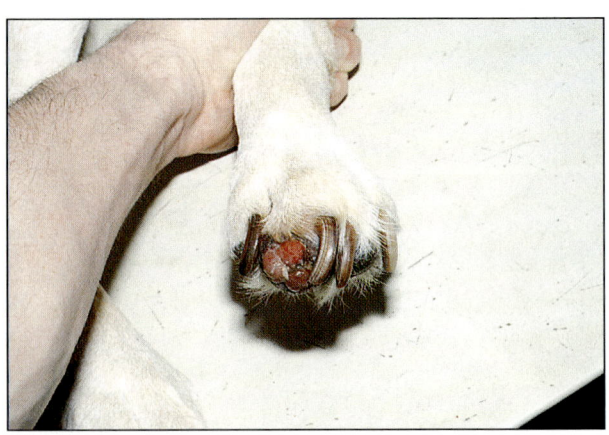

620 Squamous cell carcinoma. Solar radiation-induced tumours on the ventral abdomen of a Basset hound bitch that habitually lay with her ventrum exposed to the sun.

621 Squamous cell carcinoma. Nodular lesion on the distal limb of a Labrador retriever. Lesions in this site are very malignant and tend to demonstrate early metastasis.

productive forms are often papillomatous with a cauliflower-like appearance whereas the erosive forms commence as shallow, crusted, erosions which gradually extend to become deep, crater-like ulcers. These erosive forms are more often associated with chronic exposure to ultra violet radiation. In general, squamous cell carcinomas are of low metastatic potential but are locally invasive. An exception is the tumour which arises on the distal limb which is very malignant and has a tendency to metastasise to the lung fields (**621**).[3,11]

Tumours of mesenchymal origin

Fibromas and fibrosarcomas

These neoplasms are derived from dermal or subcutaneous fibroblasts. In general, they occur in older animals but may appear in young dogs. In kittens, multiple fibrosarcomas may be induced by a virus (Feline Sarcoma Virus, FeSV) which is a mutant of the Feline Leukaemia Virus (FeLV).[12]

Fibromas do not infiltrate neighbouring tissues and do not metastasise. They are usually solitary and appear as well circumscribed, domed or pedunculated tumours of variable texture which may, occasionally, ulcerate (**622**). Canine fibromas may be pigmented or 'pin feathered' or both. Fibrovascular papillomas ('skin tags') are uncommon benign tumours consisting of a fibrovascular core covered by an irregular hyperplastic and papillomatous epidermis. They usually appear as multiple, small (< 1cm in length) soft, variably pigmented, fingerlike projections of the skin of the ventral thorax or the extremities of large dogs (**623**). Fibrosarcomas are malignant tumours. They are usually solitary and occur in older dogs and cats showing a predilection for the trunk and limbs (**624** and **625**).[4,13] They are firm, variably sized and irregularly shaped, poorly defined tumours which are usually fixed to the overlying skin and often ulcerated (**626**). Tumour growth tends to be rapid and infiltrative, recurrence often following surgical excision. Metastasis, which is usually haematogenous, occurs in only about 25% of cases.

622 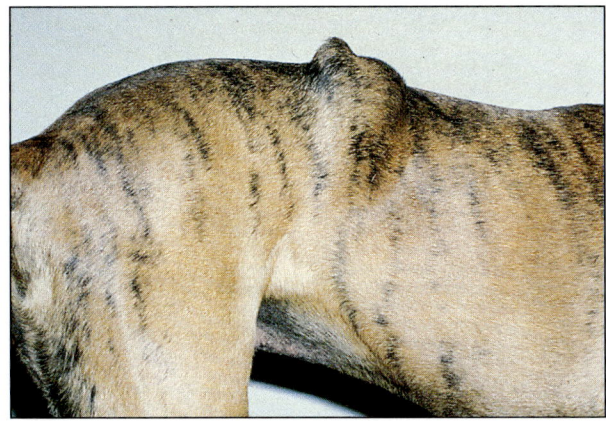 **623**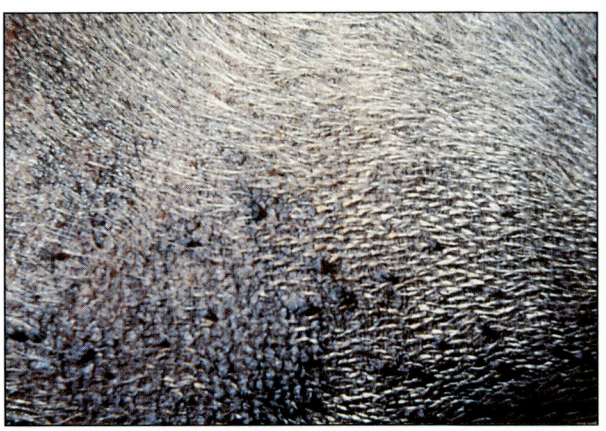

622 **Fibroma.** Large, subcutaneous fibroma in the dorsal lumbar area of a Boxer dog.

623 **Fibrovascular papillomas ('skin tags').** Pigmented skin tags on the lateral thorax of a dog.

624 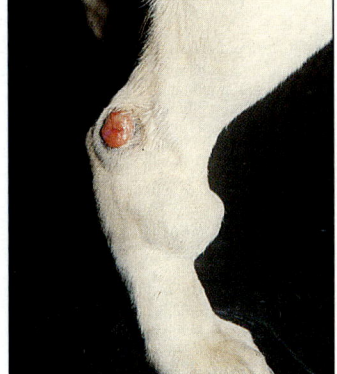 **625**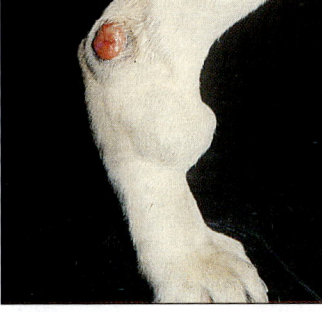

624. **Fibrosarcoma.** Locally aggressive, often ulcerated tumours. This tumour involved the hock joint of a Bull terrier and had broken through the skin anterior to the calcaneus.

625 **Fibrosarcoma.** Ulcerated tumour on the hock of a cat. Note the massive enlargement of the popliteal lymph node.

626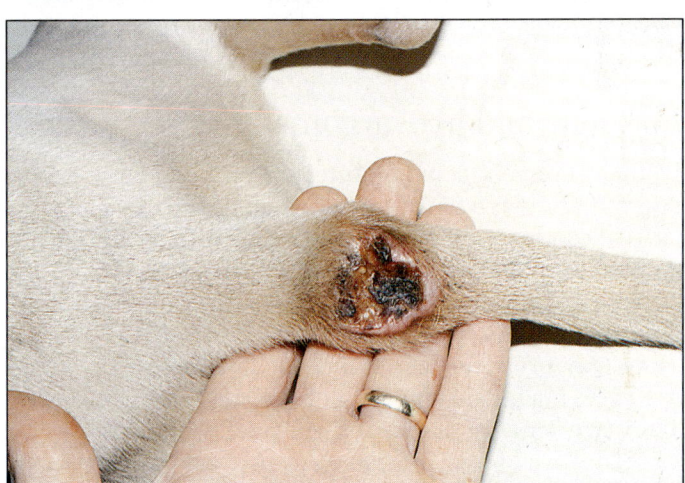

626 **Fibrosarcoma.** Ulcerated nodule on the dorsal aspect of the tail of an elderly whippet. Surgery was curative.

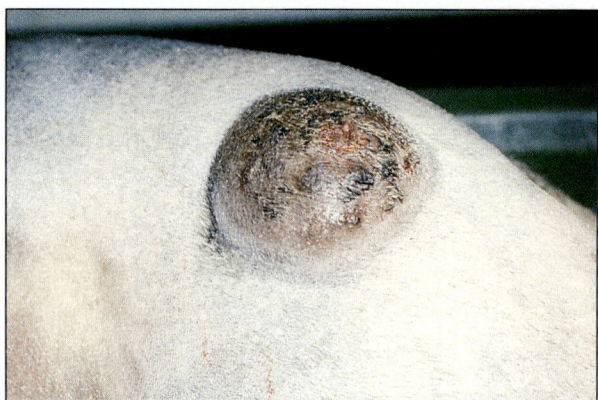

627   Lipoma. Large, well-circumscribed, mobile lipoma on the upper limb of a 6-year-old Airedale.

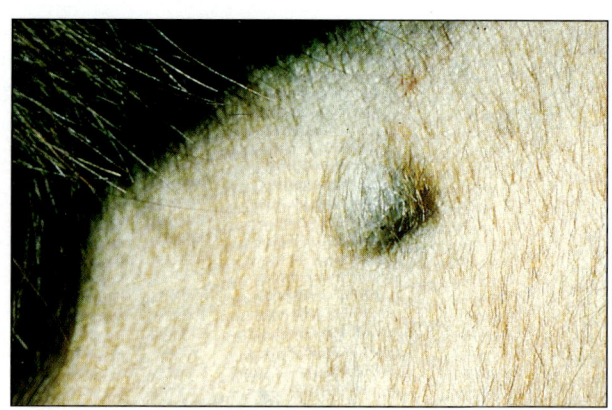

628   Haemangiosarcoma. One of a number of metastatic tumours that were spread throughout the body of a German shepherd dog. In this case, unusually, the spleen was not involved and signs were associated with disseminated intravascular coagulation.

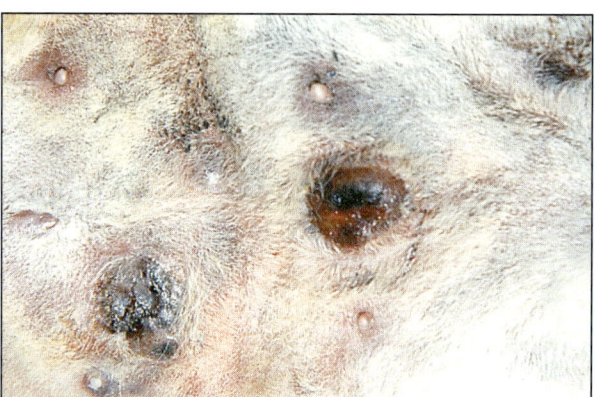

629   Haemangiosarcoma. Multiple, purple coloured, tumours on the ventral abdomen of a cat.

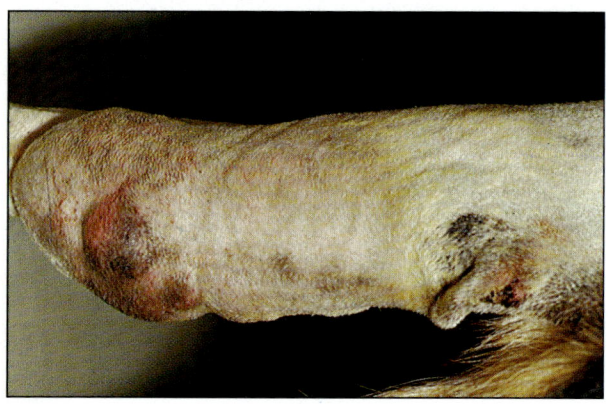

630   Haemangiopericytoma. Large, poorly-circumscribed, lobulated tumour on the leg of a dog.

Lipomas and liposarcomas

Lipomas are very common tumours of the elderly dog but are very rare in the cat. Females, particularly obese females, are predisposed.[4,15] They are derived from lipocytes and occur anywhere on the body, as single or multiple, round, ovoid or discoid, soft, well-circumscribed tumours (**627**). They may grow very large indeed. Liposarcomas are rare, malignant tumours of the dog and cat. They are usually solitary, firm, poorly-circumscribed, variably-sized tumours which are locally infiltrative but rarely metastasise.[4]

Haemangiomas, haemangiosarcomas and haemangiopericytomas

Haemangiomas are benign tumours arising from endothelial cells of blood vessels. They are uncommon in dogs and rare in cats and are usually solitary but may be multiple. Tumours may develop anywhere on the body, although there may be a predilection for the face, neck and limbs, and appear as firm to fluctuant, spherical or ovoid, well-circumscribed, bluish to reddish-black neoplasms up to 3cm in diameter.[4] Haemangiosarcomas are rare, highly invasive and malignant tumours which occur mainly in dogs and cats over nine years of age. German shepherd dogs are predisposed, males being affected more often than females. Tumours are usually solitary, poorly-circumscribed, rapidly-growing, soft and friable and cause

631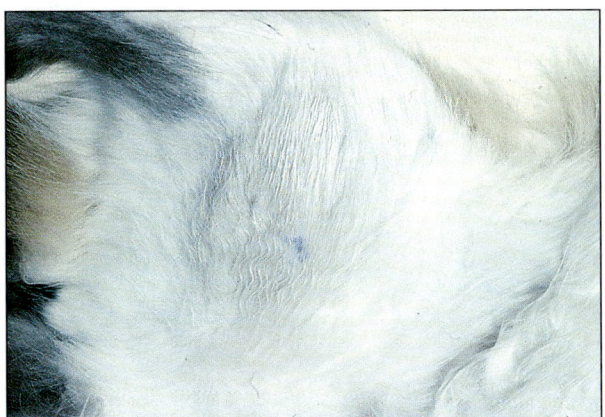

632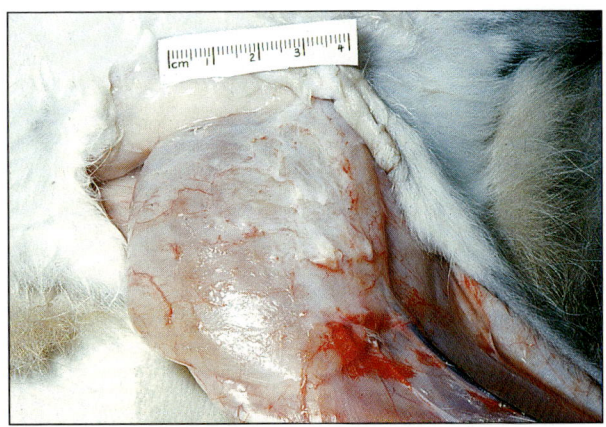

631 and 632   Lymphangioma. Large fluctuating mass on the upper median thigh of a cat and the tumour dissected out to show sac-like growth filled with clear fluid. (Illustrations courtesy of R. Sutton.)

633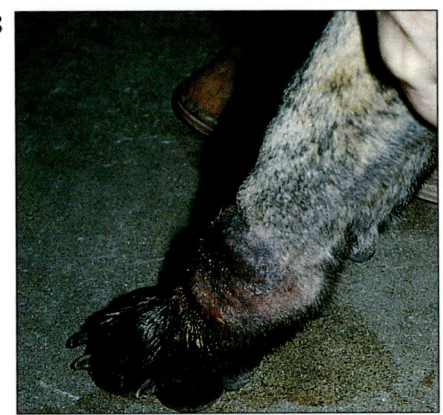

634

633 and 634   Lymphangiosarcoma. This tumour was causing gross oedema of the foreleg of a Great Dane bitch. Breakdown of the skin occurred just below the carpus and a sero-sanguinous fluid could be expressed in a jet through the resulting skin defect.

considerable inflammatory changes in neighbouring tissues (**628** and **629**). They often become ulcerated, necrotic and haemorrhage easily. Although usually solitary, canine skin tumours may be associated with visceral neoplasms showing a predilection for the right atrium of the heart and the spleen.

Haemangiopericytomas are benign tumours unique to the dog. The cell of origin is unknown but is thought to be the pericytes, which surround the capillaries. Tumours are more common in females and in dogs over six years old. German shepherd dogs, Boxers and Springer spaniels are predisposed. The neoplasms are usually solitary and mainly involve the skin over the lateral surfaces of the limbs (**630**). Small tumours appear as smooth or lobulated, firm, well-circumscribed growths over which the skin is freely movable whereas large tumours tend to infiltrate neighbouring tissues and have poorly-defined margins. Haemangiopericytomas show a high probability for recurrence following even wide surgical margins of excision[4].

Lymphangiomas and lymphangiosarcomas

Lymphangiomas are very rare tumours of the dog and cat which are thought to result from a developmental failure in lymphatic communication. They have been reported as large, solitary, fluctuant masses in the axillary and inguinal regions (**631** and **632**). Lymphangiosarcomas develop from the endothelium of lymphatics and are extremely rare (**633** and **634**).

635

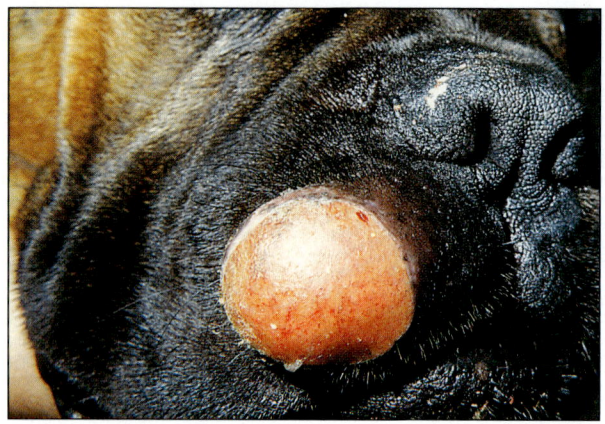

635   Mast cell tumour. Large solitary mast cell tumour on the upper lip of a Bull mastiff.

636

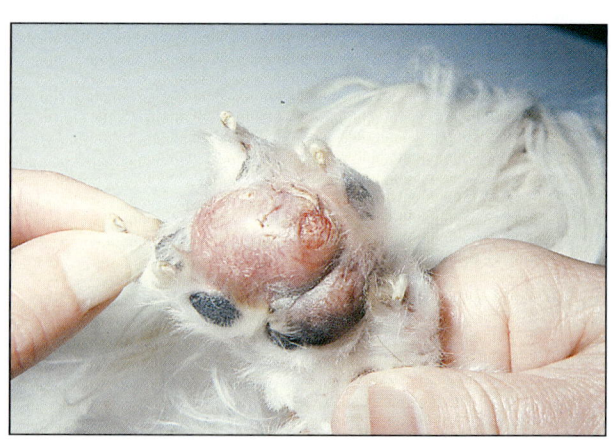

636   Mast cell tumour. Large ulcerating tumour on the foot of a Maltese terrier bitch.

637

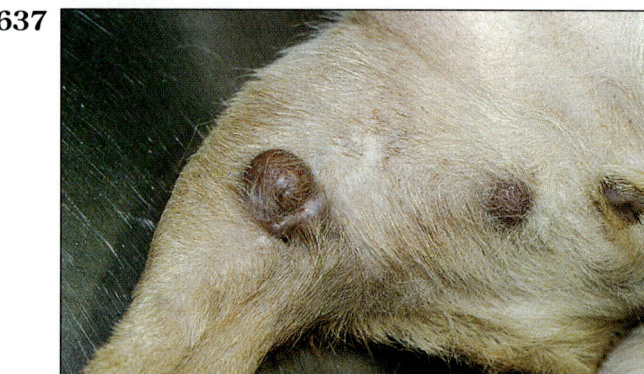

637   Mast cell tumour. Three nodular mast cell tumours on the medial aspect of the thigh of an elderly Staffordshire Bull terrier.

638

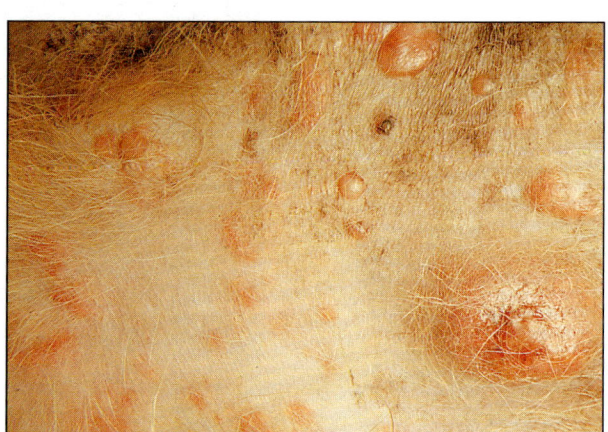

638   Mast cell tumour. Multiple tumours on the abdominal skin of a crossbred dog.

Mast cell tumours (mastocytomas, mast cell sarcomas)

Mast cell tumours are common tumours of the dog and the cat which arise from mast cells in the dermis or subcutaneous tissues.[4] Although they may be benign, they should always be regarded as potentially malignant. Boxers, English bulldogs, terriers (particularly Fox and Boston terriers), Labrador retrievers and Weimaraners are predisposed.[4] The tumours occur mainly in dogs over eight years of age. Predilection sites for the dog are the skin of the trunk, the perineal region and the extremities.[17] Feline mast cell tumours may occur anywhere on the body but the most common site is the head, particularly the base of the ear.[13] Siamese cats appear to be predisposed.[13] Canine tumours are mostly solitary (**635** and **636**) although multiple neoplasms may occur (**637–639**). Feline mast cell tumours are usually multiple (**640** and **641**). Mast cell tumours vary considerably in appearance.[11] In most cases they are small- to medium-sized (3cm or less), firm,

639

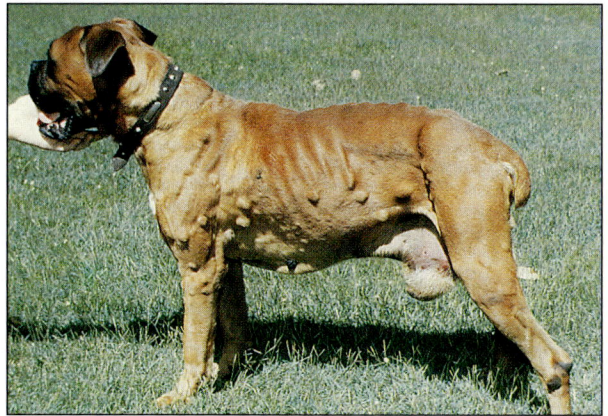

639 Mast cell tumour. Multiple tumours in a boxer dog which were associated with duodenal ulceration.

640

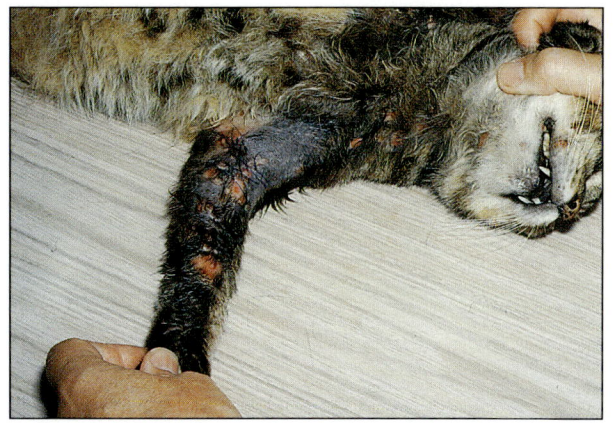

640 and 641 Mast cell tumour. Multiple erythematous tumours in the axilla, and on the medial foreleg and head of a cat.

641

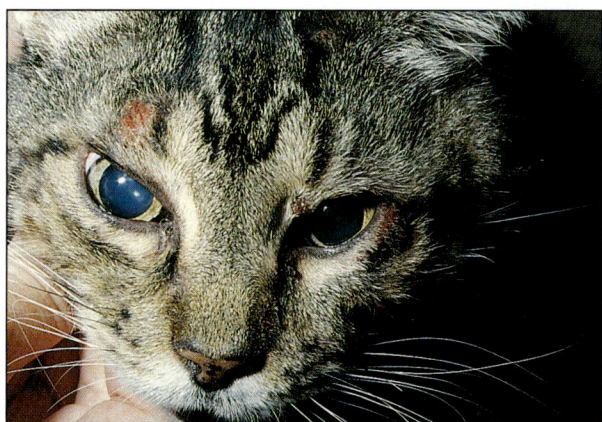

642

642 Mast cell tumour. Solitary erythematous, ulcerated mast cell tumour on the pinna of a cat.

elevated, well circumscribed, erythematous or ulcerated tumour masses (**642**).[17] Others are raised, but not ulcerated or reddened, soft and ill defined. However well defined the tumour appears, there is commonly neoplastic tissue beyond the palpable border and generous margins of excision are necessary. Paraneoplastic signs, perhaps associated with histamine and heparin release from the mast cells, include gastric and duodenal ulceration, coagulation disorders and glomerulonephritis.[11]

- Mast cell tumours are common and are impossible to rule out on the basis of clinical appearance. If cytology is not performed then treat all tumours as potential mast cell neoplasms and excise with a wide (> 2cm) margin of excision **on all aspects**.

643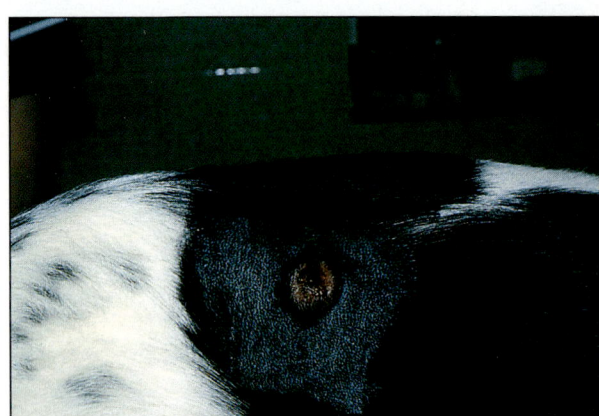

644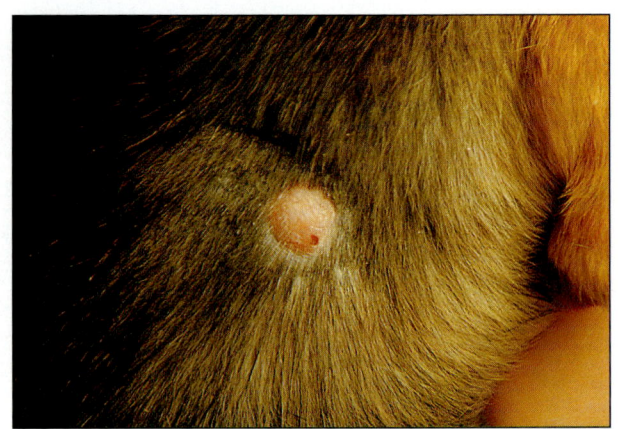

645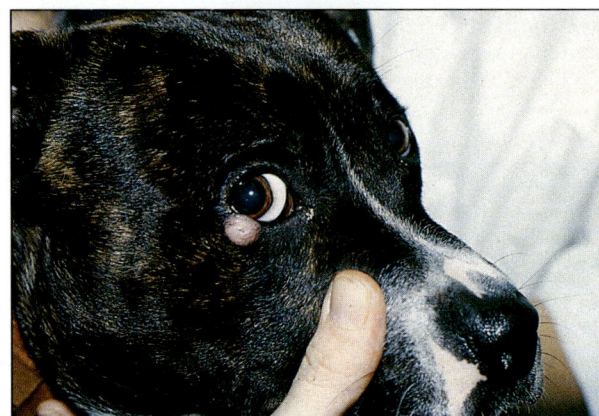

643–645   Histiocytoma. Characteristic 'button tumours' on the flank, dorsal neck and lower eyelid of three young dogs. Although of malignant appearance these neoplasms are benign and usually exhibit spontaneous regression.

Tumours of lymphohistiocytic origin

Histiocytomas ('button tumours')

Histiocytomas are common, benign skin tumours of the dog, thought to arise from Langerhans cells. They are very rare in cats. The tumours are usually solitary and are most frequently seen in young dogs, affecting mainly the head and the limbs.[6] They are small, rarely exceeding 2cm in diameter, firm, well circumscribed, domed or button-like in shape, hence the colloquial name. The overlying skin may be hairless or ulcerated **(643–645)**. The tumours are fast growing but benign and most regress spontaneously. Boxers, Cocker spaniels, Great Danes and Shetland sheepdogs are predisposed.

- Histiocytomas are common. They have a distinctive histopathological appearance to a veterinary specialist. However, a human pathologist may misinterpret the pattern and diagnose a malignant tumour.

Systemic histiocytosis

Systemic histiocytosis is a rare malignant neoplastic condition of dogs in which there is widespread infiltration of both skin and internal organs by atypical histiocytes, which often exhibit erythrophagia.[14] The Bernese mountain dog appears to be the most susceptible breed. Skin tumours are multiple, ulcerative, crusted, round and well circum-

646

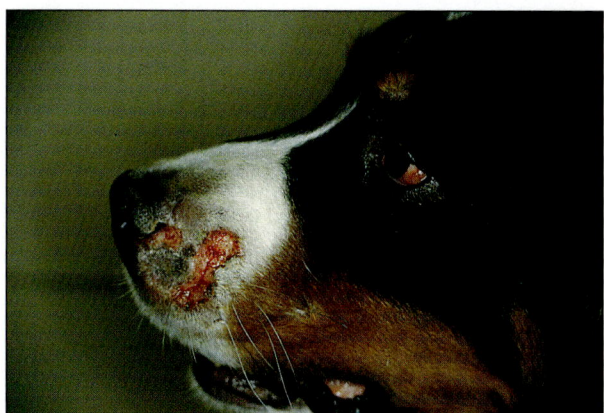

647

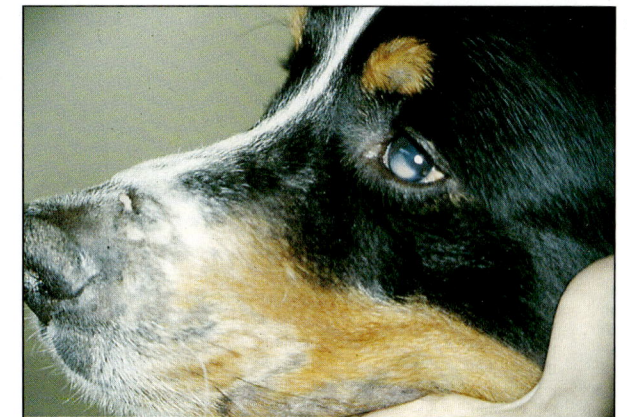

648

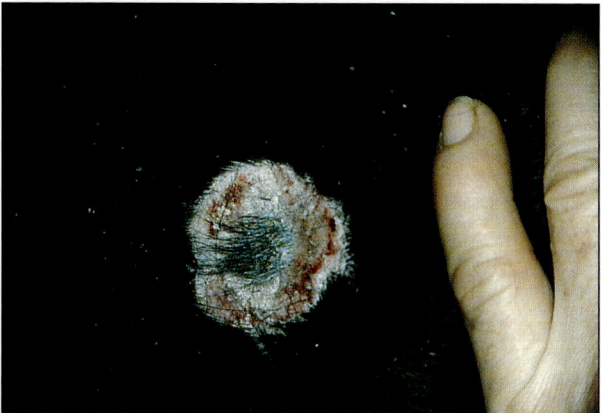

649

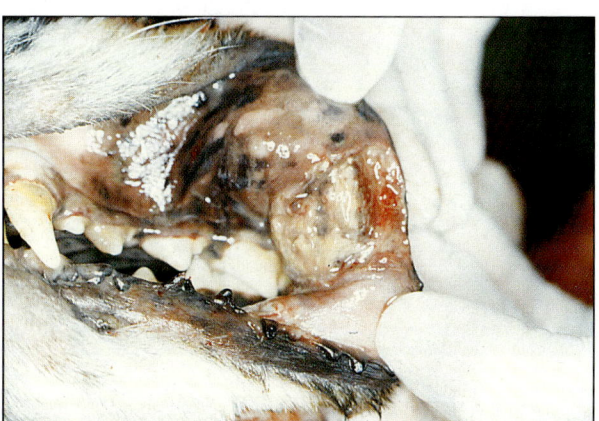

646–650 Systemic histiocytosis. Erosive lesions on the muzzle of a Bernese mountain dog (**646**) and the same dog during remission: note that the muzzle lesions have healed with some pigmented scarring (**647**). Note also the hypopyon in the anterior chamber, probably due to effusion of neoplastic histiocytes. Solitary circular lesion on shoulder region of same dog bearing a close resemblance to 'classic ringworm' lesion (**648**). Oral lesions (**649**) and lung lesions (**650**) in the same dog. (Illustrations courtesy of L. Bellstrom.)

650

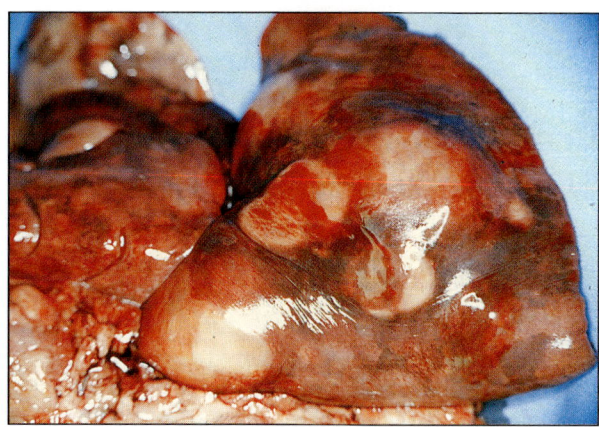

scribed. Oral involvement may occur. The lungs are the most frequently affected internal organs, the tumours appearing as large pale masses. The course of the disease is usually chronic and ultimately fatal.[14] Individual skin lesions may regress and heal but new ones appear (**646–650**).

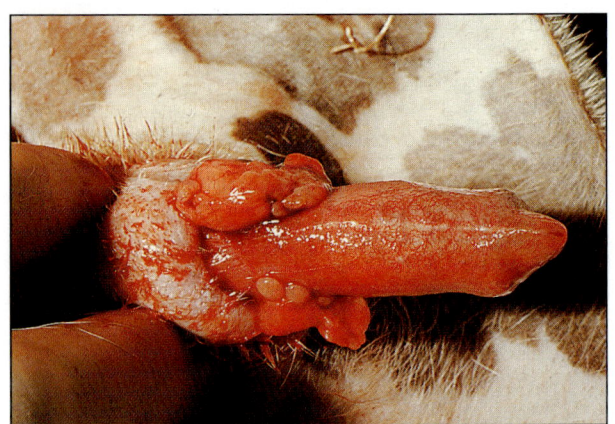

651   Canine transmissible venereal tumour. Multilobulated tumours on the penile mucosa of a Bull terrier dog.

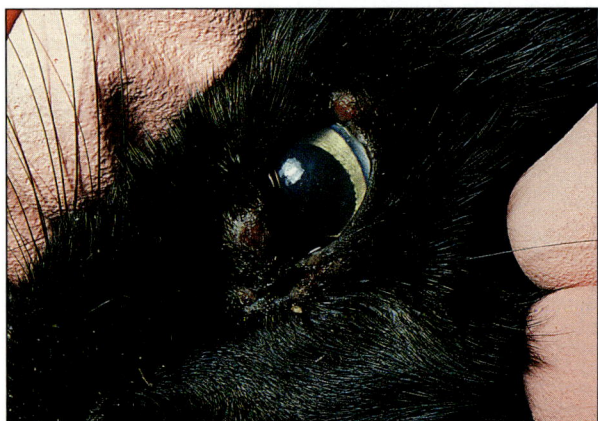

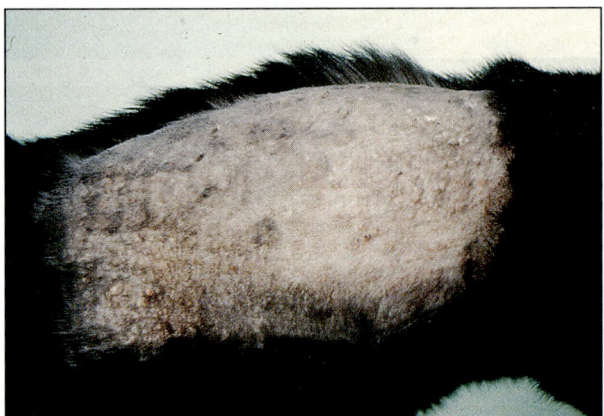

652 and 653   Cutaneous lymphoma. Multiple nodular, sometimes ulcerated lesions on the head and trunk of a cat.

Canine transmissible venereal tumours (CTVT)

CTVT are uncommon, benign to malignant, naturally occurring tumours of the dog that are transmitted by implantation of viable neoplastic cells into a susceptible host during coitus. The tumours are endemic in certain areas of the world, usually in temperate zones and in large cities. The neoplastic cells have an unusual karyotype containing 59 chromosomes instead of the usual canine complement of 78. CTVT may be solitary or multiple and almost always occur on the mucosa of the external genitalia. Occasionally, the skin of the face and limbs may be involved. The tumours are cauliflower-like, pedunculated, papillary, nodular, or multilobulated (**651**). They may be firm or friable and are often ulcerated. Recurrence after surgical removal is not uncommon.

Cutaneous lymphoma

Cutaneous lymphoma may be classified on clinical, histopathological and immunological features into two groups:

- Cutaneous B-cell lymphoma.
- Cutaneous T-cell lymphoma: comprising mycosis fungoides, Sézary syndrome and pagetoid reticulosis.

654

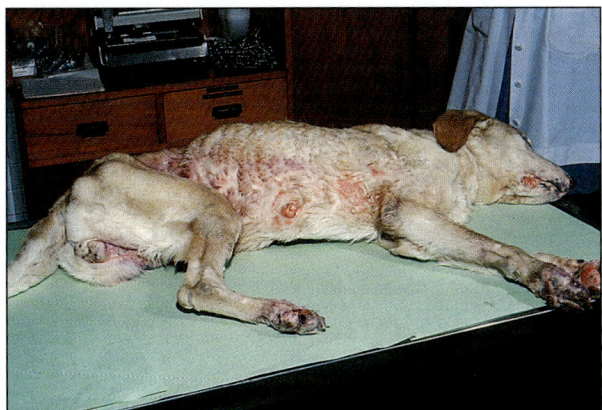

655

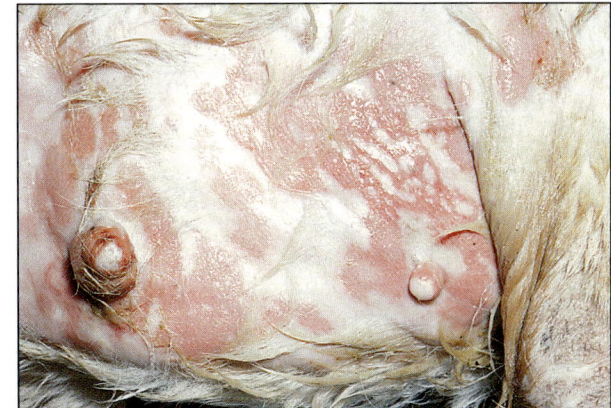

656

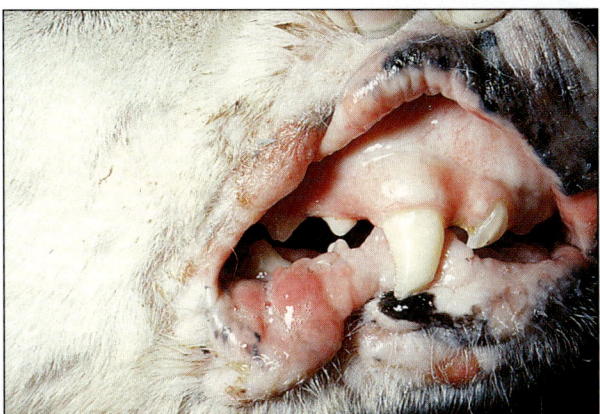

657

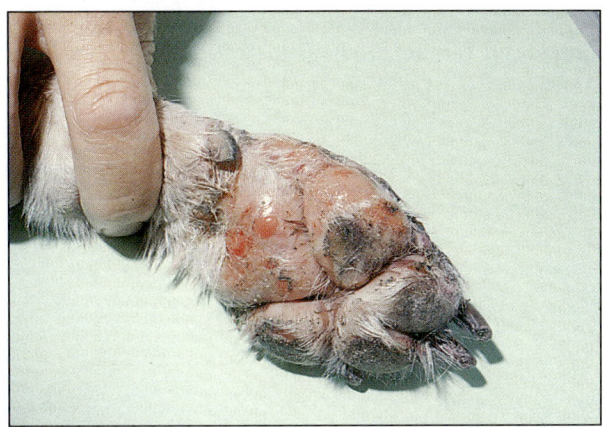

654–657 Cutaneous lymphoma. Generalised cutaneous lymphoma in a Labrador retriever bitch involving almost the whole surface of the body and the oral cavity with erythematous and proliferative lesions. Note the similarity to pemphigus vulgaris on cursory inspection.

Cutaneous B-cell lymphoma is a rare, malignant neoplasm of dogs and cats. The lesions are usually multifocal or generalised (**652–657**) although in rare cases, solitary neoplastic nodules may occur (**658**).[6] Systemic involvement is variable. In cats the feline leukaemia virus is considered to be the cause of the malignancy even though affected animals are often FeLV-negative. Tumours may present a variable appearance ranging from erythroderma and exfoliative dermatitis to ulcerated nodules and plaques which are frequently accompanied by pruritus.

658

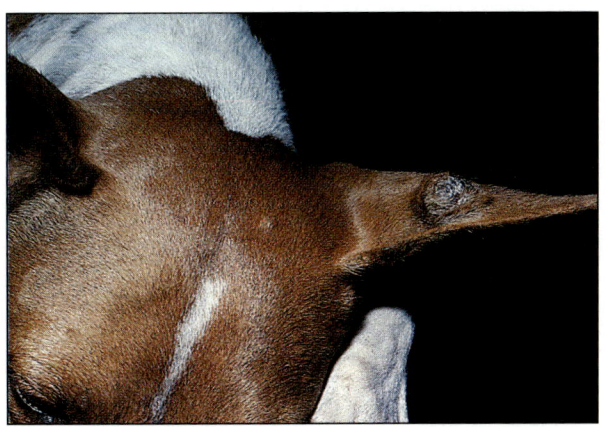

658 Cutaneous lymphoma. Rare, solitary, ulcerated tumour nodule in a crossbred terrier bitch.

659

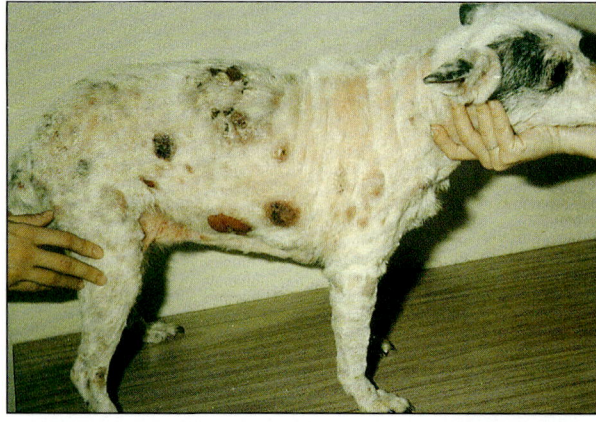

659   Mycosis fungoides. Generalised lesions in a crossbred terrier bitch. (Illustration courtesy J. A. Yager.)

660

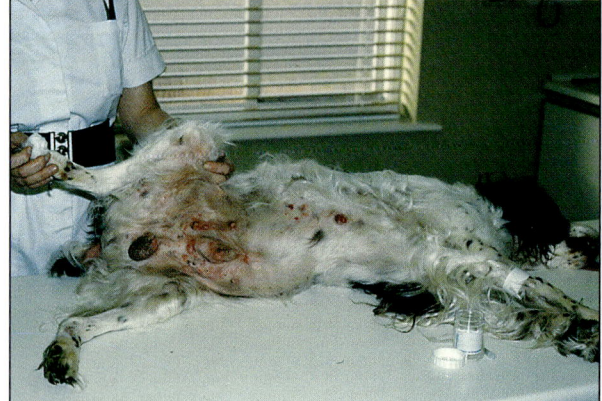

661

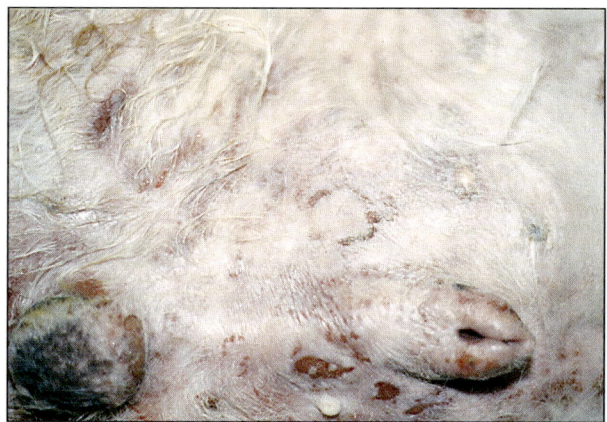

660 and 661   Mycosis fungoides. Munsterlander with extensive plaque-like lesions in the groin and on the ventral abdomen.

Mycosis fungoides is a rare, epitheliotropic T-cell lymphoma of the dog, cat and hamster.[5,7] The disease is chronic, often commencing with a pruritic erythroderma or exfoliative dermatitis (**659–664**).[19] Progression through plaque and tumour stages is variable. Oral lesions are not uncommon (**665** and **666**). and the prognosis is grave.

- Lymphoma is often diagnosed at a late stage. The early signs of pruritus and exfoliative dermatitis are not recognised as indications of neoplastic change.

662 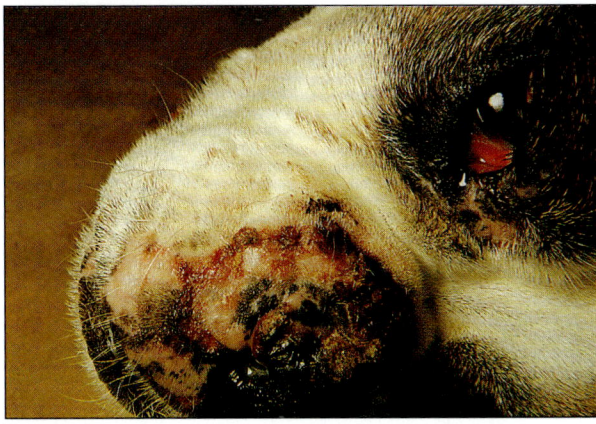 **663**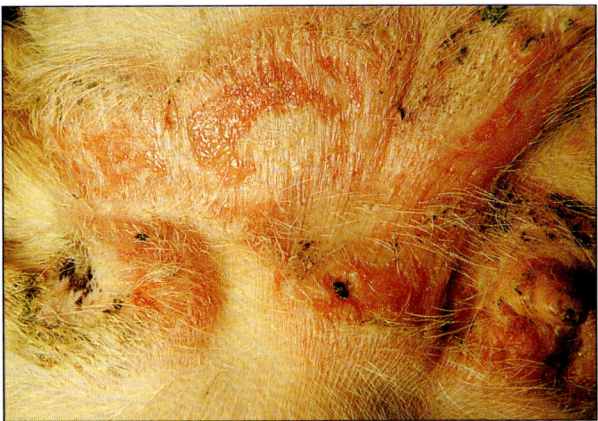

662 and 663   Mycosis fungoides. Infiltrated and crusted plaque-like lesions in a Boxer bitch.

664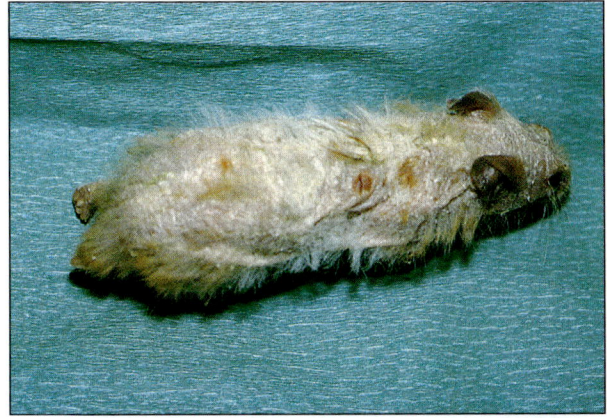

664   Mycosis fungoides. An elderly Syrian hamster with pruritic exfoliative dermatitis due to mycosis fungoides. The major differential in this species is demodicosis.

65 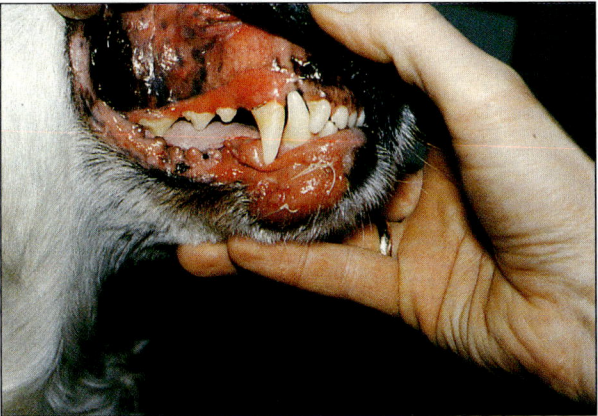 **666**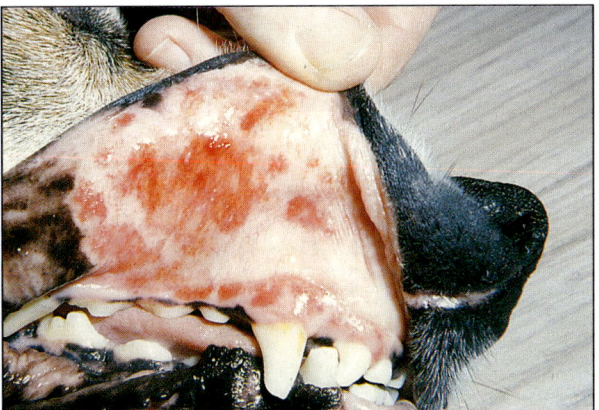

665 and 666   Oral lesions are not uncommon in mycosis fungoides. Note the nodular mass in the oral cavity of the Golden retriever and the erosive, erythematous lesions in the mouth of the crossbred terrier (in which the lesions extended through the fauces to involve the larynx).

667

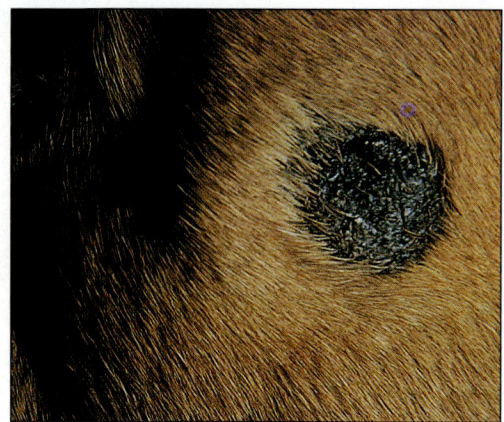

667   Melanoma. Benign melanoma on upper thigh of a Boxer dog.

668

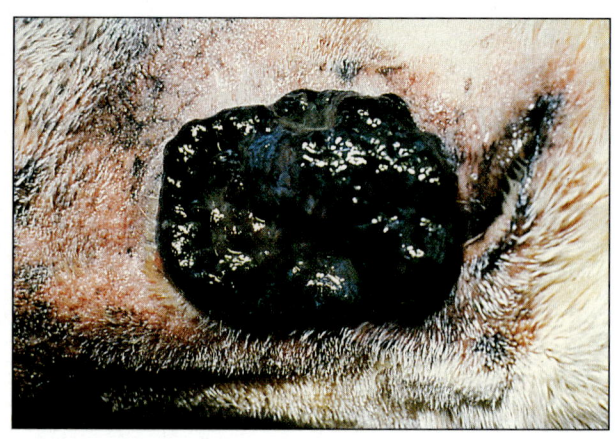

668   Melanoma. Malignant tumour on the forehead of a cross-bred dog.

669

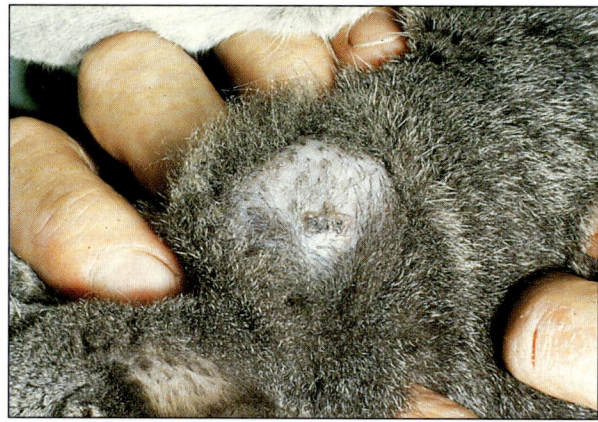

669   Melanoma. A rare malignant tumour in a cat.

Melanocytic neoplasms

Melanomas

Melanomas are relatively common in dogs but rare in cats and may be benign or malignant. They arise from melanocytes and melanoblasts and occur most commonly in animals between seven and 14 years of age. Scottish and Boston terriers, Airedales and Cocker spaniels are most often affected.[11] There may be a predilection for male animals.[6] Melanomas of the skin are usually solitary, occurring on the face, especially the eyelids, the trunk and the limbs. They appear as small black macules or as black, dark brown, grey or non-pigmented nodules or masses (**667**). In malignant tumours the overlying skin is often ulcerated (**668** and **669**). Most skin melanomas are benign but those arising from the mucocutaneous junction of the oral cavity, the scrotum or from the digits tend to be malignant[11, 15], metastasising early to regional lymph nodes and distant visceral sites.[1,6]

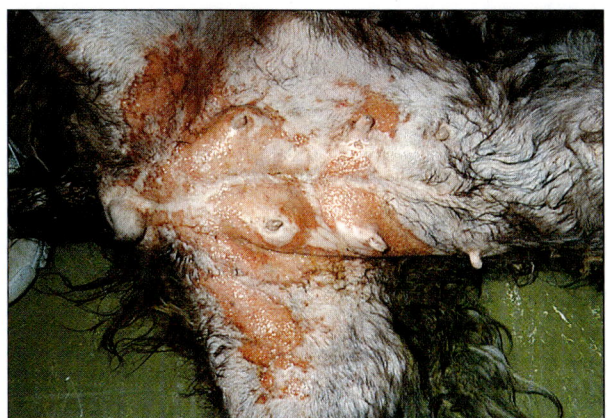
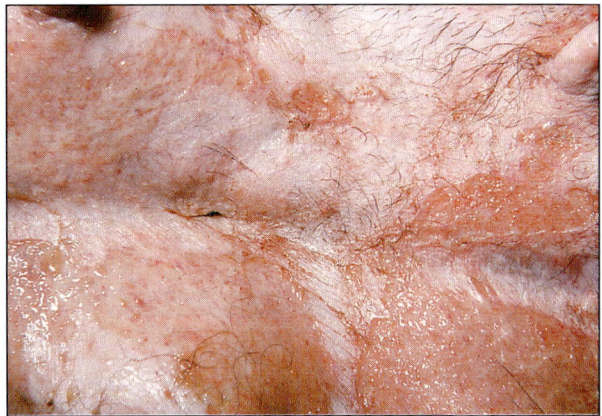

670 and 671 Metastatic anaplastic carcinoma. These pruritic, erythematous and erosive lesions on the ventral abdomen, inguinal region and inner thighs of an Afghan bitch were due to metastatic deposits of an anaplastic carcinoma. It had spread throughout the body and was thought to originate in the colon.

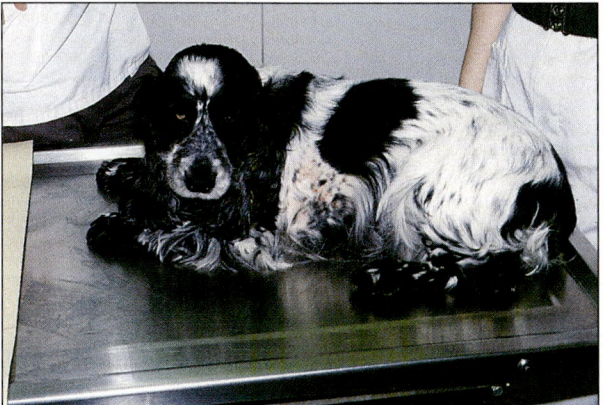
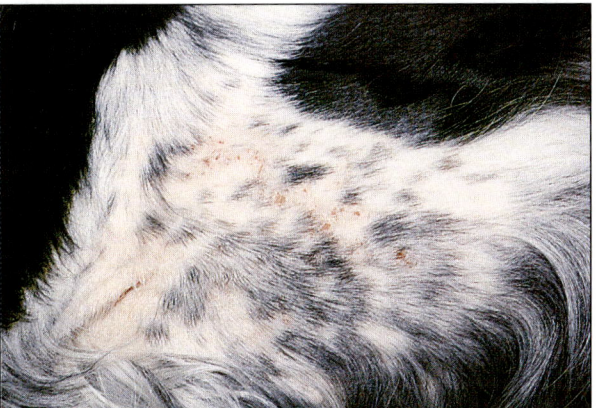

672 and 673 Metatastatic pulmonary adenocarcinoma. This Cocker spaniel presented with a few discrete, ulcerated, crusted nodules on the lateral thorax. Biopsy suggested that these were metastases and thoracic radiography demonstrated pulmonary neoplasia.

Cutaneous metastases of internal neoplasms

Any internal tumour which produces metastases has the potential to produce cutaneous lesions and carcinomas, in particular, spring to mind. Although these are rare they should be considered in the differential of eruptive, ulcerative or focal lesions (**670–673**). Diagnosis is based on histopathological examination of biopsy samples.

References

1. Aronsohn, M. G. and Carpenter, J. L. (1990). Distal extremity melanocytic nevi and malignant melanomas in dogs. *Journal of the American Animal Hospital Association*, **26**: 605–612.

2. Barton, C. L. (1987). Cytologic diagnosis of cutaneous neoplasia: an algorithmic approach. *Compendium on Continuing Education*, **9**: 20–33.

3. Bevier, D. E. and Goldschmidt, M. H. (1981a). Skin tumors in the dog. Part I: Epithelial tumors and tumorlike lesions. *Compendium on Continuing Education*, **3**: 389–400.

4. Bevier, D. E. and Goldschmidt, M. H. (1981b). Skin tumours in the dog. Part II: Tumors of the soft (mesenchymal) tissues. *Compendium on Continuing Education*, **3**: 506–516.

5. Collins, R. E. (1987). Dermatologic disorders of common small nondomestic pets. In: Nesbitt, G. E. (Ed.) *Contemporary Issues in Small Animal Practice No. 8 Dermatology* pp. 235–294. Churchill Livingstone, New York.

6. Goldschmidt, M. H. and Bevier, D. E. (1981). Skin tumors in the dog. Part III: Lymphohistiocytic and melanocytic tumours. *Compendium on Continuing Education*, **3**: 588–594.

7. Harvey, R. G., Whitbread, T. J., Ferrer, L. and Cooper, J. E. (1992). Epidermotropic cutaneous T-cell lymphoma (mycosis fungoides) in Syrian hamsters (*Mesocricetus auratus*). A report of six cases and the demonstration of T-cell specificity. Veterinary Dermatology, **3**: 13–19.

8. Henderson, R. A. (1986). Recent advances in surgical control and management of neoplasia. In: Gorman, N. T. (Ed.) *Contemporary Issues in Small Animal Practice No. 6 Oncology* pp. 45–69. Churchill Livingstone, New York.

9. Kalaher, K. M., Anderson, W. I. and Scott, D. W. (1990). Neoplasms of the apocrine sweat glands in 44 dogs and 10 cats. *Veterinary Record*, **127**: 400–432.

10. Keller, E. T. and Madewell, B. R. (1992). Locations and types of neoplasms in immature dogs: 69 cases (1964–1989). *Journal of the American Veterinary Medical Association*, **200**: 1530–1532.

11. Kwochka, K. W. (1986). Clinical diagnosis and management of cutaneous neoplasia in the dog. In: Gorman, N. T. (Ed.) *Contemporary Issues in Small Animal Practice No. 6 Oncology* pp. 195–212. Churchill Livingstone, New York.

12. Macy, D. W. and Reynolds, H. A. (1981). The incidence, characteristics and clinical management of skin tumours of cats. *Journal of the American Animal Hospital Association*, **17**: 1026–1034.

13. Miller, M. A., Nelson, S. L., Turk, J. R., Pace, L. W., Brown, T. P., Shaw, D. P., Fischer, J. R. and Gosser, H. S. (1991). Cutaneous neoplasia in 340 cats. *Veterinary Pathology*, **28**: 389–395.

14. Rosin, A., Moore, P. and Dubielzig, R. (1986). Malignant histiocytosis in Bernese mountain dogs. *Journal of the American Veterinary Medical Association*, **188**: 1041–1045.

15. Rothwell, T. L. W., Howlett, C. R., Middleton, D. J., Griffiths, D. A. and Duffs, B. C. (1987). Skin neoplasms of dogs in Sydney. *Australian Veterinary Journal*, **64**: 161–164.

16. Scott, D. W. and Anderson, W. I. (1990). Canine sebaceous gland tumours: a retrospective analysis of 172 cases. *Canine Practice*, **15**: 19–27.

17. Tams, T. R. (1981). Canine mast cell tumours. *Compendium on Continuing Education*, **3**: 869–882.

18. Vail, D. M., Withrow, S. J., Schwartz, P. D. and Powers, B. E. (1990). Perianal adenocarcinoma in the canine male: a retrospective study of 41 cases. *Journal of the American Animal Hospital Association*, **26**: 329–334.

19. Wilcock, B. P. and Yager, J. A. (1989). The behaviour of epidermotropic lymphoma in twenty-five dogs. *Canadian Veterinary Journal*, **30**: 754–756.

Chapter 15:

Non-neoplastic papules, nodules and tumours

Introduction

Not all lumps are neoplasms. Non-neoplastic lesions may be of varied origin and may be difficult to differentiate on clinical examination. Lesions may be solitary or multiple, haired, ulcerated or fistulous. Unless the cause is readily apparent (for example a sebaceous cyst) then suspect lesions should be treated with suspicion. Cytological samples should be examined (see Chapter 3), particularly for evidence of an infectious agent. If doubt still remains as to the cause then biopsy or surgical excision are indicated in order to aid the definitive diagnosis. Histopathological examination of biopsy material may not yield definitive results but it will identify the process taking place. Thus, identification of a granulomatous reaction warrants identification of the cause and, if not apparent, further samples should be taken for submission for bacteriological, mycobacterial and fungal culture and sensitivity (see Chapter 3).

Non-neoplastic papules, nodules and tumours may have many causes:

- Developmental; naevi.
- Association with internal neoplasia; nodular dermatofibrosis of the German shepherd dog.
- Infectious agents; abscess, botriomycosis, nocardiosis, mycobacterial infection, pseudomycetoma, sporotrichosis, mycetoma.
- Foreign bodies; endogenous, i.e. calcium, keratin, lipid, urate, saliva; exogenous, i.e. sutures, plant awns, silica, remnants of biting or stinging insects, components of injected substances.
- Cysts of epidermal and adnexal origin and cutaneous horn.
- Traumatic lesions; haematomas, neurotropic dermatitis.
- Psychodermatoses; acral lick granuloma.
- Benign mammary hypertrophy.
- Idiopathic disease; nodular panniculitis and sterile pyogranuloma.

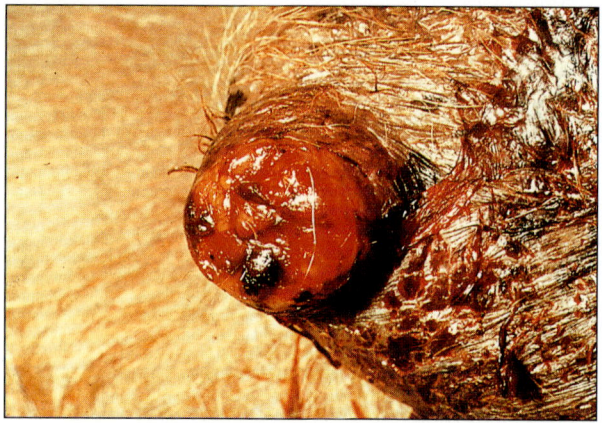

674 **Vascular naevus.** Ulcerated lesion on the scrotum of a Labrador retriever.

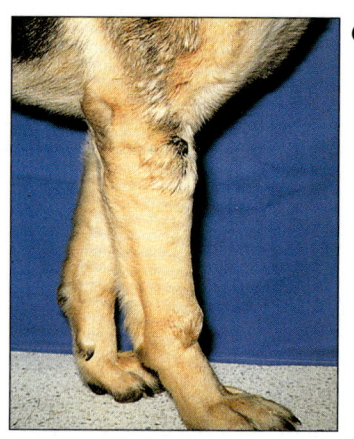

675 **Collagenous naevus.** Multiple nodular lesions on the foreleg of a German shepherd dog. (Illustration courtesy J. A.Yager.)

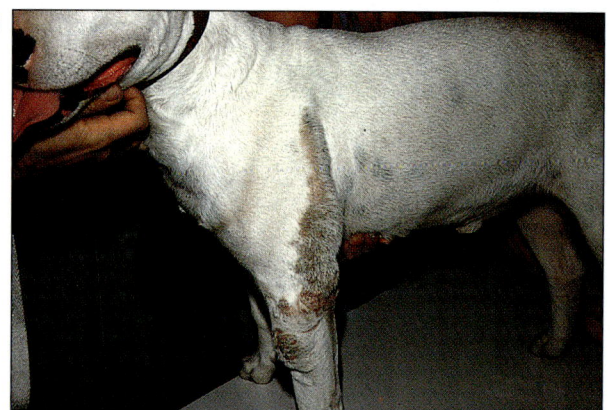

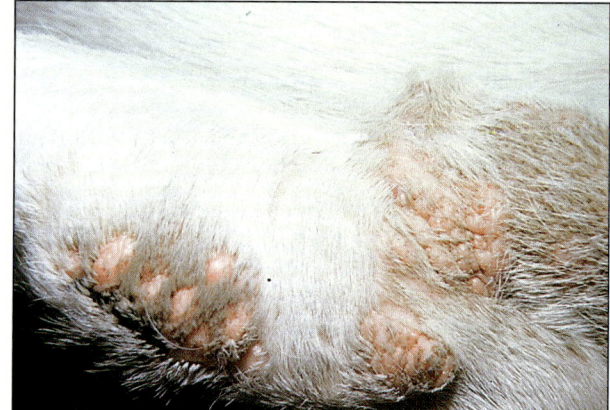

676 and 677 **Collagenous naevus.** Linear form on the shoulder and upper foreleg of a young Bull terrier.

Naevi

Naevi are congenital or acquired, circumscribed, developmental defects of the skin which may arise from any component of the skin or combination thereof. The developmental defect takes the form of hyperplasia of the affected tissue. The condition is rare. Several types of naevi have been described.

678

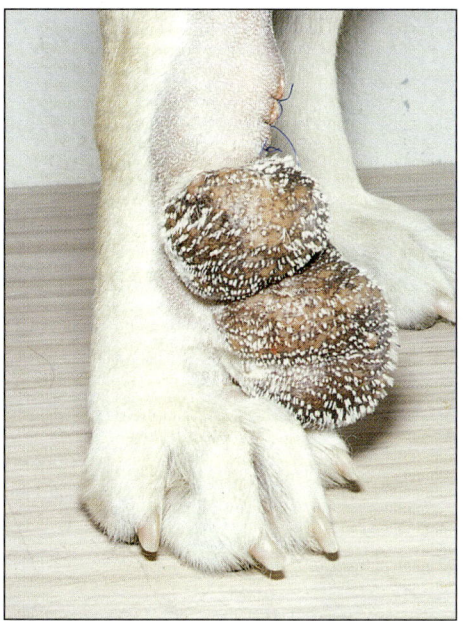

679

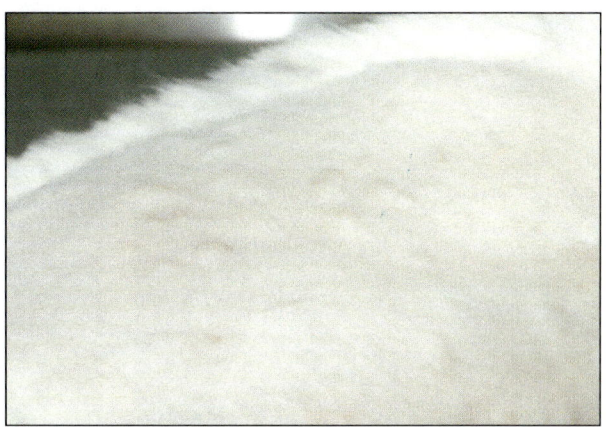

679   Collagenous naevi on the ventral abdominal wall of a New Zealand white rabbit.

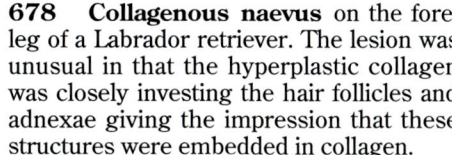

678   Collagenous naevus on the foreleg of a Labrador retriever. The lesion was unusual in that the hyperplastic collagen was closely investing the hair follicles and adnexae giving the impression that these structures were embedded in collagen.

Vascular naevus

This condition occurs in the scrotum of dogs (**674**) and constitutes one of the few emergency skin conditions. On occasion it may be life-threatening. It is characterised by the formation of hyperpigmented elevated plaques in the scrotal skin which may become ulcerated, either spontaneously or through the trauma of the dog continually licking the area, and give rise to profuse and sometimes fatal haemorrhage. The syndrome is seen most frequently in middle-aged or more elderly dogs, particularly in those breeds with pigmented skins, such as black Labrador retrievers, Scottish terriers and Airedale terriers.

The basic pathological change in this condition is the presence in the dermis of collections of collapsed capillaries forming potential vascular spaces initially devoid of blood. These spaces become progressively filled with blood from a large central artery, eventually to form cavernous haemangiomas which bulge the epidermis and produce the clinically appreciable plaques. Ulceration of the overlying epidermis may broach the large central artery and the dog can exsanguinate within a comparatively short space of time.

Collagenous naevus[3,10]

This is a not uncommon condition of dogs in which focal accumulations of collagen present as solitary or multiple, dome-shaped papules and nodules (**675–678**). Multiple collagenous naevi have been reported in the dog, particularly the German shepherd.[10] This condition appeared to be benign, in contrast to nodular dermatofibrosis (see below). Naevi are painless on palpation and are variably alopecic. They may also occur in other animals, such as the rabbit (**679**).

680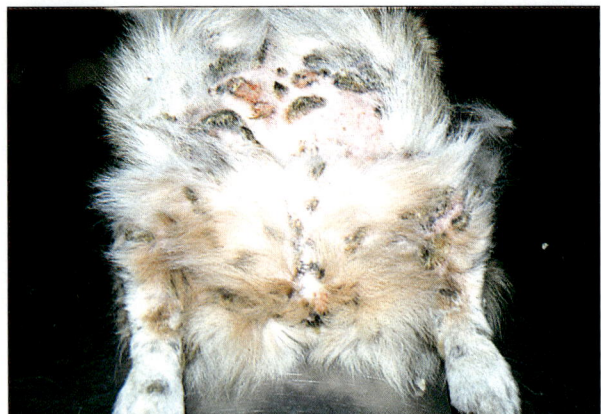

681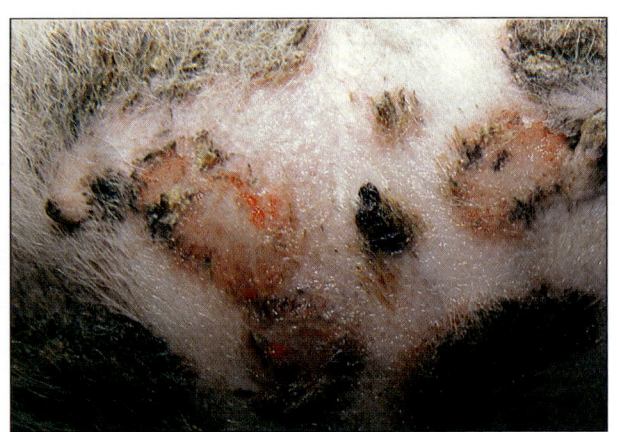

682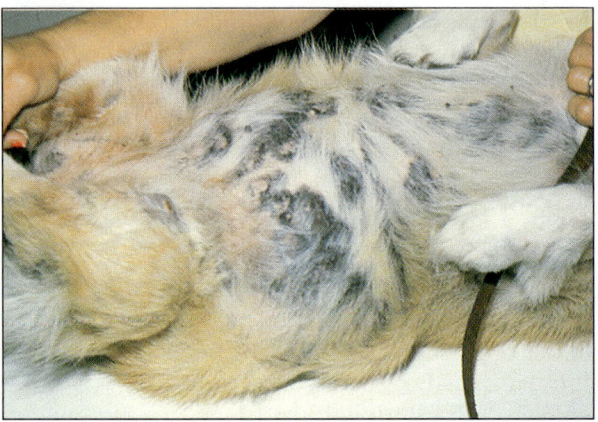

683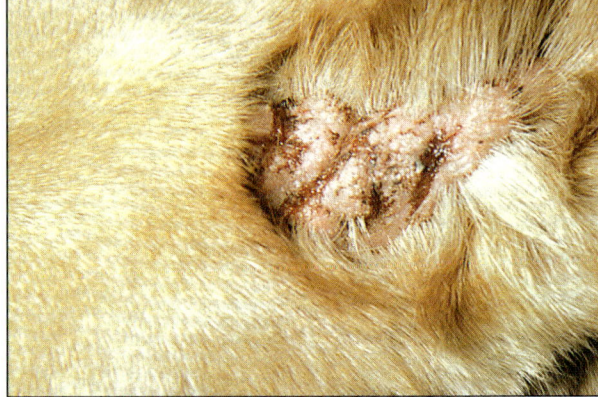

680–682 Epidermal naevus. Orthokeratotic hyperkeratotic and papillomatous hyperplastic lesions on the abdomen of an elderly Pembroke corgi bitch. The lesions healed with hyperpigmentation after a four-week course of cyclophosphamide and prednisolone.

683 Organoid (mixed) naevus. Papillomatous hairy lesion on the occipital region of a Labrador retriever.

Epidermal naevus

In this condition there are hyperpigmented, hyperkeratotic plaques over the trunk (**680–682**). Histologically, the lesion is characterised by orthokeratotic hyperkeratosis and papillomatous hyperplasia.

Hair follicle naevus

(Organoid or mixed naevus, hamartoma). In this form of naevus there is hyperplasia of hair follicles, sebaceous and, more rarely, epitrichial glands. The condition has been reported mainly as occurring on the face and head of cats, and appearing as single or multiple, dome-shaped or pedunculated, papillomatous, hairy lesions (**683**).

684

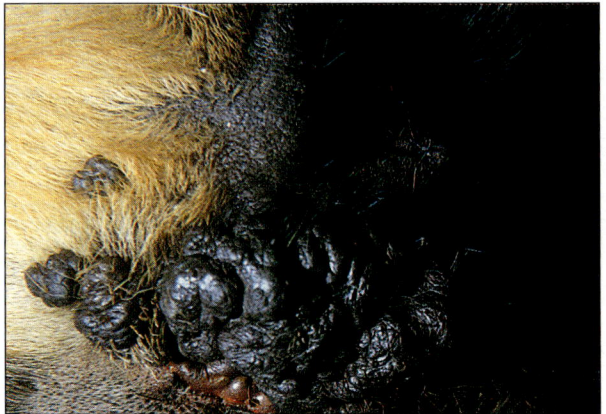

684   Melanocytic naevus. Large heavily pigmented lesions in the perivulvar region of a Rottweiler bitch.

685

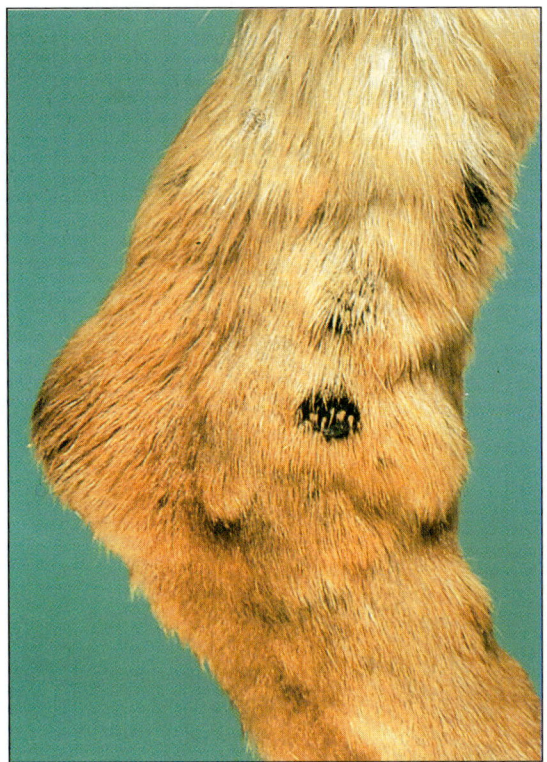

685   Nodular dermatofibrosis. Note the presence of multiple nodules around the hock of this German shepherd dog. This apparently benign presentation is associated with malignant neoplasia of the renal epithelium. Nodular dermatofibrosis must be distinguished from that of multiple collagenous naevi, a benign disorder. (Illustration courtesy of C. Griffin.)

Melanocytic naevus

These lesions (**684**) present a similar appearance to benign melanomas and are seen most commonly in the skin of the abdomen.

Infectious agents

The clinical features and approach to infectious causes of granulomatous dermatoses such as bacteria, mycobacteria and fungi are covered in Chapters 5–7.

Lesions associated with internal neoplasia

Nodular dermatofibrosis is a dermatosis characterised by multiple, discrete fibrous nodules most often situated on the limbs and head (**685**). Nodular dermatofibrosis has been described in the German shepherd and may have an hereditary basis.[6] These lesions are associated with renal neoplasia, particularly renal cystadenocarcinoma and, in some cases, uterine leiomyoma.

686

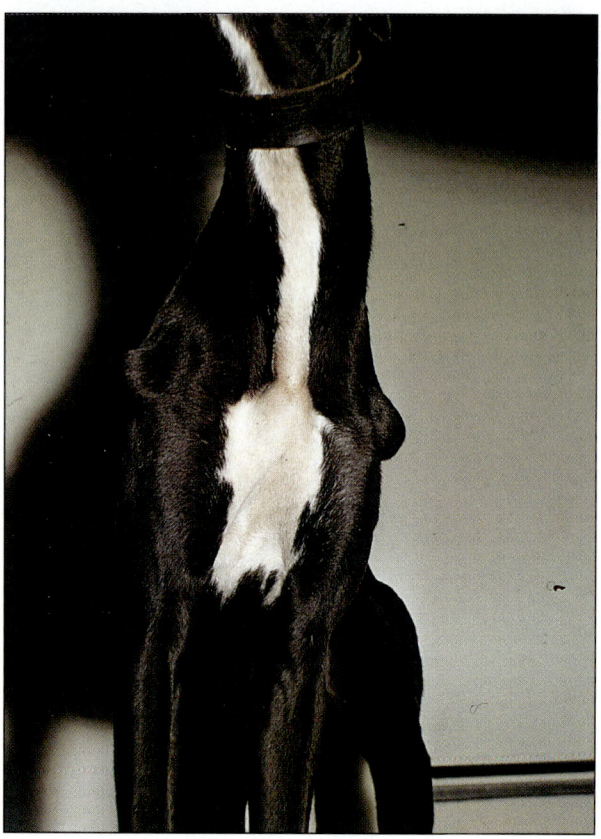

687

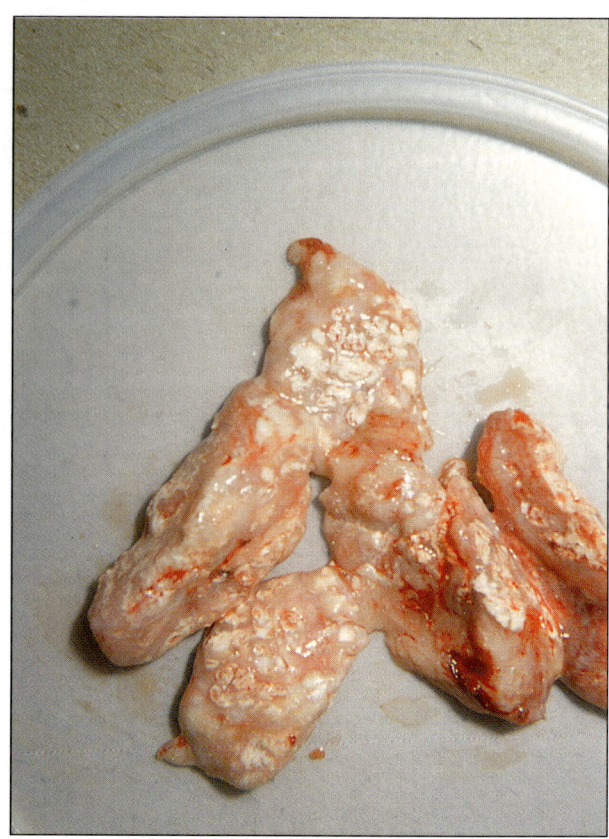

686   Calcinosis circumscripta. Bilateral lesions overlying the shoulder joints of a young Greyhound.

687   Calcinosis cutis. Excised lesion sectioned to show foci of chalky material surrounded by granulomatous inflammation separated by fibrous trabeculae.

Foreign bodies

Endogenous substances

Free calcium may provoke an intense inflammatory reaction in some instances (calcinosis cutis) but may also be seen in more discrete, minimally-inflammatory lesions such as calcinosis circumscripta. These lesions are localised areas of calcification of the skin occurring most commonly in younger dogs of the large breeds, especially German shepherd dogs.[9] The lesions are dome-shaped, firm to hard, single or multiple and may be ulcerated. They may discharge a chalky-white, pasty, gritty material. Predilection sites are over bony prominences and around joints (**686**). A section of a lesion shows foci of white, chalky material surrounded by granulation tissue and separated by fibrous trabeculae (**687**). The cause of the condition is unknown but trauma is suspected of playing a part in the aetiology.

Keratin may reach the dermis from ruptured hair follicles in diseases such as demodicosis or in conditions associated with folliculitis and deep pyoderma. The dermo-epidermal compartmentalisation is compromised and follicular contents enter the dermis where they provoke an inflammatory reaction. Keratin may also be inoculated by grass awns resulting in inflamed, erythematous nodules, typically found in the interdigital web (**688–690**).

688

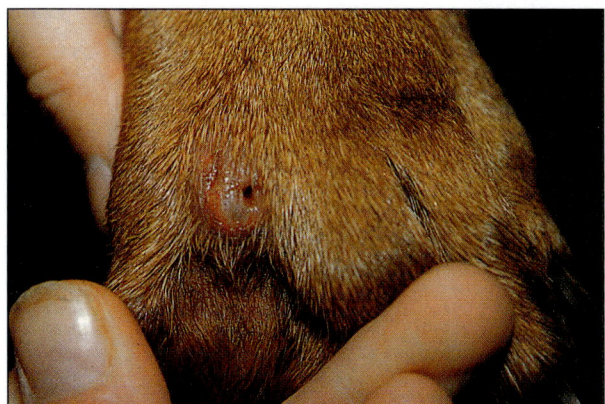

689

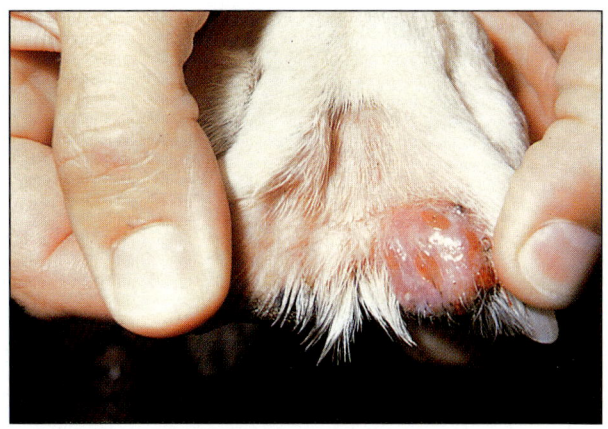

690

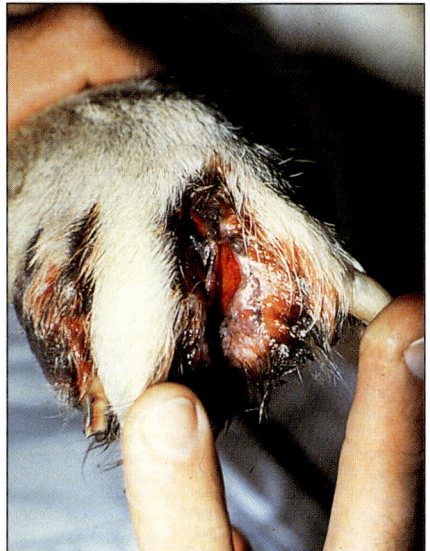

688–690 **Foreign body reactions to penetrating grass awn** in the interdigital region. These are not cysts. Failure to demonstrate a foreign body should prompt treatment with broad spectrum antibacterial agents rather than systemic glucocorticoids.

691

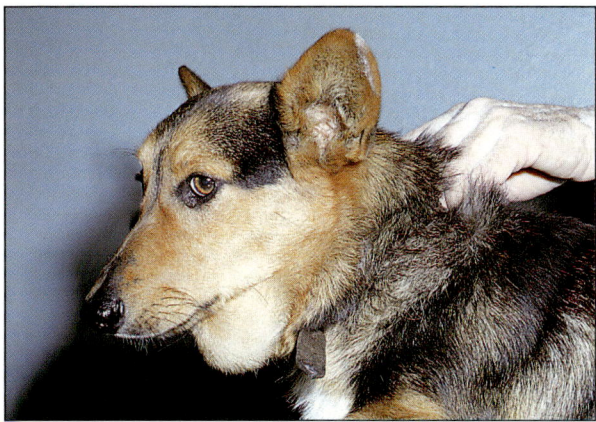

691 **Salivary mucocoele** in a German shepherd dog.

Free lipid also may provoke an inflammatory granulomatous reaction and may result in fistula formation. Reaction to free lipid may be found in a number of uncommon dermatoses such as xanthomas (usually accompanying dyslipoproteinaemia), pansteatitis (Chapter 11) and nodular panniculitis (see below).

Other components of the body may provoke distension of the skin or inflammation within or below the skin when free within the dermis or subcutis. Salivary mucocoeles are not uncommon in the dog but are rare in the cat. There is a fluctuant swelling under the tongue, in the submandibular space or in the parotid region. The swelling results from accumulation of saliva in the subcutis from blockage and rupture of a salivary gland duct (**691**).

Exogenous substances

Substances such as suture material may occasionally provoke granulomatous reactions, nodules or even calcinosis cutis[4], particularly if non-absorbable sutures are placed subcutaneously. Penetrating grass awns[1], silica, fibreglass fibres, insect stings and mouth parts (particularly from ticks) are occasionally causes of cutaneous nodules, granulomatous reactions or fistulae.

692

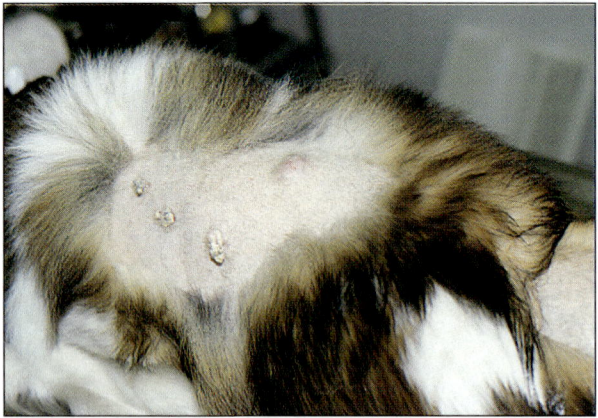

692   Epidermal cysts on the trunk of a Shetland sheepdog. Multiple lesions such as this may be difficult to manage as excision is tiresome and new lesions frequently occur.

693

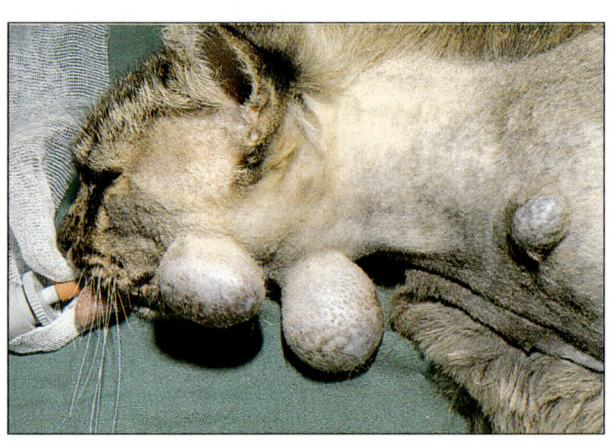

693   Epitrichial sweat gland cysts are rare in the cat. This illustration shows a number of pedunculated epitrichial sweat gland cysts on the neck of a cat.

694

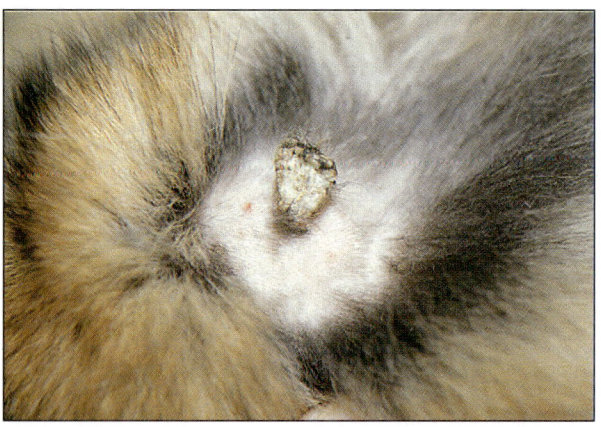

694   Solitary cutaneous horn on the head of a Shetland sheepdog.

695

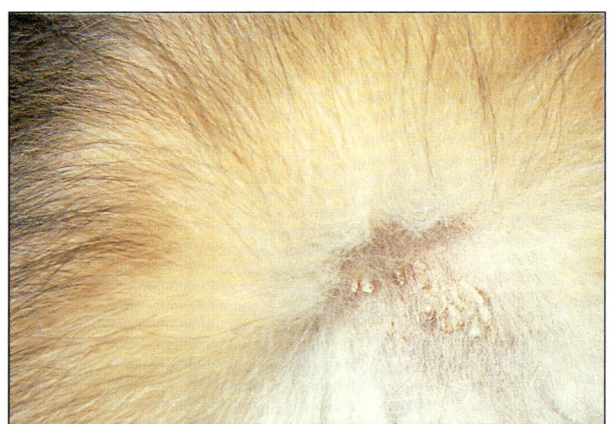

695   Cutaneous horn. Cluster of slender cutaneous horns in a Shetland sheepdog.

Cysts of epidermal and adnexal origin and cutaneous horn

Epidermal and sebaceous cysts are common. They present as soft to firm nodules, commonly on the dorsal trunk or base of the tail (**692**). Occasionally cysts may be pedunculated (**693**). Many of the epidermal and sebaceous cysts have a crusted fistulae at their peak, an indication that spontaneous rupture has taken place. Some individuals suffer from multiple, recurrent cysts which may make management difficult.

Cutaneous horns are firm, horn-like projections from the skin that may be up to 5 cm in length (**694**). Sometimes a small group of slender cutaneous horns may be formed (**695**). The horn may result from papillomas or keratoses and if broken off it may regrow from its base in the skin. The lesions may be single or multiple and have no apparent age, sex or site predilections.

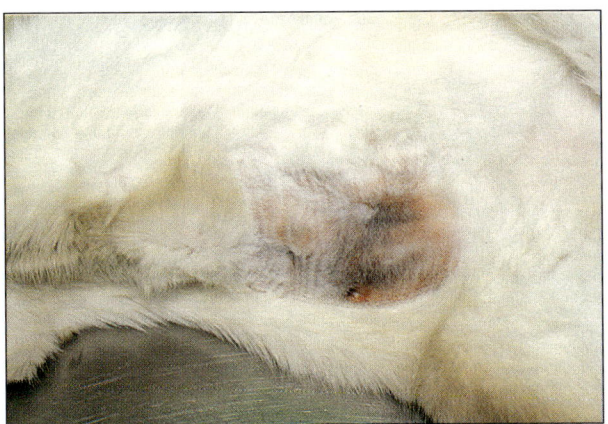

696   Traumatic penetration by an air gun pellet. There is a bruised nodule on this cat. The entry wound is visible.

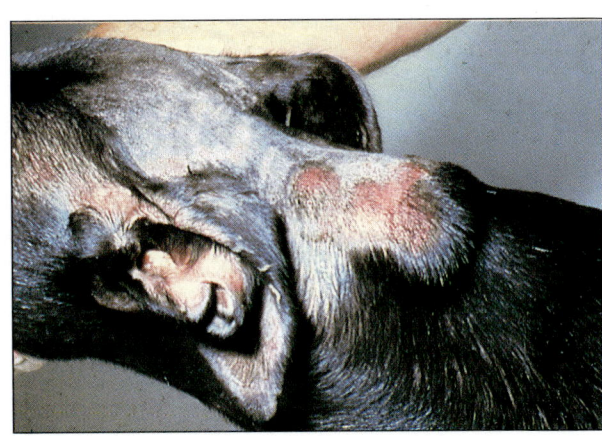

697   Sterile abscess formation at the site of a subcutaneous injection into the dorsal neck of a dog.

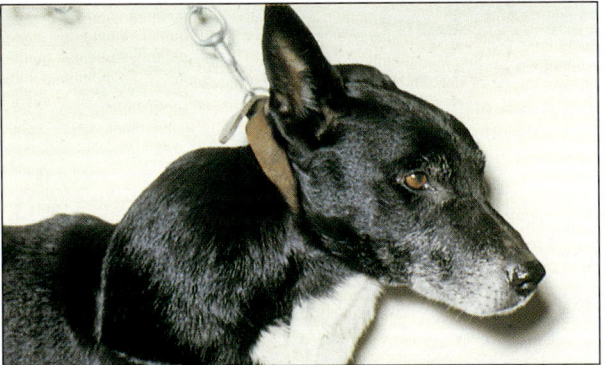

698   Subcutaneous haematoma on the back of the neck of a crossbred dog resulting from a fight injury.

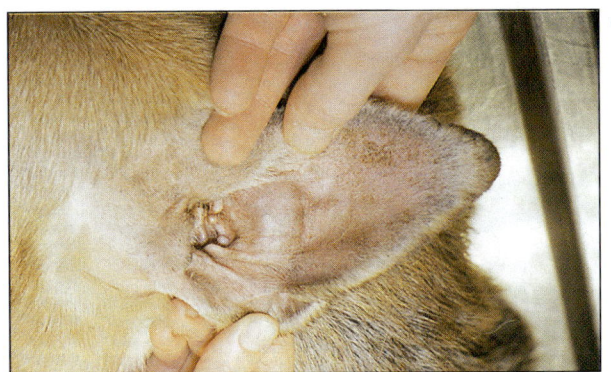

699   Aural haematoma at the base of the pinna.

Traumatic lesions

Trauma from penetrating air gun pellets or darts may result in swollen, bruised and painful nodules (**696**). Sterile abscesses may occur at the site of subcutaneous injections (**697**).

Haematomas are usually the result of accidental or surgical trauma. These lesions are usually in the subcutis and can form quite large, slightly fluctuant, tumour-like masses which enlarge rapidly (**698**). Aural haematomas occur on the pinnae (**699**). Self trauma has been considered the most common cause, often a result of otodectic mange or atopy. However, the presence of autoantibodies suggests that in some cases there may be an autoimmune aetiology.[5]

Neurotropic dermatitis may result in ulcerated nodules and areas of chronic self trauma similar in appearance to canine acral lick granuloma. However, in neurotropic dermatitis the self trauma is a reaction to abnormal sensation resulting from damage to afferent nerves (**700**).

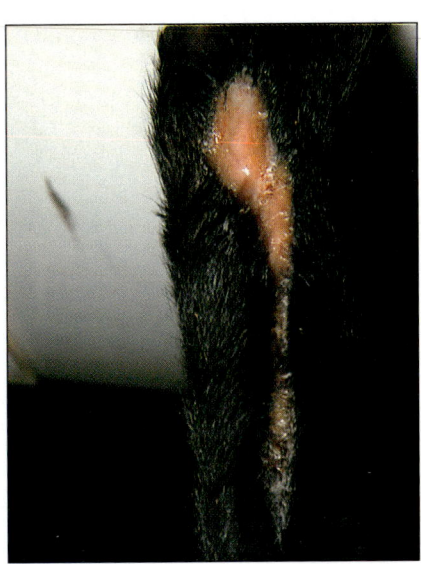

700   Neurotropic dermatitis. Non-healing lesion on the foreleg of a dog following brachial plexus avulsion.

701

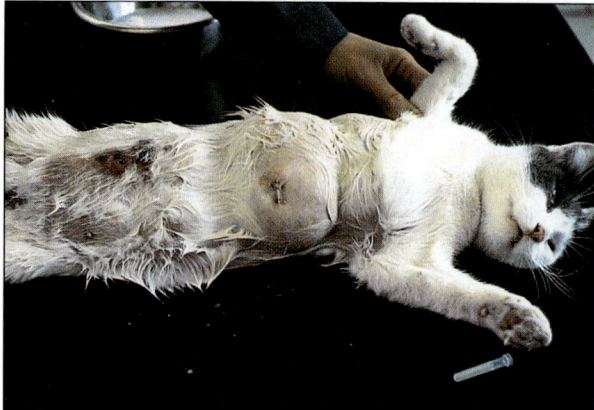

701   Benign mammary hypertrophy. Note traumatic lesions due to contact with the ground.

702

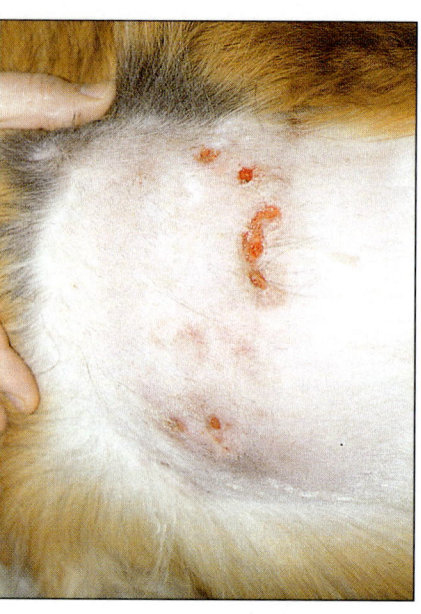

702   Sterile nodular panniculitis. Nodules and discharging fistulae on the lateral thoracic wall of a Shetland sheepdog.

703

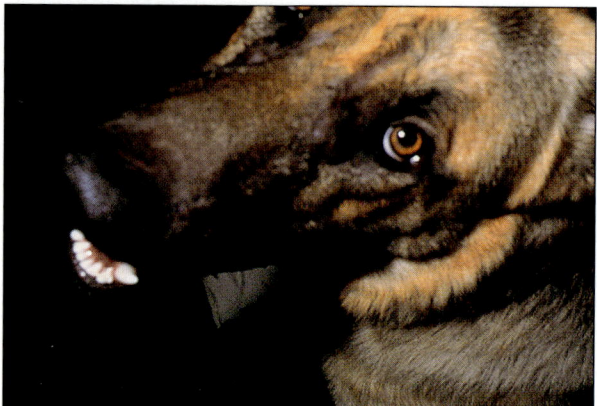

703   Sterile pyogranuloma on the face of a German shepherd dog.

704

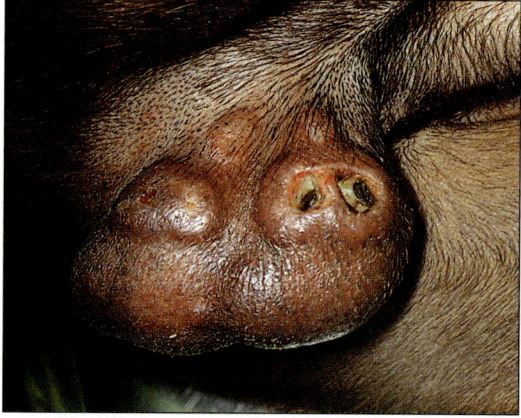

704   Sterile pyogranuloma. Ulcerated lesions on the scrotum of a Doberman pinscher dog.

Psychodermatoses

Acral lick granuloma presents as an erythematous nodule or plaque (see Chapter 16).

Benign mammary hypertrophy

A condition seen in young female cats, which appears to be progesterone-dependent. It has been reported in cats in the early stages of pregnancy, and also in spayed cats treated with progestagens, notably megestrol acetate.[2] Histologically, there is pronounced fibro-adenomatous hypertrophy of the affected mammary gland(s). The hypertrophied glands may be sufficiently large as to sustain superficial trauma by contact with the ground (**701**).

Idiopathic disease

A number of dermatoses presenting as papules, nodules and discharging fistulae have no identified cause even though the clinical features are well characterised. In some cases a definitive diagnosis may be made whereas in others the diagnosis is made by exclusion of all known causes.

Nodular panniculitis is an uncommon condition in which there is sterile inflammation of the subcutaneous fat.[8] The cause is unknown. There is no breed, age or sex predisposition. Clinical signs are confined to the skin in most cases and consist of nodules and fistulae, particularly on the neck and lateral thoracic wall (**702**). The discharge is thin oily and often yellow-brown in colour. A variation of this clinical picture has been reported in the German shepherd dog. Individuals of this breed exhibit small fistulae on the plantar aspects of the feet, in the metacarpal and metatarsal region in particular.

Sterile pyogranulomata present as single or multiple papules or nodules found principally on the feet but also on the head and elsewhere on the body (**703** and **704**). Chronic pododermatitis is often complicated by the introduction of keratin into the dermis which results in granulomatous inflammation which is refractory to antibacterial therapy. There is a predisposition on males, particularly in certain breeds such as Boxer, Golden retriever, Great Dane and Weimaraner.[7] Although some of the pedal lesions may show a limited response to systemic antibacterial therapy, the resolution is minimal and systemic glucocorticoids may be indicated.

References

1. Brennan, K. E and Ihrke, P. J. (1983). Grass awn migration in dogs and cats: a retrospective study of 182 cases. *Journal of the American Veterinary Medical Association*, **182**: 1201–1204.

2. Chen, J. C. and Bellenger, C. R. (1987). Obese appearance, mammary development and retardation of hair growth following megestrol acetate administration to cats. *Journal of Small Animal Practice*, **28**: 1161–1167.

3. Jones, B. R., Alley, M. R. and Craig, A. S. (1985). Cutaneous collagen nodules in a dog. *Journal of Small Animal Practice*, **26**: 445–451.

4. Kirby, B. K., Knoll, J. S., Manley, P. A. and Miller, L. M. (1989). Calcinosis circumscripta associated with polydioxanone suture in two young dogs. *Veterinary Surgery*, **18**: 216–220.

5. Kuwahara, J. (1986). Canine and feline aural haematoma: clinical, experimental and clinicopathologic observations. *American Journal of Veterinary Research*, **47**: 2300–2308.

6. Lium, B and Moe, L. (1985). Hereditary multifocal renal cystadenocarcinoma and nodular dermatofibrosis in the German shepherd dog: macroscopic and histopathologic changes. *Veterinary Pathology*, **22**: 447–455.

7. Panic, R. (1992). Sterile pyogranulomatous and granulomatous disorders of the dog and cat. In: Kirk, R. W. and Bonagura, J. D. (Eds.). *Current Veterinary Therapy XI*, pp. 536–539. W. B. Saunders, Philadelphia.

8. Scott, D. W. and Anderson, W. I. (1988). Panniculitis in dogs and cats: a retrospective analysis of 78 cases. *Journal of the American Animal Hospital Association*, **24**: 551–559.

9. Scott, D. W. and Buerger, R. G. (1988). Idiopathic calcinosis circumscripta in the dog: a retrospective analysis of 130 cases. *Journal of the American Animal Hospital Association*, **24**: 651–658.

10. Scott, D. W., Yager-Johnson, J. A., Manning, T. O., Walton, D. K., Johnson, R. P., Parker, V. M. and Carman, P. S. (1984). Nevi in the dog. *Journal of the American Animal Hospital Association*, **20**: 505–511.

Chapter 16

Psychogenic dermatoses

Introduction

These dermatoses are regarded as examples of stereotypic behaviour in which there is constant repetition of a meaningless gesture or behaviour pattern. When carried out to excess they often result in self-injury.[1] In dogs, the behaviour may involve continued licking, scratching or chewing at one, or several, areas of the body resulting in lick granulomas. In the cat the typical presentation is one of chronic overgrooming resulting in areas of alopecia.[5,7] Although in some cases there is an underlying cause of chronic pruritus such as atopy, pyoderma or underlying disease[2,5], the self trauma is perpetuated as a habit. In the true psychodermatosis, no discernible cause is identified[5], although an abnormal neurological function has been reported in the sensory nerves of dogs with acral lick granuloma.[3]

- The diagnosis of a psychogenic dermatosis is usually achieved by exclusion.

Canine acral lick dermatitis (acral pruritic nodule, 'lick granuloma')

This is a relatively common condition in which a firm, thickened, oval plaque of skin is formed on the lower foreleg or hindleg as a result of persistent licking (**705**). The constant licking causes and maintains ulceration of the surface of the plaque but also prevents secondary, surface bacterial infection. The condition occurs most commonly in male dogs.[2,5] Labrador retrievers, Golden retrievers, German shepherd dogs, Doberman pinschers and both English and Irish setters are predisposed.[2,5] There is no age predisposition.

The most frequent sites affected are the anterior aspect of the metacarpal region, the carpus and the lateral tarso-metatarsal area (**706**).[2,4,5]

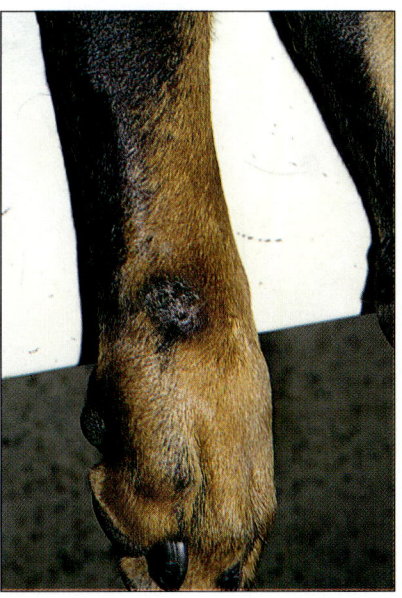

705 **Canine acral lick dermatitis.** Classic presentation of a discrete, ulcerated, raised nodule overlying the metacarpals on a Doberman pinscher.

706 **Canine acral lick dermatitis.** Acral pruritic nodule on lateral metatarsal area of Dalmatian bitch.

705

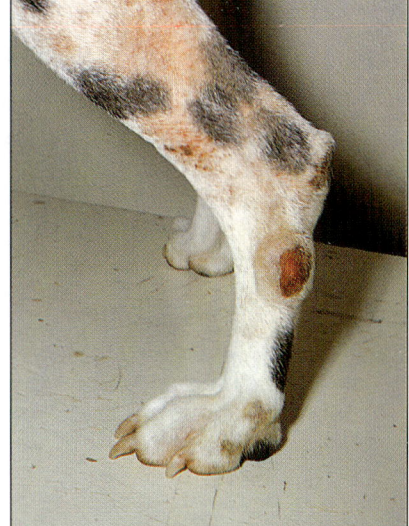

706

707

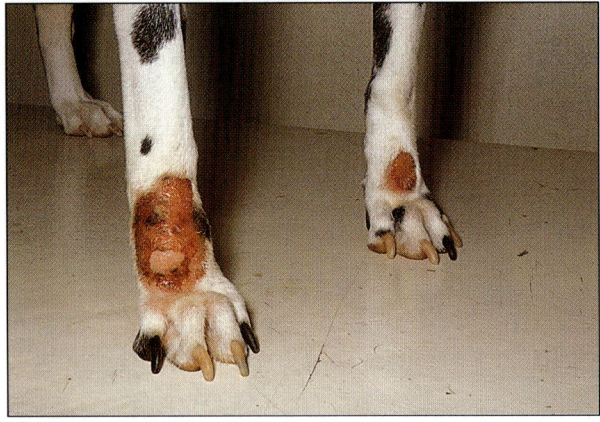

707   Canine acral lick dermatitis. More severe, bilateral lesions on the anterior aspects of the metacarpal regions of a Dalmatian bitch.

Lesions are usually unilateral although more than one limb can be affected (**707**), in which case the prognosis is poorer.[5]

The condition is commonly thought to be psychogenic in origin, resulting from boredom in dogs left to their own devices while their owners are out at work or otherwise occupied. However, in many cases the condition reflects an underlying organic cause such as arthritis, a chronic slow healing wound, bacterial infection or hypersensitivity reactions such as atopy or dietary intolerance. Neurotropic dermatitis should also be considered.

Acral lick dermatitis is characterised by:
- Pruritic plaque-like thickening of the skin of the limbs.

Differential diagnoses include:
- Deep folliculitis.
- Hypersensitivities and underlying skeletal abnormalities.
- Foreign body granulomas.
- Neurotropic dermatitis.
- Neoplasia.

Diagnosis is made by:
- Consideration of the history and clinical signs.
- Rule out of differentials.
- Histopathological examination of biopsy samples.

- Many cases of apparent psychogenic acral lick granuloma respond to long courses of systemic antibacterial treatment. Lesions should always be biopsied to assess the degree of bacterial folliculitis.
- Rule out underlying bone or joint disease, atopy and dietary intolerance before diagnosing psychogenic acral lick granuloma as these conditions may respond to specific therapy or management.

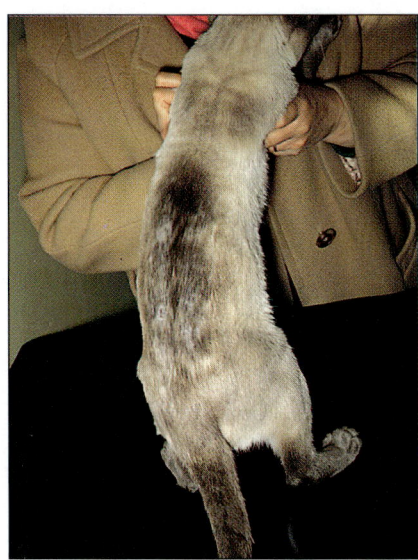

708

708 Feline psychogenic alopecia. Characteristic lesion overlying the dorsal thoracolumbar area of a Siamese cat. Note the dark colouration of the regrown hair.

709

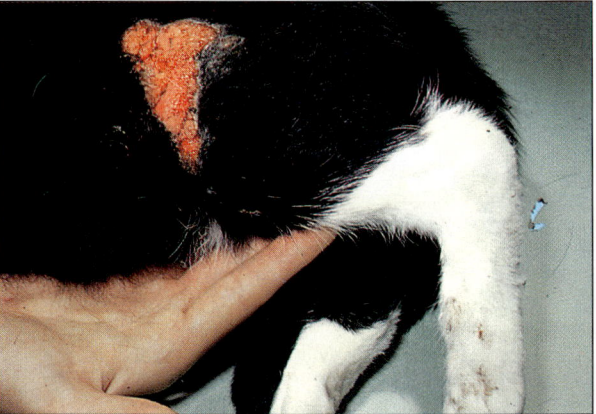

710

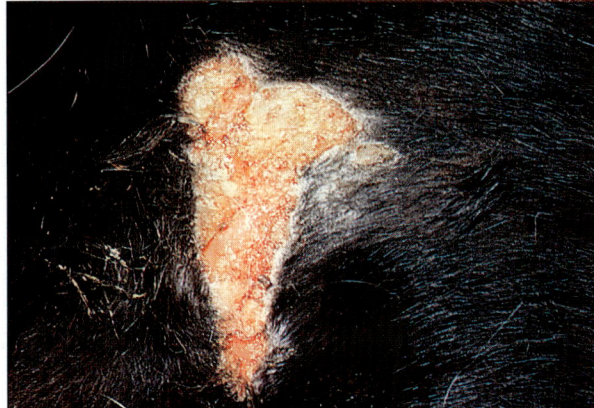

709 and 710 Feline psychogenic dermatosis. Dermatitic form showing chronic severe erosion and ulceration in the flank of a cat. This lesion had recurred twice following radical excision but resolved after a course of X-ray therapy.

Feline psychogenic alopecia (trichotillomania)

This condition, which is the feline equivalent of canine acral lick dermatitis, is characterised by alopecia. The cat licks and chews at areas within easy reach, such as the medial thighs, the ventral abdomen and dorsal lumbosacral region, causing bilaterally symmetrical loss of hair (**708**). As is the case in the dog, there may be a discernible underlying cause such as flea bite hypersensitivity, atopy or dietary hypersensitivity. The psychodermatosis occurs spontaneously in some cats. Although Oriental cats have been cited as predisposed[5], European short-haired cats are also affected.[7]

The condition may result from displacement phenomena, triggered by a new baby in the house, new furniture or carpets, noisy visiting children, moving feeding dishes or sanitary trays from their usual location or threats to territory due to a new cat moving in nearby. The cat becomes 'uptight' and retires to a place of concealment where it proceeds to vent its frustrations by licking at one particular spot or area. Such licking and biting may be quite gentle and produce only hair loss but may be more vigorous and obsessive resulting in erosion and ulceration, the dermatitic form.[5]

Often the owners will assert that the cat does not lick or bite the affected area, but microscopic examination of trichogram preparations will reveal that hairs have been subjected to trauma (see Chapter 3). Siamese, Siamese crosses and Burmese cats will sometimes remove the hair from the middle of the back without damaging the skin. As the hair colour is temperature dependent in these cats the affected area is delineated by regrowth of darker hair coat.

In the more severe dermatitic form ('licker's skin') the vigorous licking and biting at one particular spot may cause a severe dermatitis with erosion and ulceration (**709** and **710**). Some of these lesions are thought to be the result of a neuritis, as they are sometimes situated along the course of a major nerve branch. Occasionally an eosinophilic granuloma may develop at the site.

Feline psychodermatoses are characterised by:
- Hair loss in the absence of any observable cause.
- Bilaterally symmetrical alopecia.
- Occasionally focal erosion and ulceration.

Main differential diagnoses are:
- Flea bite hypersensitivity, atopy and dietary intolerance.
- Dermatophytosis.
- Eosinophilic plaque.

The diagnosis is made by:
- Consideration of the history and clinical signs.
- Elimination of other causes of pruritus or alopecia.

References

1. Dodman, N. H., Shuster, L., White, S. D., Court, M. H., Parker, D. and Dixon, R. (1988). Use of narcotic antagonists to modify stereotypic self-licking, self-chewing, and scratching behavior in dogs. *Journal of the American Veterinary Medical Association*, **193**: 815–819.

2. Scott, D. W. and Walton, D. K. (1984). Clinical evaluation of a topical treatment for canine acral lick dermatitis. *Journal of the American Animal Hospital Association*, **20**: 565–570.

3. van Ness, J. J. (1986). Electrophysiological evidence of sensory nerve dysfunction in 10 dogs with acral lick dermatitis. *Journal of the American Animal Hospital Association*, **22**: 157–160.

4. Veith, L. (1986). Acral lick dermatitis in the dog. *Canine Practice*, **13**: 15–22.

5. Walton, D. K. (1986). Psychodermatoses. In: Kirk, R,. W. (Ed.), *Current Veterinary Therapy IX*, pp. 557–559. W. B. Saunders, Philadelphia.

6. White, S. D. (1990). Naltrexone for treatment of acral lick dermatitis in dogs. *Journal of the American Veterinary Medical Association*, **196**: 1073–1076.

7. Willemse, T., Spruijt, B. M. and van Osterwyck, A. (1989). Feline psychogenic alopecia and the role of the opioid system. In: von Tscharner, C. and Halliwell, R. E. W. (Eds.), *Advances in Veterinary Dermatology, 1*, pp. 195–198. Baillière Tindall, London.

Chapter 17:

Congenital and hereditary dermatoses

A number of dermatological conditions can be shown to have a heritable basis on the strength of the analysis of test breeding programmes and heritance studies. A larger number of more common dermatoses, such as atopy, generalised demodicosis or mast cell neoplasia, for example, can be shown to exhibit breed or familial predispositions which suggest, in part, a heritable factor. This chapter will concentrate on the former diseases as the latter group have been covered in the relevant sections earlier in the book.

Congenital dermatoses are present at birth and do not always reflect a heritable cause. Heritable defects may be congenital (i.e. present at birth) or tardive (apparent some time after birth). Not all defects are regarded as worrying by the breeder. Some, such as the feline rex mutation and the hairless characteristics of Mexican or Chinese crested dogs are regarded as desirable.

Heritable and congenital dermatoses are refractory to treatment.[14] Patently, an animal with an ectodermal defect cannot be treated and hair or teeth will not appear if the basic elements are not in place at birth. However, in the more complex disorders such as icthyosis or familial dermatomyositis some of the more severe signs may be ameliorated by treatment.

- Many of these dermatoses are self-evident but some, such as colour dilute alopecia or dermatomyositis, have important differential diagnoses. Histopathological examination of representative punch biopsy samples is a cost-effective diagnostic tool.

711

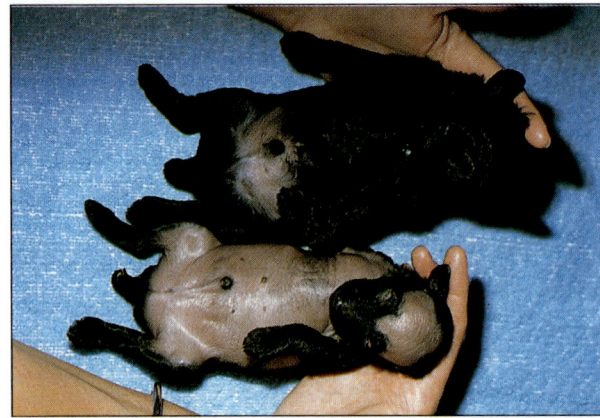

711   Congenital ectodermal defect. Miniature Poodle littermate puppies showing extensive alopecia on the ventral surface of the trunk and the head of the affected animal. (Illustration courtesy K. V. Mason.)

712

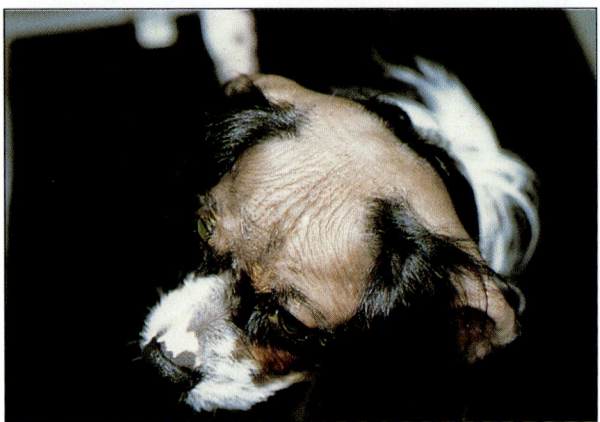

713

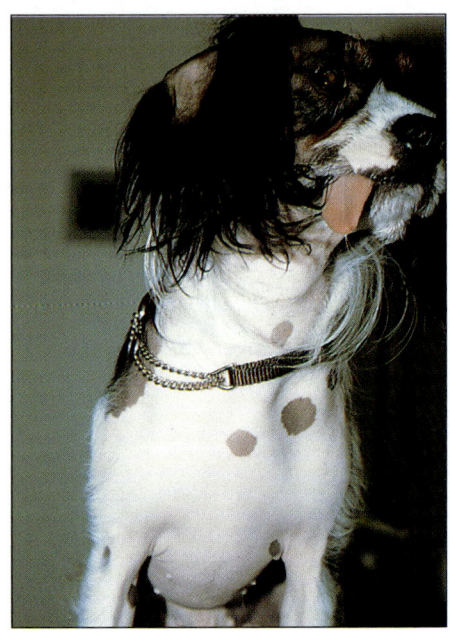

712 and 713   Congenital ectodermal defect in a dog. Note the areas of alopecia. This dog had more extensive ectodermal problems than the one illustrated in **711**. Note the inability to contain the tongue within the oral cavity, a result of an absence of dentition. (Illustration courtesy I. S. Mason.)

Epithelial and adnexal defects

Epitheliogenesis imperfecta, ectodermal defect, ectodermal dysplasia

These diseases reflect abnormalities in the embryological development of the skin. Epitheliogenesis inperfecta is extremely rare and usually fatal.[7] All epithelial components are absent from affected areas. These defects are clinically apparent as variably sized patches of exudative ulceration. Animals are at risk from bacteraemia and septicaemia. Less serious defects are termed ectodermal defects or dysplasias and reflect an absence of adnexal components rather than absolute absence of epithelium. Many of these animals exhibit an absence of hair as a consequence of an absence of hair follicles in affected areas (**711**). Alopecia universalis is regarded as desirable by breeders of certain breeds of dog and cat although it may also occur as a spontaneous mutation. Some animals present with variably-sized patches of alopecia and exhibit other ectodermal deficiencies such as an absence of dentition (**712** and **713**).

714 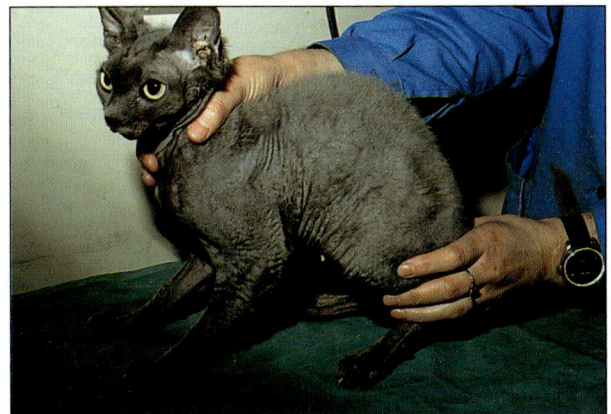 **715**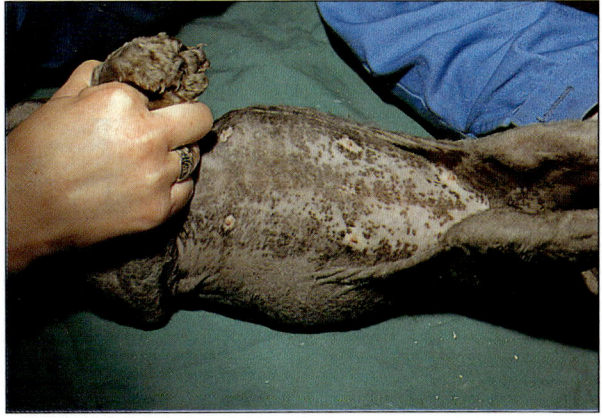

714 and 715   Congenital hypotrichosis in a Devon rex cat. Note the areas of alopecia on the thoracic wall and on the ventral trunk. (Illustrations courtesy K. L. Thoday.)

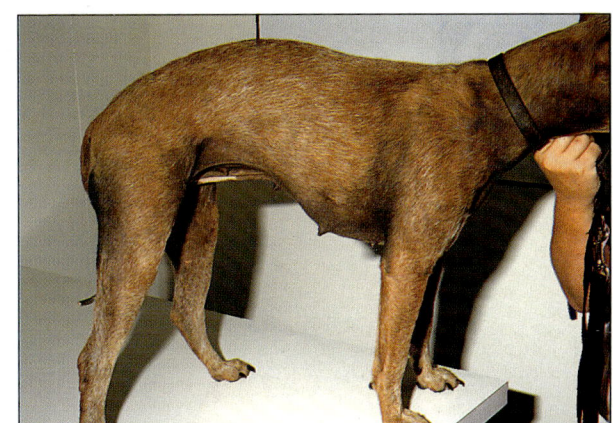 **716**

716   Congenital hypotrichosis in an Australian kelpie bitch. This is a tardive condition becoming apparent during the first year of life. There is hypotrichosis of the neck and trunk.

Alopecic disorders

Alopecia is not always associated with an absence of hair follicles. In congenital or hereditary conditions exhibiting alopecia in the presence of hair follicles the term hypotrichosis or follicular dysplasia is used. In these animals there are hair follicles within the epidermis or dermis but either no hair is produced or, if it is produced, some or all of the hair is abnormal. This is in contrast to alopecia associated with an ectodermal defect where there are no hair follicles at all in affected skin.

Hypotrichosis and **follicular dysplasia** occur in both the cat and the dog and result in thinning of the coat and possibly alopecia. The Devon rex cat has a tendency to lose its fur, especially older cats. The condition is part of the rex syndrome for the rex coat is itself abnormal with an absence of primary hairs and a decreased number of thin secondary hairs. In some individuals the abnormality is intensified and there is a more severe deficiency of the secondary hairs. This, and the tendency of these abnormal hairs to fracture, results in patchy or generalised alopecia (**714** and **715**).

Follicular dystrophy is well recognised in some breeds of dog, for example the tardive hypotrichosis seen in the Australian kelpie (**716**). Occasional cases of congenital follicular dysplasia

717

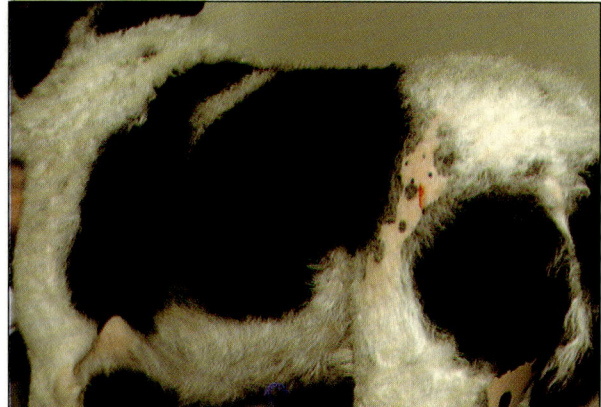

718

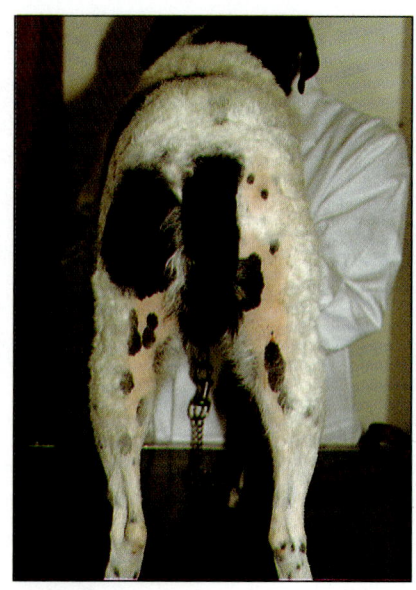

717–719 Follicular dysplasia in a cross-breed. The dog exhibited patches of alopecia over the hind-quarters. Examination of the hairs from these areas revealed abnormal shafts (**719**).

719

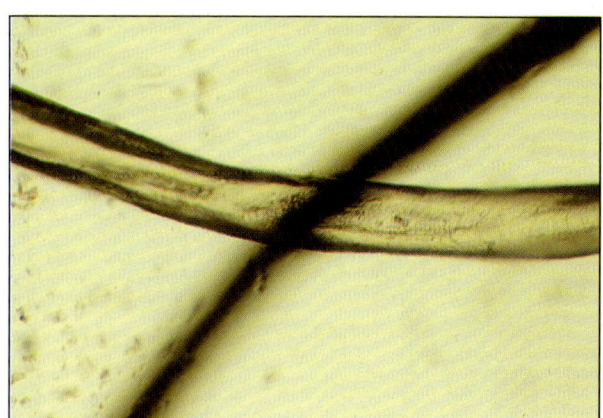

720

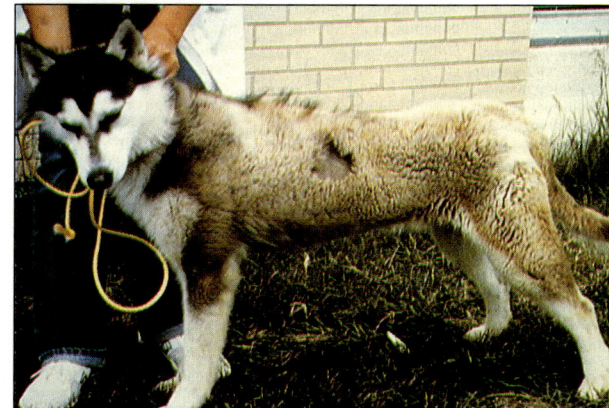

720 Hair follicle dysplasia of Siberian huskies. Note the rust coloured, woolly puppylike coat, the clipped patch on which the hair has failed to regrow and the normal appearance of the head and lower limbs. (Illustration from: Post, K., Dignean, M. A. and Clark, E. G. [1988]. Hair follicle dysplasia of Siberian huskies. *Journal of the American Animal Hospital Association*, **24**: 659–662.)

will be encountered and can be expected to occur in any breed (**717** and **718**). Clues to the diagnosis can be obtained from the examination of tricho-grams (see Chapter 3) which may reveal shaft abnormalities (**719**). In some instances the follicular abnormality is restricted to black hairs (**black hair follicle dysplasia**).

A tardive follicular dysplasia of unknown aetiology has been described in Siberian huskies.[16] Until the age of three or four months, affected animals have an apparently normal hair coat.

Between that age and two years old, the guard hairs fail to shed, deteriorate, break and fail to regrow. The head may remain unaffected but the remainder of the body coat consists of secondary hairs, which have a woolly texture with a rusty colour (**720**). There is arrest of the hair cycle in the catagen stage, primarily affecting the primary follicles. It is thought that the rusty colour of the remaining secondary hairs may be due to abnormal exposure to ultra violet radiation.

Colour dilute alopecia may be associated with

721 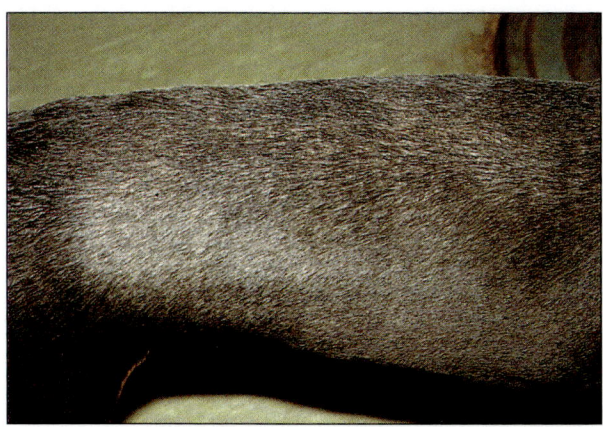 722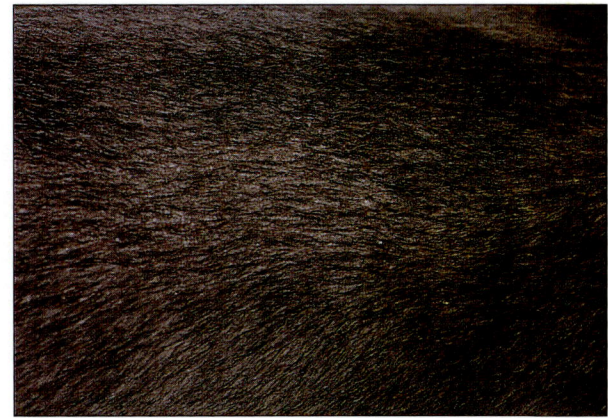

723 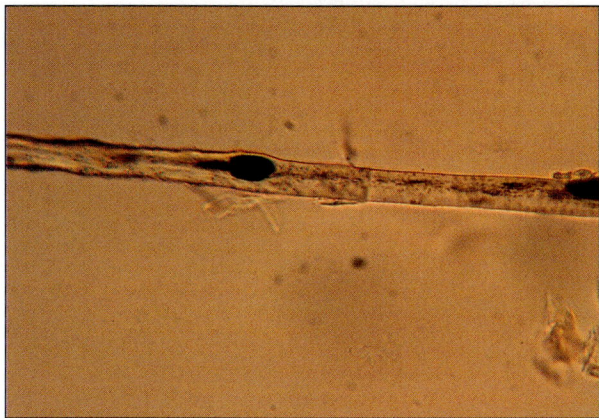 724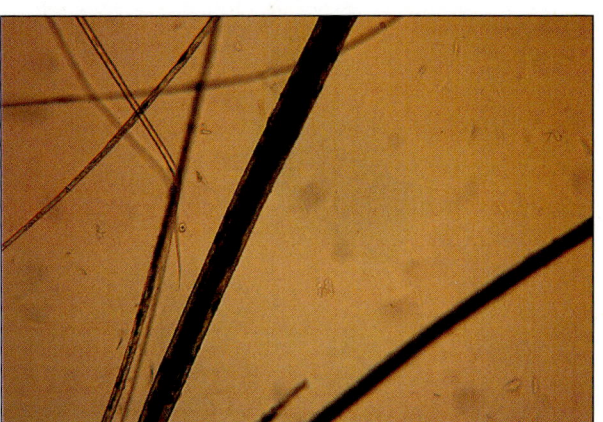

721–724   Colour dilute alopecia in a blue Doberman pinscher. Note the sparse hair and the focal sites of alopecia which result from either hyperkeratotic follicles or a secondary superficial pyoderma. Trichogram preparation of hair from a colour dilute Doberman pinscher (**723**). Note the irregular clumps of melanin within the hair shaft and compare with the hair shaft from a normal Doberman pinscher (**724**). In the normal hair the pigment is distributed evenly along the shaft. (Illustration courtesy D. Bentley.)

alopecia in certain individuals. The condition is usually tardive and is characterised by the production of abnormal, rather wiry hairs and alopecia.[10] Although most common in breeds such as the blue Doberman pinscher and fawn Irish setter it has been reported in other breeds[12] (**721** and **722**). In addition to the abnormal coat there may also be papules which arise as a result of follicular hyperkeratosis. Microscopic examination of hair shafts reveals abnormal clumping of melanin granules (**723** and **724**) and, occasionally, shaft defects.

- Not all colour dilute dogs have follicular dysplasia. Secondary superficial pyoderma is a common complication (see Chapter 5) and is a prime differential diagnosis, as is hypothyroidism (Chapter 10).

725

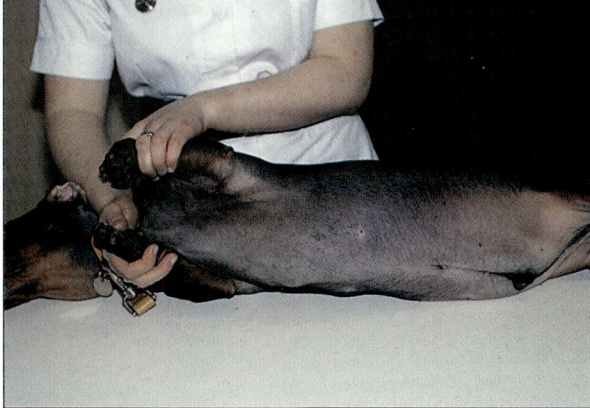

726

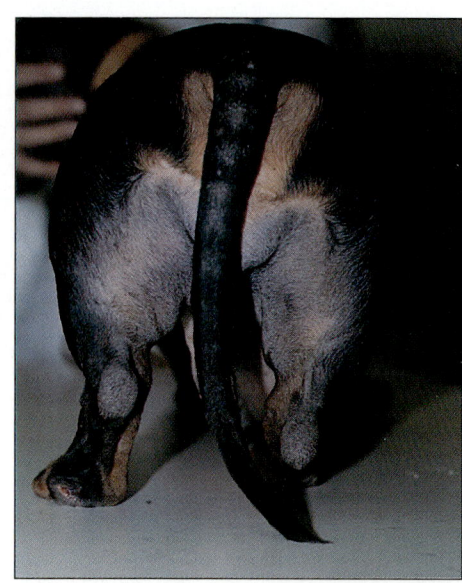

725 and 726   Pattern baldness in a Dachshund.

727

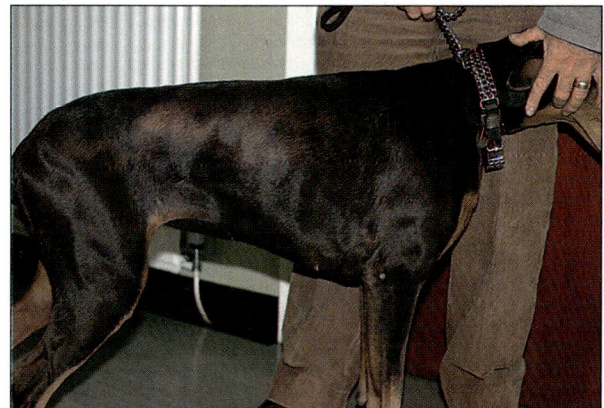

728

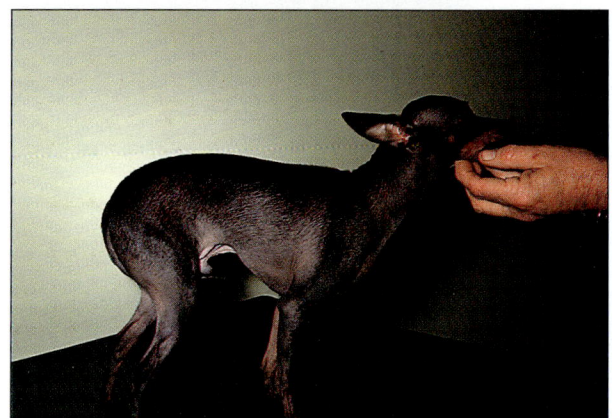

727 and 728   Follicular dysplasia in a red Doberman pinscher and a miniature pinscher. The condition is refractory to treatment.

Pattern baldness is a tardive follicular dysplasia that is particularly seen in miniature dachshunds. The condition is characterised by a progressive loss of hair along the ventrum of the trunk (**725** and **726**). The major differential diagnosis is hypo-oestrogenism (see Chapter 10).

A clinically well-recognised follicular dysplasia is seen in Doberman pinschers, particularly the red variety[11], the miniature pinscher and the Manchester terrier. There is a very sparse hair coat amounting to alopecia in certain areas, especially the flanks, caudomedial and caudolateral thighs, the ventral surface of the neck and thorax and the caudal surface of the pinnae (**727** and **728**).

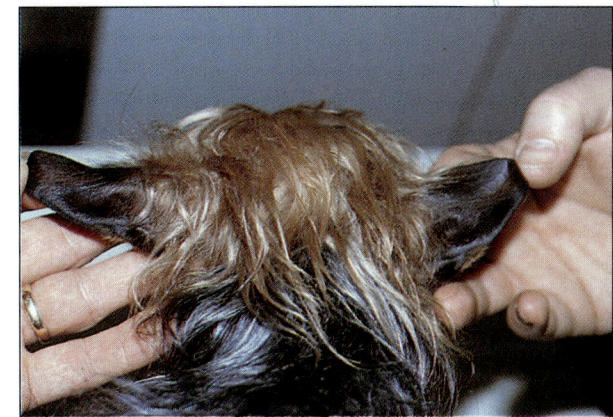

729

729 **Pinnal alopecia** in some breeds may be accompanied by hyperpigmentation. The cause is unknown.

730

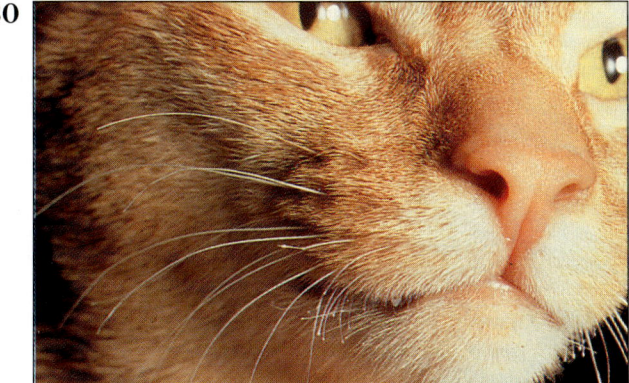

731

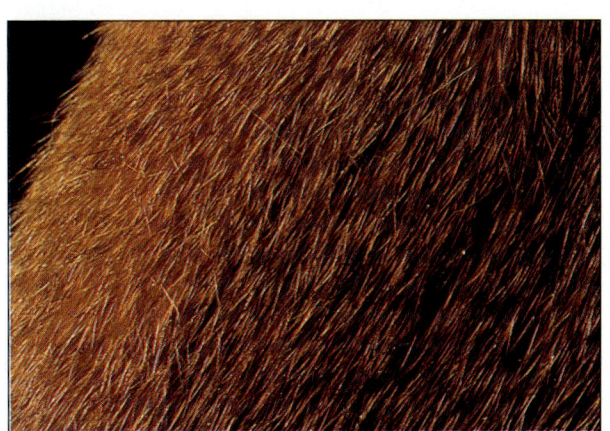

730 and 731 **'Onion-tipped whiskers/hairs' in Abyssinian cats.** Note how the affected whiskers end in a round bulb compared with the tapering point of the normal ones. Note the rough appearance of the coat in an affected cat. (Illustrations from: Wilkinson, G.T. and Kristensen, T.S. [1989]. A hair abnormality in Abyssinian cats. *Journal of Small Animal. Practice*, **30**: 27–28.)

Pinnal alopecia: Some individuals of certain breeds such as Yorkshire terriers, Dachshunds and Doberman pinchers develop an idiopathic pinnal alopecia commencing when the animal is less than one year old with a fine hair covering or partial alopecia of the ear flap then proceeding slowly to complete baldness over the ensuing years. There may be dense hyperpigmentation (**729**). Miniature Poodles may develop a similar condition which, however, is intermittent with recovery occurring within a few months.

Occasional abnormalities of the hair shaft have been reported such as *pili torti* and 'onion-tipped' hairs.[3,22] In the latter condition the whiskers and coat hairs end in an onion-shaped enlargement instead of tapering to a fine point. This unusual feature imparts a rough look to the coat and a rather singed look to the whiskers (**730** and **731**). The anomaly has been reported in Danish and Australian Abyssinian cats.

732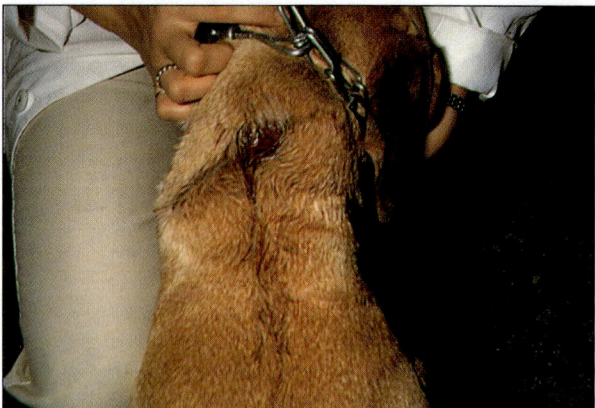

733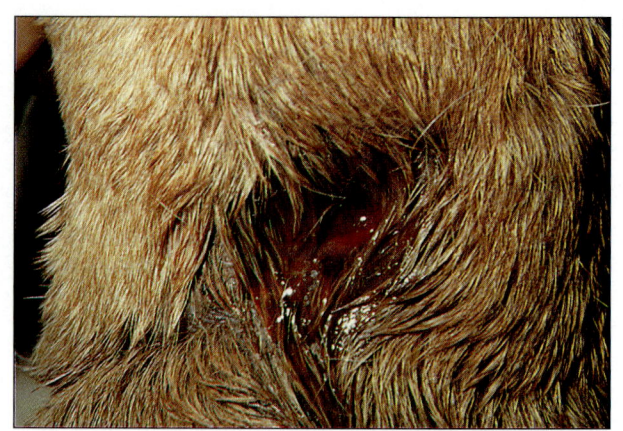

734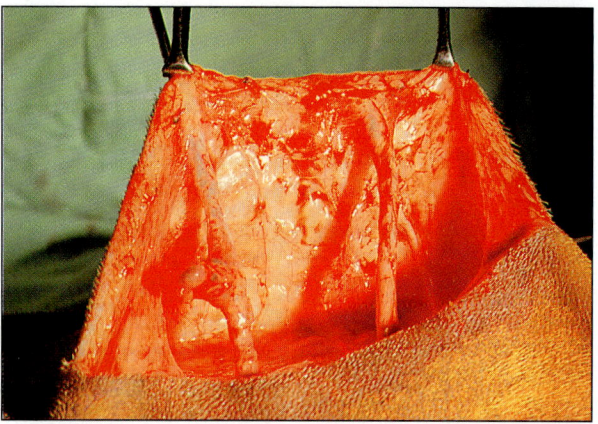

735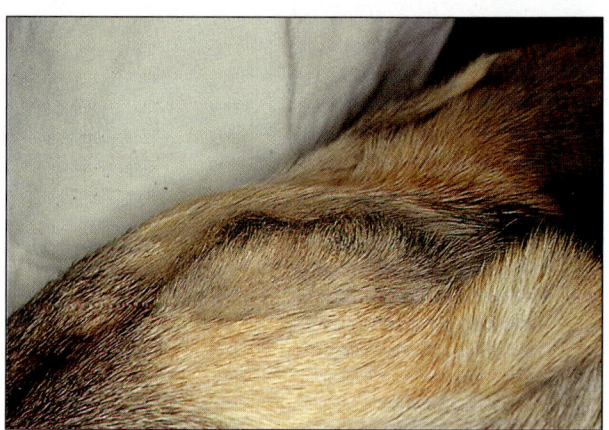

732–734   Dermoid sinus in a Rhodesian Ridgeback dog is typically found on the dorsal midline of the neck in the cervicothoracic region. Close examination may reveal a funnel-shaped sinus opening (**733**) and dissection of the sinus tracks displays their tube-like nature (**734**).

735   Dermoid cyst. Cyst in the region of the nuchal crest of a young German shepherd dog.

Dermoid sinus in Rhodesian Ridgeback dogs

A condition occurring in some Rhodesian Ridgeback dogs in which discharging funnel-shaped sinus openings, which may be single or multiple, appear in the skin of the midline of the caudal portion of the neck or in the sacral region. It is thought that the condition is inherited as a simple recessive gene. It is due to failure of separation between the embryonic ectoderm and the neural tube. The sinuses consist of tube-like tracks lined by epithelium containing hairs, sebaceous and sweat glands which may extend down to the dura mater, to the periosteum of the vertebral superior spines, or may end blindly before reaching the spine (**732–734**). Hair, sebum, and keratin debris may fill the sinus which often becomes cystic or inflamed as a consequence.

Dermoid cysts are not uncommon in the region of the nuchal crests of young dogs, especially of the German shepherd and setter breeds. The cysts usually remain static in size and seldom discharge (**735**). They usually contain keratin, cartilage and sometimes bone.

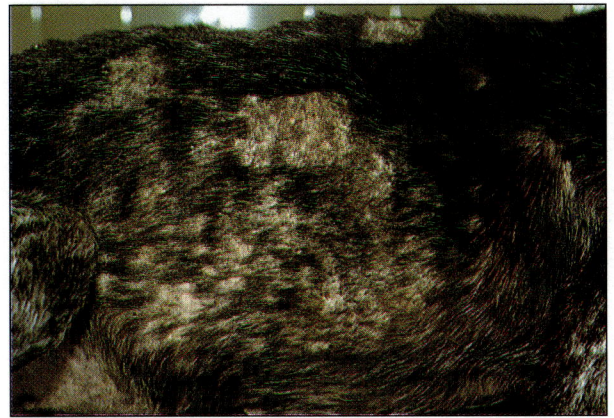 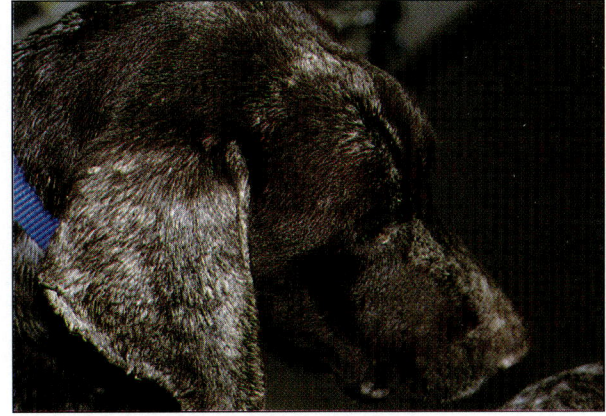

736 and 737 Ichthyosis. German short-haired pointer with congenital defect. Note the severe crusting on the pinnae and flanks.

Defects in keratinisation and ichthyosis

Keratinisation refers to the entire process of transforming a viable keratinocyte into a flattened, tough, impermeable squame within a lipid domain and the subsequent desquamation of these squames in an orderly fashion. The term is not confined to the sequential synthesis of various types of keratin. A defect in any part of this process of keratinisation may result in varying degrees of clinical disease. Signs vary from moderate accumulation of lipid scale in intertriginous regions such as the lip fold and around the nipples, to extensive areas of papules, crusting, scale, grease and alopecia. An inevitable consequence of this change in cutaneous homeostasis is inflammation which is manifest as erythema and pruritus. Secondary pyoderma and overgrowth of *Malassezia pachydermatis* contributes to the pruritus and results in further deterioration in the clinical signs.

Ichthyosis

This is a rare dermatosis. A number of ichthyoses have been described in the human literature and in some cases specific defects in enzyme activity have been documented. Some canine cases may represent animal models of the human disorder, for example of lamellar ichthyosis. Affected individuals exhibit severe scale and crust formation, often with an underlying erythema (**736** and **737**). Hyperkeratosis of the foot pads may be so severe that weight bearing and locomotion are difficult.

- Most cases characterised by crust and scale feature the triad of the keratinisation defect itself, inflammation and secondary infection. It may prove difficult to establish whether the defect is the primary problem or is secondary to inflammation or infection.
- Most cases characterised by crust and scale are associated with secondary changes in keratinisation. The principal causes are ectoparasites, bacterial infections, hypersensitivities and endocrinopathies. These must be ruled out before the diagnosis of an idiopathic defect in keratinisation (primary seborrhoea) is made.

738

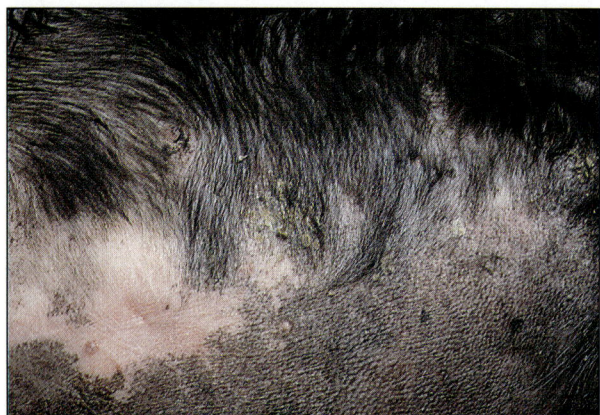

739

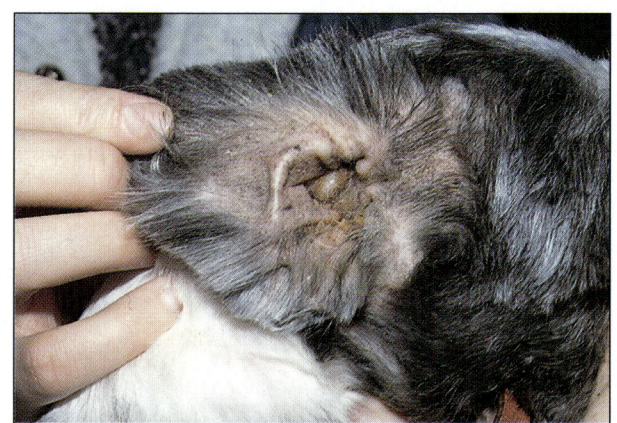

740

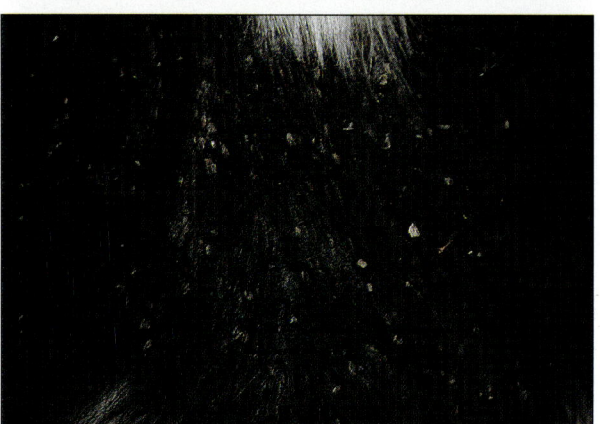

741

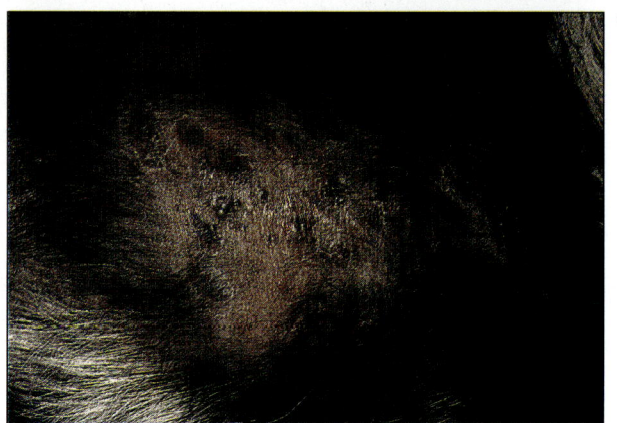

742

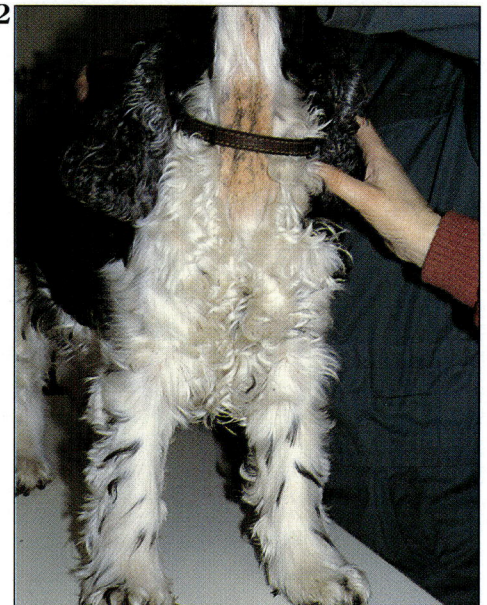

738–742   Defect of keratinisation in Cocker spaniel. Animals exhibit a variety of signs ranging from a fine scale to papules, crusts, greasy scale and alopecia.

Defects in keratinisation

Individuals from a number of breeds of dog suffer from defects in keratinisation which present as varying combinations of scale, crust, lipid scale and inflammation. In cocker spaniels it is regarded as an heritable dermatosis and the same may well be true of similar syndromes in Springer spaniels and Basset hounds, Doberman pinschers, Shar pei, Irish setters and German shepherds. All of these animals may, equally well, suffer secondary defects in keratinisation, and it behoves the clinician to investigate properly all of these cases rather than condemn the animals to a lifetime of symptomatic therapy on the basis of a cursory examination.

Clinical syndromes vary. Cocker spaniels exhibit variations on a theme. Moderate cases may have an accumulation of lipid confined to the lip folds, the external ear canals and around the nipples (**738** and **739**). More severe cases exhibit scale formation on the trunk and this may be accompanied by papules and crusting (**740** and **741**). There may be erythema, particularly in the intert-

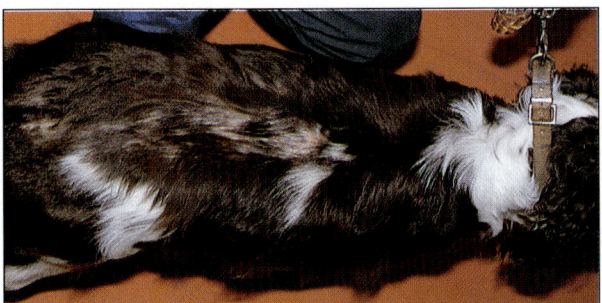

743 **Dorsal pruritus and alopecia** in Springer spaniels. In these animals it is predominantly accompanied by scale and crust formation.

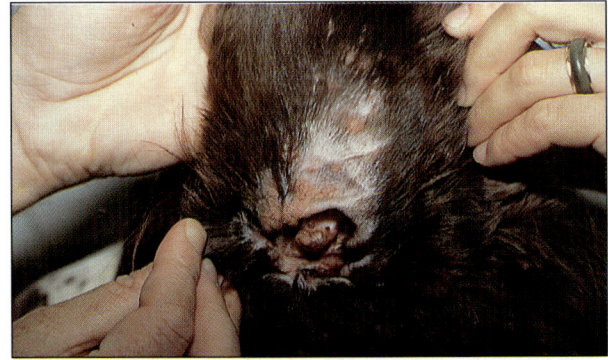

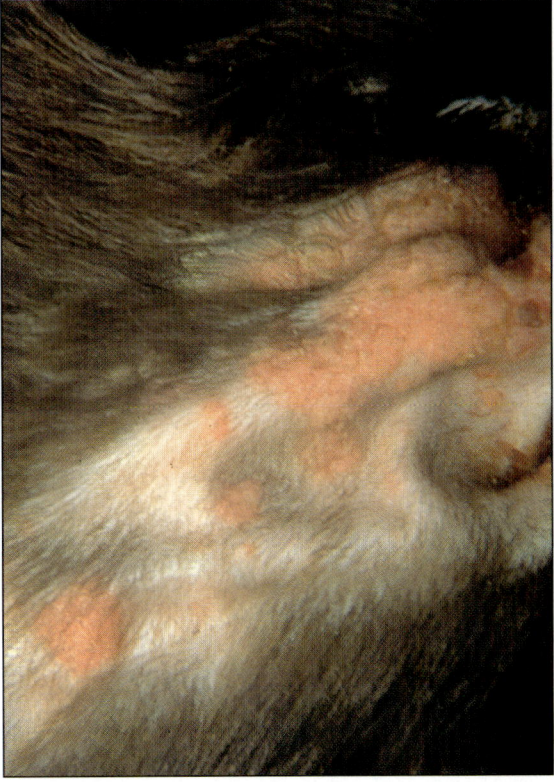

744 and 745 **Lichenoid-psoriasiform dermatosis.** (Illustrations courtesy R. E. W. Halliwell.)

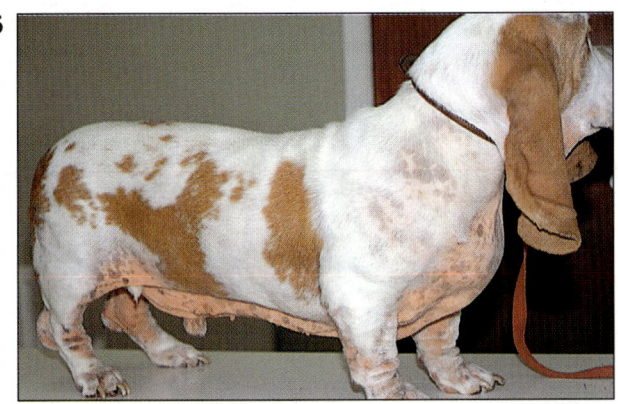

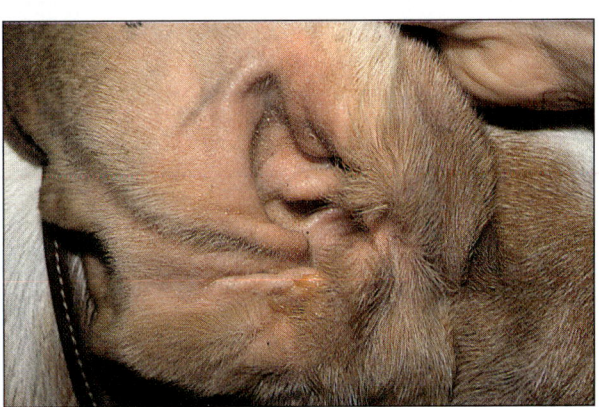

746 and 747 **Defect of keratinisation on a Basset hound.** Note the predominantly ventral distribution of erythema and alopecia.

rigines, hyperkeratotic plaques and secondary infection (**742**). Generalised disease is not uncommon.

Springer spaniels exhibit dorsal scale, pruritus and alopecia (**743**) Generalised disease is uncommon. Springer spaniels also have been reported to suffer lichenoid-psoriasiform dermatosis. This presents initially as symmetrical erythematous plaques in the groin and inguinal region, the exter-nal ear canal and ventral pinnae[9] (**744** and **745**).

Basset hounds typically exhibit a ventral dermatosis characterised by erythema and accumulation of lipid scale in the external ear canals, ventral neck, axillae, ventral trunk and groins (**746** and **747**). Lesions may also be present in the intertriginous areas between skin folds on the legs.

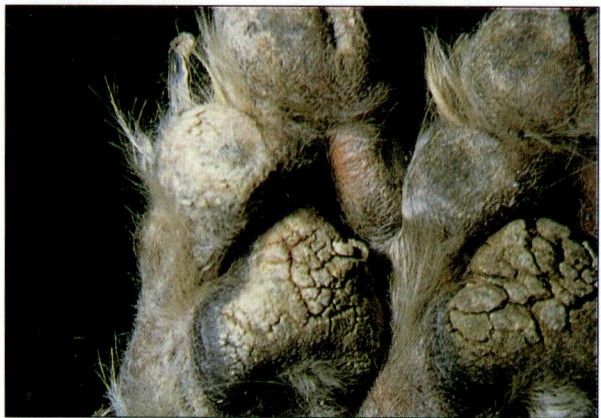

748   Hyperkeratosis of pads.

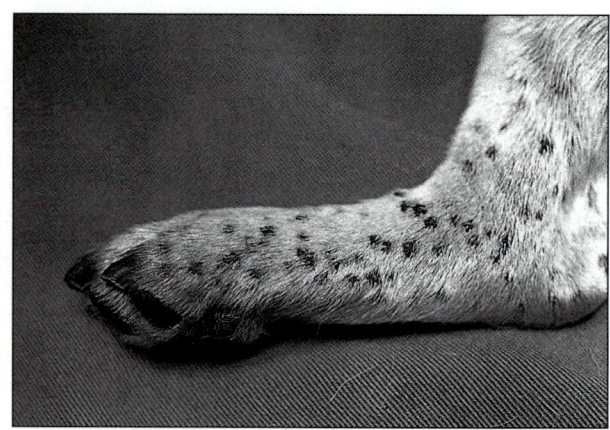

749   Hereditary   lentiginosis   profusa.
Hyperpigmented macules on a Pug. (Illustration courtesy O. M. Briggs.)

Nasodigital hyperkeratosis

Hyperkeratosis of the nasal planum and foot pads may occur in the same individual or as a single entity. Hyperkeratosis of the foot pad is regarded as hereditary in Irish terriers and, perhaps, in Dogues de Bordeaux[15], but may also occur in other breeds of dog. There is excessive horny overgrowth of the papillae of the pads which may be sufficient to cause lameness (**748**). In other individuals corns, or deep circular plaques of excess keratin, form in the pads.

- Many factors can alter the degree of cutaneous pigmentation. Chronic inflammation and endocrinopathies are the most common causes of hyperpigmentation.

Pigmentary defects

Melanin pigment is produced from dopa by the action of tyrosinase on tyrosin. The process takes place in melanosomes. When fully melanised the melanosome is referred to as a melanin granule and it is this organelle which is taken up by the keratinocyte. Thus, lack of pigment may reflect a lack of melanocytes, an inability to synthesise adequate melanin or an inability to store or transfer the melanin granules. Similarly, excess pigmentation may be a result of an increased number of functional melanocytes or from increased numbers of melanin granules within keratinocyte.

Hyperpigmentation

Hereditary lentiginosis profusa has been reported in pugs.[1] A lentigo is a hyperpigmented macule that is characterised by an increase in the number of melanocytes and in the amount of melanin within the epidermis. The dermatosis in pugs is characterised by hyperpigmented macules that are particularly visible on the distal limbs although the head and ventral abdomen were occasionally involved (**749**). There were no associated signs of dermatological disease.

Lentigo simplex in orange cats similarly has no associated dermatological disease although in this case the lentigines are found on the lips, gingivae, eyelids and nose.[18]

750

751

752

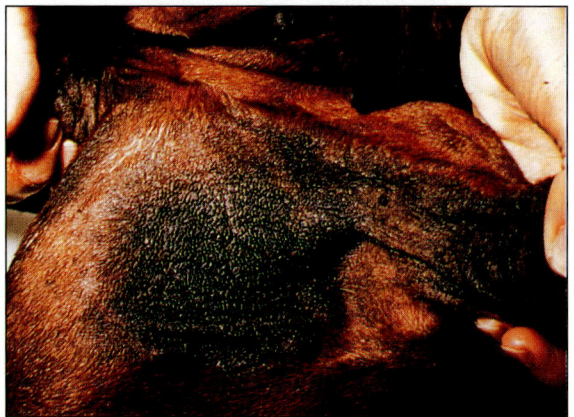

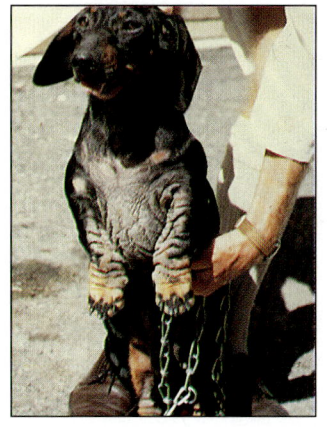

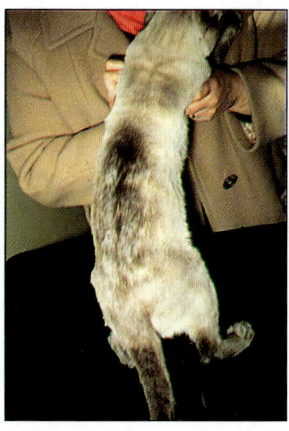

750   Acanthosis nigricans in a smooth-coated Dachshund showing marked hyperpigmentation in the axillae.

751   Acanthosis nigricans in a smooth-haired Dachshund showing more severe lesions with marked thickening of the skin and formation of folds, especially on the forelegs.

752   Acromelanism. Siamese cat showing regrowth of dark hair following psychogenic alopecia.

Acanthosis nigricans is an uncommon canine dermatosis the primary form of which appears to be a genodermatosis seen almost exclusively in smooth-haired Dachshunds.[20] The disease is probably best regarded as a skin reaction pattern characterised by hyperpigmentation, lichenification and alopecia of the axillae, the pathogenesis of which has not yet been elucidated. Primary acanthosis nigricans first appears in Dachshunds aged between six months and one year as a bilateral, small, hyperpigmented area in the axillae. Initially the condition evokes little or no discomfort, but as the disease progresses the axillary skin becomes thickened, hyperpigmented (**750**) and lichenified, and develops a greasy appearance (**751**) and a rancid, seborrhoeic odour. Secondary bacterial infection usually occurs giving rise to erythema and tenderness. The condition slowly extends to involve the ventral chest, abdomen, groins and the anterior and medial surfaces of the limbs. On the latter the thickened skin becomes thrown into folds, which may form unsightly flaps in the tarsal region of the hindlimbs.

> • Chronic cutaneous changes such as hyperpigmentation and lichenification can occur in many dermatoses, particularly in hypersensitivities and endocrinopathies. These changes appear to mimic acanthosis nigricans.

Acromelanism is used to describe the temperature-dependent pigmented coat colour of the points of Siamese and colourpoint (Himalayan) and to a lesser extent of Burmese cats. High temperatures produce a light coloured coat and low temperatures a dark one. The points, being on the extremities, are at a lower temperature than the rest of the body and are dark. If the cat is kept in a high ambient temperature the points tend to merge into the light body colour, but in cats kept outdoors throughout the winter the body hair grows dark and merges with the points. These effects can be seen in alopecia and following preoperative clipping of the hair where the hair loss lowers the skin temperature and the hair grows back dark (**752**). It is believed the phenomenon is due to the activity of a temperature-dependent enzyme involved in melanin synthesis.

753

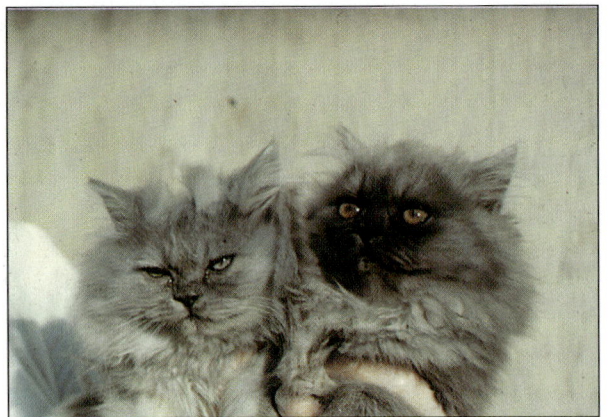

754

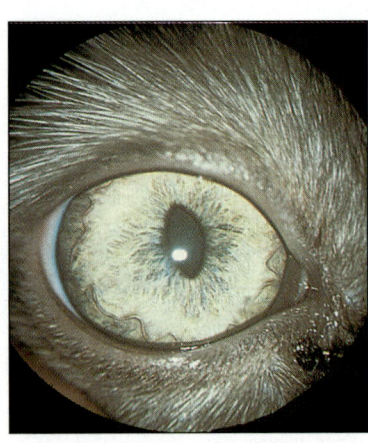

753 and 754   Chediak–Higashi syndrome. Affected and normal Persian cat littermates. Affected animals possess light yellow irises and light blue smoke coat colour in comparison with the rich copper coloured iris and dark coat of normal Persian littermates. (Illustrations courtesy D. J. Prieur and L. L. Collier.)

Hypopigmentation

Albinism is very rare in dogs and cats.[5,14] It is an autosomal recessive condition which may be classified as tyrosinase-negative or positive. In the former instance melanin cannot be synthesised whereas in the latter there is an inability to transfer melanin granules to the keratinocyte. Ocular defects are rare and the classic pink eye is unusual in dogs and cats, the iris usually remaining a pale blue.[6] In cats exhibiting the Maltese dilution (black coat to blue and orange to cream), there are no ocular pigmentary defects at all.[17]

Chediak–Higashi syndrome is a rare condition occurring in long-haired (Persian) cats which has an autosomal recessive mode of inheritance. The salient features of the syndrome include a partial albinism of the eyes and the coat (**753**). The irises are yellow instead of the normal rich gold or copper colour and the coat is a lighter version of the 'blue smoke' colour of normal Persians (**754**). These cats exhibit a susceptibility to bacterial infection due to neutrophil defects.

Cyclic neutropaenia is a condition of grey collies. These animals develop signs of immunoincompetence at an early age with pyrexia, pyoderma, enteritis, keratitis and respiratory infections. Affected animals exhibit cyclic neutropaenia with a frequency of approximately 12 days.

Vitiligo is a depigmenting disorder caused by a selective destruction of melanocytes. There is evidence to suggest that the loss of pigment is a result of an autoimmune process in some cases although others are hereditary.[13] Vitiligo has been reported in Rottweilers, Belgian tervuren, German shepherd dogs and Siamese cats. The loss of pigment is tardive and in Rottweilers[19] for example, usually begins between one and a half and three years of age. The loss of pigment commonly affects the nose, lips, eyelid and nails (**755–758**).

Dudley nose refers to leukoderma confined to the planum nasale, usually seen in German shepherd dogs and Doberman pinschers (**759**).

755

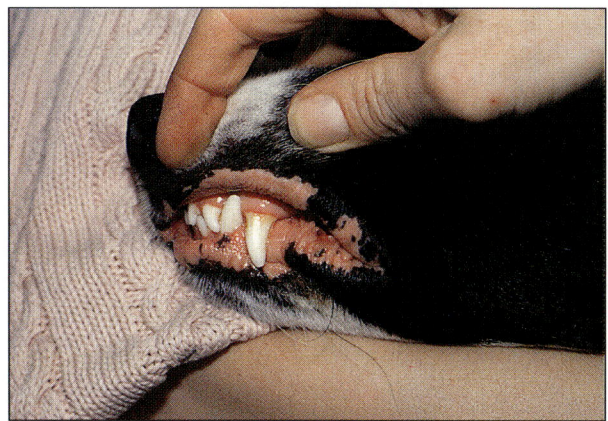

755 Vitiligo. Note the depigmentation of the lips on this Border collie. This was a tardive dermatosis and further progression was not noted.

756

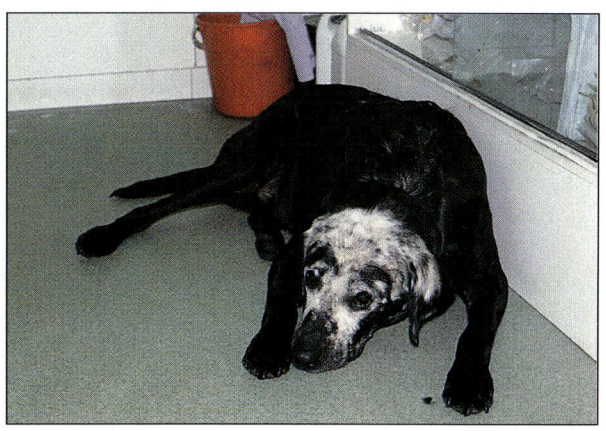

756 Vitiligo. More extensive loss of pigment in a Labrador retriever.

757

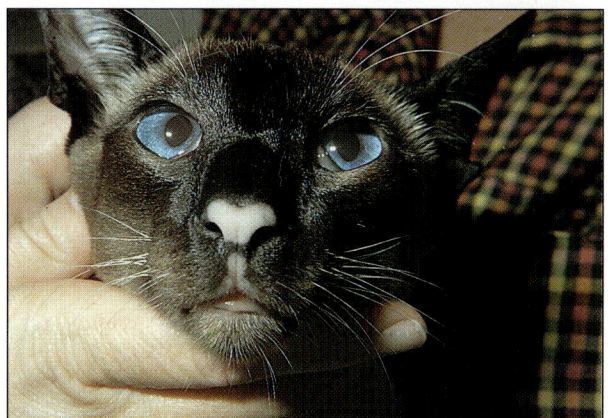

758

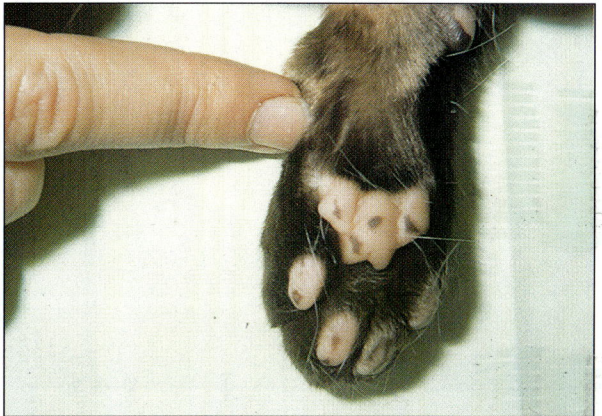

757 and 758   Vitiligo. Hypopigmentation of the foot pads and planum nasale in a Siamese cat. The loss of pigment occurred over a period of a few weeks. Note the symmetrical pattern and the sparing of the centre of the pads.

759

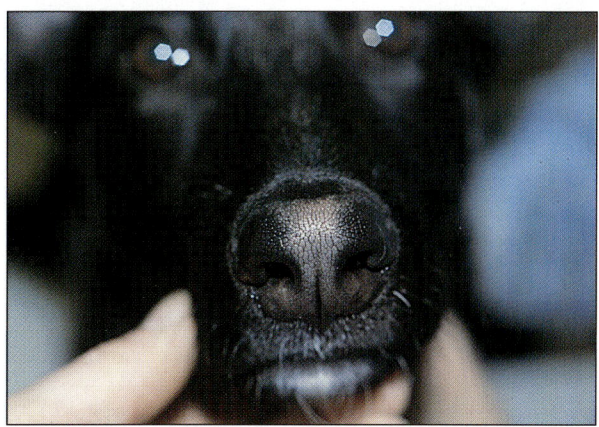

759   Leukoderma confined to the nasal rhinarium is a common defect in German shepherds.

760

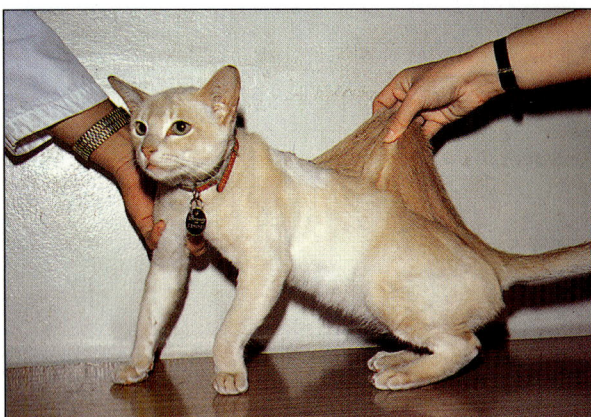

761

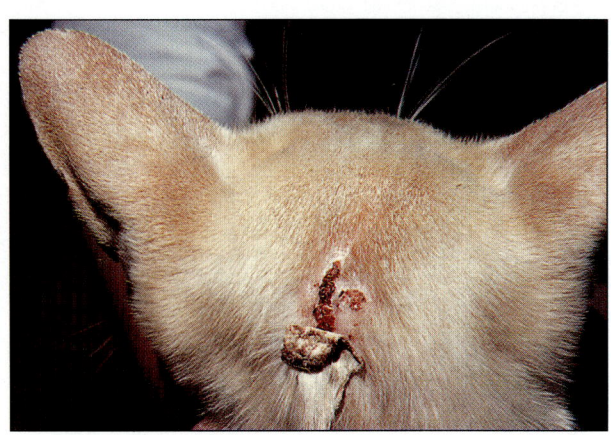

760 and 761 **Cutaneous asthenia.** A cream Burmese male cat showing characteristic hyperelasticity of the skin. **761** illustrates a traumatic lesion on the head showing sloughing of necrotic skin. The necrosis resulted from local ischaemia following shearing of blood vessels in the subcutis after mild skin trauma.

762

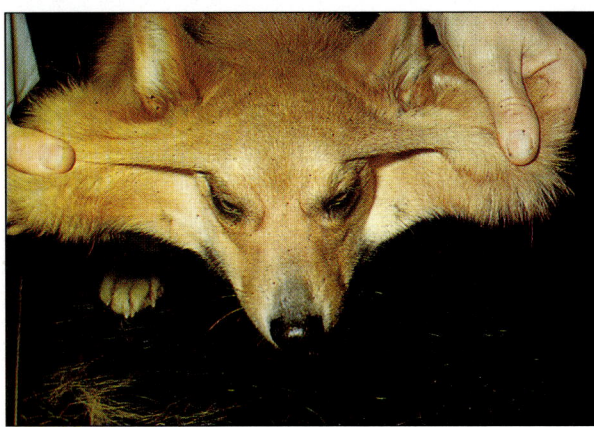

763

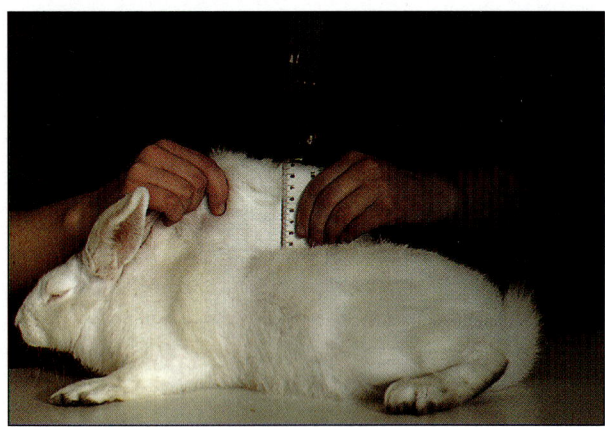

762 **Cutaneous asthenia.** Pembroke corgi dog showing hyperelasticity of the skin. (Illustration courtesy J. M. Keep.)

763 and 764 **Cutaneous asthenia in a rabbit.** Note the hyperextensible skin and (**764**) the gaping, 'fish mouth' wound on the dorsum.

764

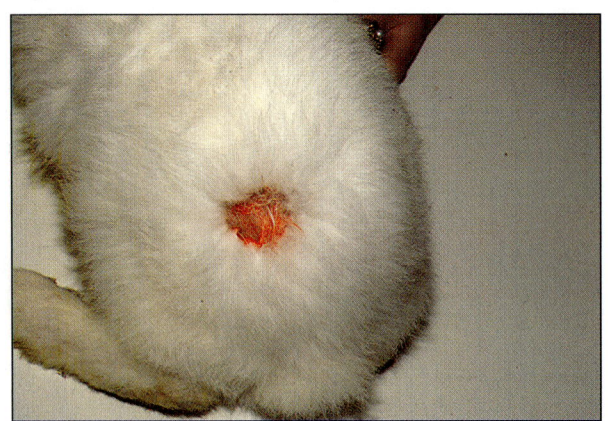

Other hereditary defects

Cutaneous asthenia (Ehlers–Danlos syndrome, Dermatosparaxis)

This is a rare, inherited, congenital complex of connective tissue disorders in which there are variable defects in collagen. These defects result in signs of disease which may be confined to the skin or reflect internal damage to the joints or blood vessels. Cutaneous signs include abnormally loose skin, hyperextensible skin which is fragile and tears easily with very little bleeding, leaving gaping 'fish mouth' lesions (**760–764**). These heal

765 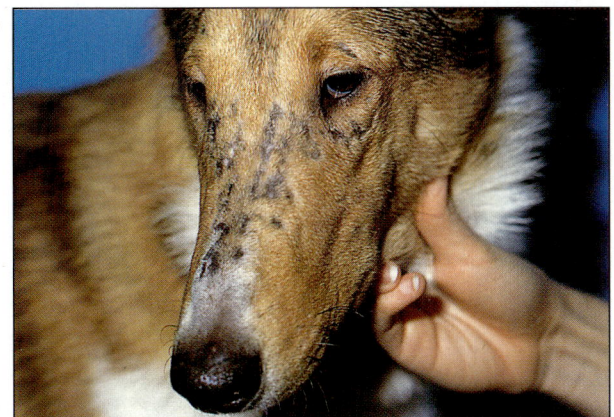 766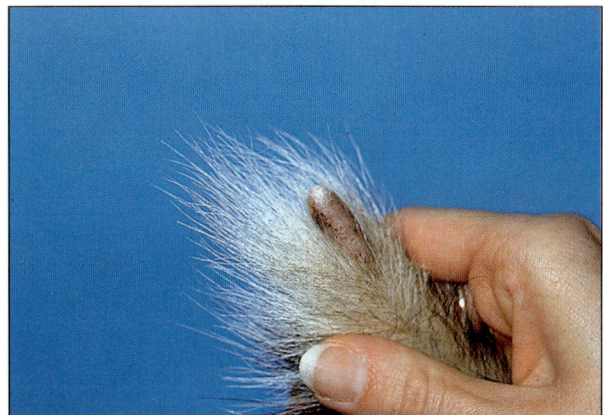

767 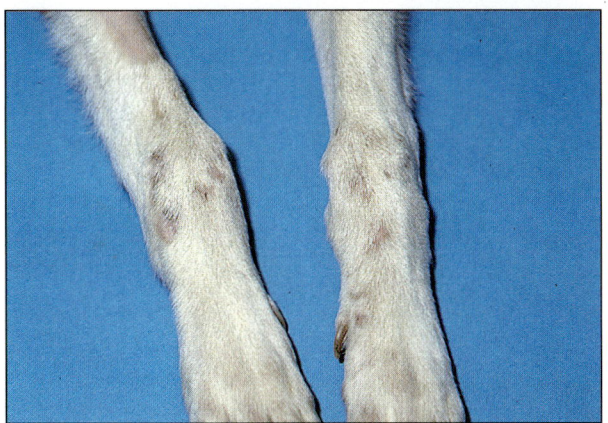 768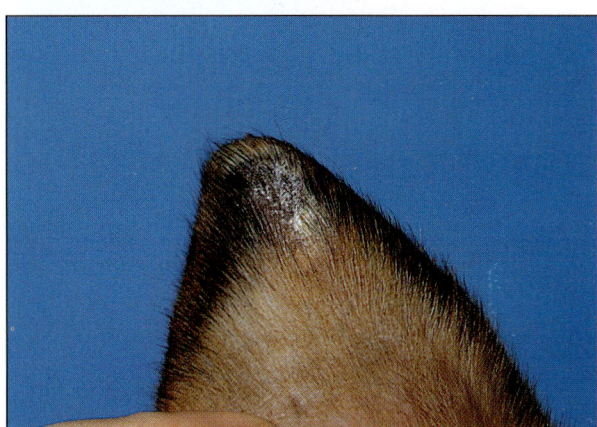

765–768 **Dermatomyositis.** These illustrations depict the classical lesions of the condition in a seven-month old collie pup. (Illustrations courtesy G. A. Kunkle.)

fairly readily with the production of weak 'tissue paper' scars. The condition may be inherited as a recessive or a simple dominant autosomal trait.

Familial dermatomyositis

This is an autosomal dominant disease of rough collies and Shetland sheep dogs with variable expression. The cause of the lesions is unknown but they may result from immune complex deposition.[6] The disease presents as a dermatosis in pups as young as 7 to 12 weeks of age. Lesions consist of papules, vesicles and crust with focal alopecia. Lesions most commonly affect the face, pinnae, tip of the tail and distal limbs.[8] The severity of the disease is variable and lesions may resolve completely in some animals. In others the course of the disease is chronic. Most animals also show evidence of muscle damage at the time of the appearance of cutaneous lesions although this may be detectable only on histopathological examination of biopsied tissue. In some dogs there is temporal and masseter atrophy although dysphagia is rare[4] (**765– 768**).

769

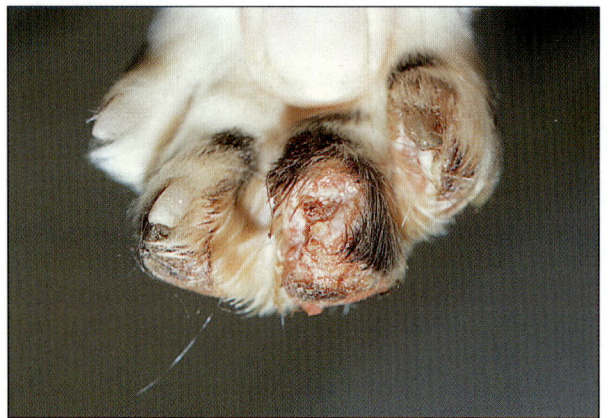

770

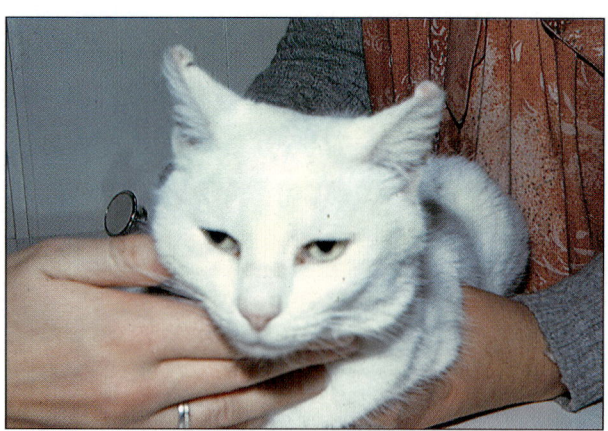

769   Acral mutilation. This English Springer spaniel was one of two littermates affected. Both dogs exhibited severe pedal self-trauma necessitating amputation of one toe in one instance. Note the degree of damage to the digit. The self-trauma is prevented by use of Elizabethan collars and leather boots.

770   Folded ear tips on a cat.

Acral mutilation

This is a rare autosomal recessive syndrome of dogs in which severe self trauma to the distal limbs occurs.[2] The affected dogs lick, chew and gnaw their digits and feet (**769**). Auto-amputation may occur and in some cases surgical removal of affected digits may be indicated. Clinical diagnosis is one of exclusion aided by the lack of response to noxious stimuli applied to the affected feet. *Post mortem* examination of the spinal roots of sensory nerves will demonstrate changes in ganglia and associated neurones and degeneration of nerve fibres.

Acrodermatitis

This is a rare autosomal recessive disorder of English Bull terriers associated with deficiencies in zinc metabolism, possibly at the cellular level[21] (see Chapter 11, **530–532**).

Folded ear tips in cats

This is a condition in which the tips of both ears are folded medially (**770**). Some cases appear to be congenital but others are acquired and have been associated with excess glucocorticoid administration and solar radiation damage.

References

1. Briggs, O. M. (1985). Lentiginosis profusa in the pug: three case reports. *Journal of Small Animal Practice*, **26**: 675–680.

2. Cummings, J. F., de Lahunta, A. and Winn, S. S. (1981). Acral mutilation and nocioceptor loss in English pointer dogs. *Acta Neuropathologica*, **53**: 119–127.

3. Geary, M. R. and Baker, K. P. (1986). The occurrence of pili torti in a litter of kittens in England. *Journal of Small Animal Practice*, **27**: 85–88.

4. Gross, T. L. and Kunkle, G. A. (1987). The cutaneous histology of dermatomyositis in collie dogs. *Veterinary Pathology*, **24**: 11–15.

5. Guagere, E. and Alkaidari, Z. (1989). Disorders of melanin pigmentation in the skin of dogs and cats. In: Kirk, R. W. (Ed.), *Current Veterinary Therapy, X*, pp. 628–632. W. B. Saunders, Philadelphia.

6. Haupt, K. H., Prieur, D. J., Moore, M. P., Hargis, A. M., Hegreberg, G. A., Gavin, P. R. and Johnson, R. S. (1985). Familial canine dermatomyositis: clinical, electrodiagnostic and genetic findings. *American Journal of Veterinary Research*, **46**: 1861–1869.

7. Jayasekara, U. (1982). Congenital defects of the skin. *Veterinary Medicine and Small Animal Clinician*, **77**: 1461–1475.

8. Kunkle, G. A., Gross, T. L. and Fadok, V. (1985). Dermatomyositis in collie dogs. *Compendium on Continuing Education*, **7**: 185–192.

9. Mason, K. V., Halliwell, R. E. W. and McDougal, B. J. (1986). Characterisation of lichenoid-psoriasiform dermatosis of Springer spaniels. *Journal of the American Veterinary Medical Association*, **189**: 897–901.

10. Miller, W. H. (1990). Color dilution alopecia in doberman pinschers with blue or fawn coat colors: a study in the incidence and histopathology of this disorder. *Veterinary Dermatology*, **1**: 113–122.

11. Miller, W. H. (1990). Follicular dysplasia in adult black and red doberman pinschers. *Veterinary Dermatology*, **1**: 181–187.

12. Miller, W. H. (1991). Alopecia associated with coat colour dilution in two Yorkshire terriers, one saluki and one mix-breed dog. *Journal of the American Animal Hospital Association*, **27**: 39–43.

13. Naughton, G. K., Mahaffey, M. and Bystryn, J-C. (1986). Antibodies to surface antigens of pigmented cells in animals with vitiligo. *Proceedings of the Society for Experimental Biology and Medicine*, **181**: 423–426.

14. O'Neill, C. S. (1981). Hereditary skin disease in the dog and cat. *Compendium on Continuing Education*, **3**: 792–800.

15. Paradis, M. Footpad hyperkeratosis in a family of Dogues de Bordeaux. *Veterinary Dermatology*, **3**: 75–78.

16. Post, K., Dignean, M. A. and Clark, E. (1988). Hair follicle dysplasia of Siberian huskies. *Journal of the American Animal Hospital Association*, **24**: 659–662.

17. Prieur, D. J. and Collier, L. L. (1984). Maltese dilution of domestic cats. *The Journal of Heredity*, **75**: 41–44.

18. Scott, D. W. (1987). Lentigo simplex in orange cats. *Companion Animal Practice*, **1**: 23–25.

19. Scott, D. W. (1990). Vitiligo in the rottweiler. *Canine Practice*, **15**: 22–25.

20. Scott, D. W. and Walton, D. K. (1985). Clinical evaluation of oral vitamin E for the treatment of primary canine acanthosis nigricans. *Journal of the American Animal Hospital Association*, **21**: 345–349.

21. Smits, B., Croft, D. L. and Abrams-Ogg, A. C. G. (1991). Lethal acrodermatitis in bull terriers: a problem of defective zinc metabolism. *Veterinary Dermatology*, **2**: 91–96.

22. Wilkinson, G. T. and Kristensen, T. S. (1989). A hair abnormality in Abyssinian cats. *Journal of Small Animal Practice*, **30**: 27–28.

Chapter 18

Miscellaneous dermatoses

Feline

Feline Indolent Ulcer

Indolent ulcer may be uni- or bilateral. The mildest lesions appear as a shallow, pink erosion of the upper lip, usually in the region of the median raphe but sometimes opposite the tip of the lower canine tooth (**771** and **772**). More severe erosions with loss of deeper tissue are associated with a chronic, often crusted, inflammatory thickening of the affected portion of the upper lip. Sometimes the ulceration is sufficiently deep to expose the upper incisors and the gum. Occasionally, indolent ulcers may be found on the lower lip or elsewhere on the body. The origin of indolent ulceration is not understood and the contribution of persistent licking to the development of the lesion is difficult to establish as most cases are not pruritic. Indolent ulcer may co-exist with eosinophilic plaque in some cats.

Indolent ulceration is characterised by:
- Non-pruritic ulceration of the upper lip.

Differential diagnoses include:
- Traumatic ulceration.
- Squamous cell carcinoma.
- Pox virus infection.

Diagnosis is made by:
- Consideration of the history and clinical signs.
- Histopathological examination of biopsy material.

- The term eosinophilic granuloma complex has been traditionally applied to the indolent ulcer, eosinophilic granuloma and collagenolytic granuloma. However, although two or even all three lesions may coexist on the same cat, their relationship is difficult to define.[10]

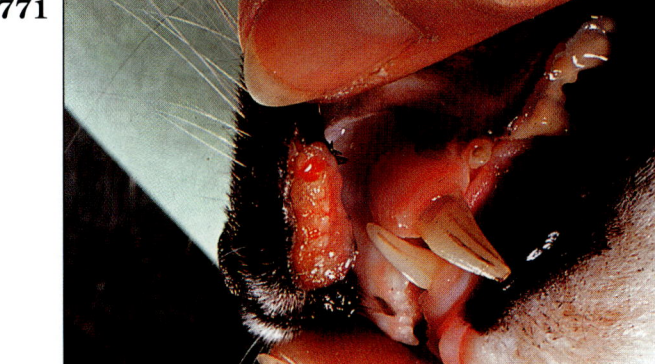

771   **Indolent Ulcer.** Unilateral lesion originating opposite tip of lower canine tooth. Note line of necrotic foci within the lesion.

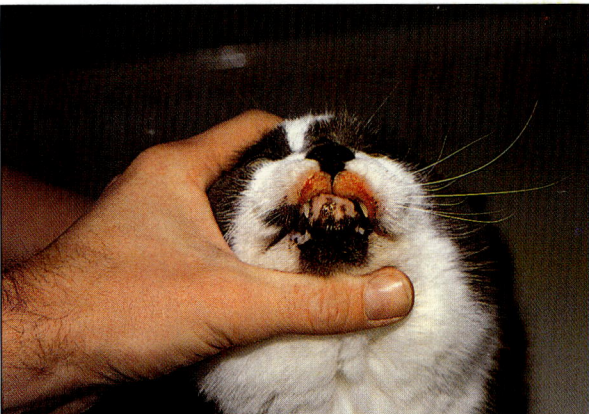

772   **Indolent Ulcer.** Bilateral lesions originating opposite tips of lower canine teeth.

773

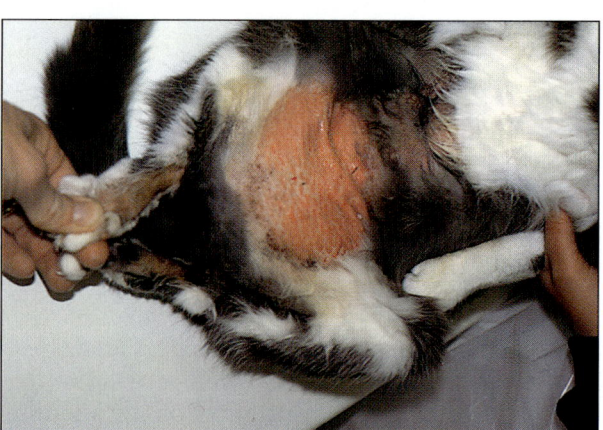

773   Eosinophilic plaque. Multiple nodular lesions on the medial thigh. Note the rough surface of the lesions and the hyperpigmentation of the skin around them, an indication of the chronicity of the condition.

774

774   Eosinophilic plaque. Large plaque-like area on the ventral abdomen formed by coalescence of multiple papular lesions. Note also the saliva staining on the medial aspects of the hocks.

775

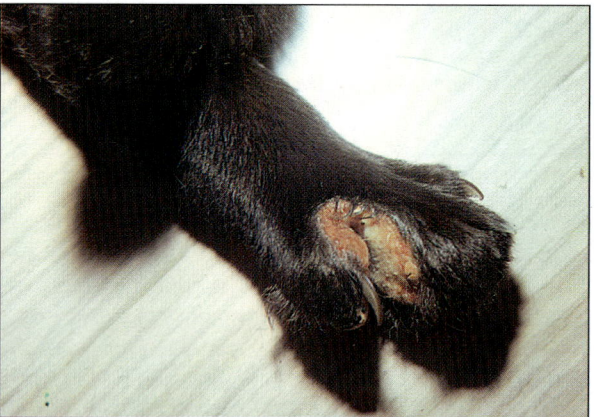

775   Eosinophilic plaque. Severely inflamed and markedly pruritic lesion in the interdigital skin of the hind foot.

776

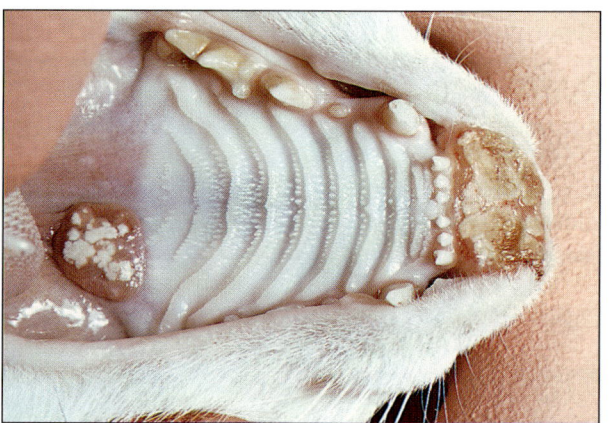

776   Eosinophilic plaque. Large characteristic nodule occurring on the soft palate. Note the large crusted indolent ulcer on the upper lip.

Eosinophilic plaque

Lesions may be single or multiple, usually the latter, and consist of highly pruritic, raised, well circumscribed, red papules or plaques. Some lesions possess a rough, necrotic-looking surface and small necrotic foci are often visible on the surface of the lesions within the nodules. Predilection sites are the skin of the medial thighs (**773**) and the abdomen (**774**) although other sites, including the oral cavity and foot may be involved (**775** and **776**). Occasionally, neighbouring lesions may coalesce to form large, plaque-like areas.

Eosinophilic plaque is characterised by:
- Pruritus.
- Well demarcated, alopecic, ulcerated nature of the lesion.

Differential diagnoses include:
- Mast cell neoplasia.
- Dermatitic variant of a psychodermatosis.

Diagnosis is made by:
- Consideration of the history and clinical signs.
- Histopathological examination of biopsy material.

777

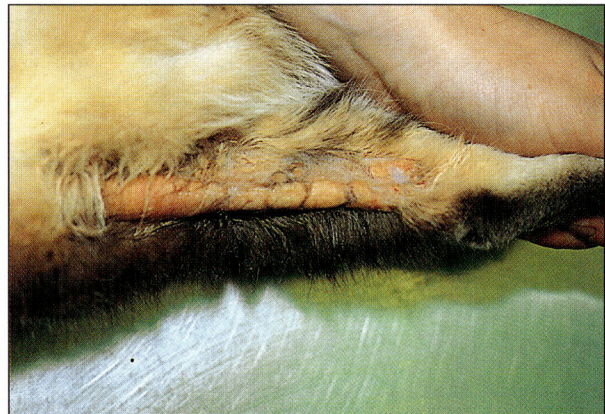

777   Linear granuloma. Typical site on posterior aspect of hind leg.

778

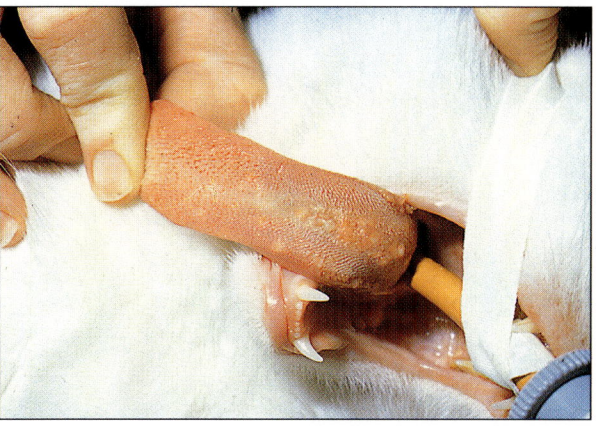

778   Linear granuloma. Oral form appearing as nodules on the dorsum of the tongue.

779

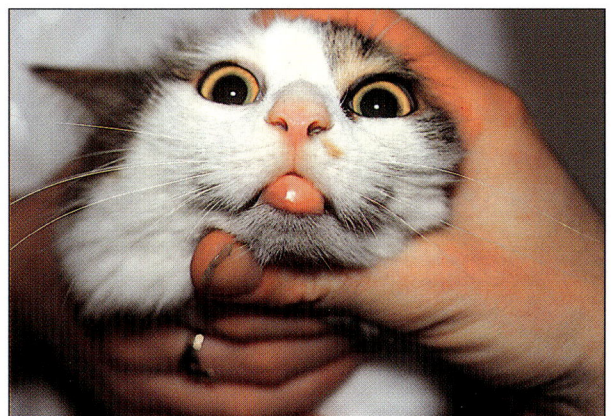

780

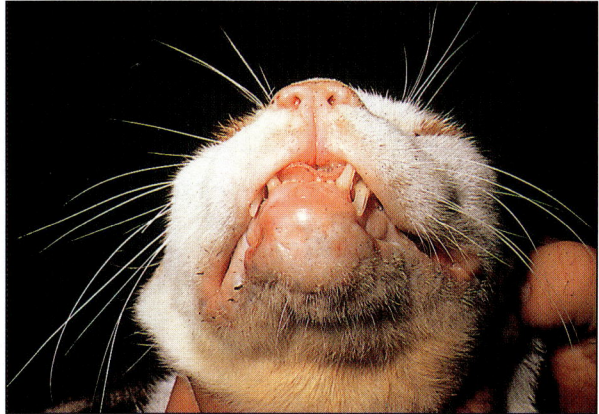

779 and 780   'Fat chin'. Note the hairless, shiny, swollen and erythematous appearance of the point of the chin. (**780** courtesy of J. M. Keep.)

- Underlying hypersensitivity such as atopy, food hypersensitivity, flea bite and mosquito-bite hypersensitivity have been documented or proposed as underlying causes of these conditions.[9] However, not all cases, by any means, respond to specific treatment of the coexistent hypersensitivity and some cases respond to non-specific immunotherapy.[2] Furthermore, indolent ulceration and eosinophilic plaque have both been reported in SPF cats in which hypersensitivities could not be demonstrated.[8]

Collagenolytic granuloma

Collagenolytic granuloma occurs most commonly as a well circumscribed, raised, firm, yellowish to pink, linear lesion on the skin of the medial and posterior aspects of the thighs (**777**). It may also occur as nodules within the oral cavity, usually on the palate and tongue (**778**). A rarer variant manifests as a swollen, shiny chin known colloquially as 'fat chin' (**779** and **780**). Lesions are painless and rarely pruritic and are usually discovered by chance.

781

782

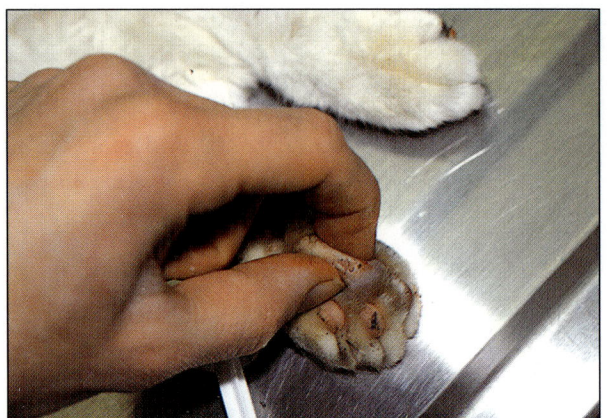

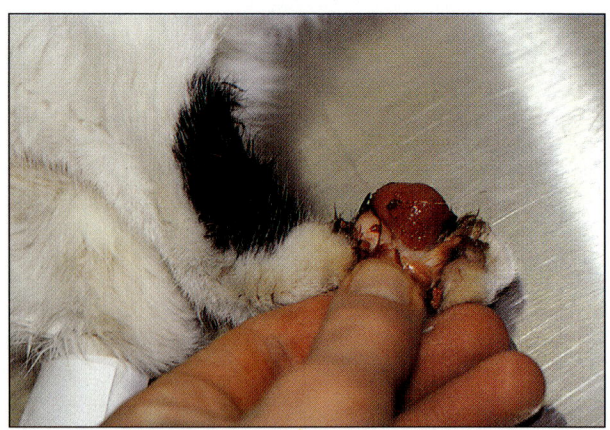

781 and 782   Feline plasma cell pododermatitis. Affected digital pads in a short-haired cat. Note the very soft texture of the affected pad (**781**) and the domed ulcerated nature of a more severe case (**782**).

Feline plasma cell pododermatitis

A distinct clinical entity believed to be immune-mediated in origin.[1] The condition commences as a soft, non-painful swelling, usually of the central metacarpal and metatarsal pads, although the digital pads may be affected occasionally (**781** and **782**). Ulceration exposing exuberant granulation tissue may follow, possibly with secondary bacterial infection. The ulcerated areas often bleed but affected cats are not usually lame and there is no self-inflicted trauma. Immune-mediated renal disease may accompany the pedal lesions.

Plasma cell pododermatitis is characterised by:
- Non-painful swelling and possible ulceration of the pads.

Differential diagnoses include:
- Trauma.
- Infection.
- Eosinophilic granuloma complex.

Diagnosis can be made by:
- Consideration of the history and clinical signs.
- Histopathological examination of biopsy material.
- Little or no response to glucocorticoid therapy.

783

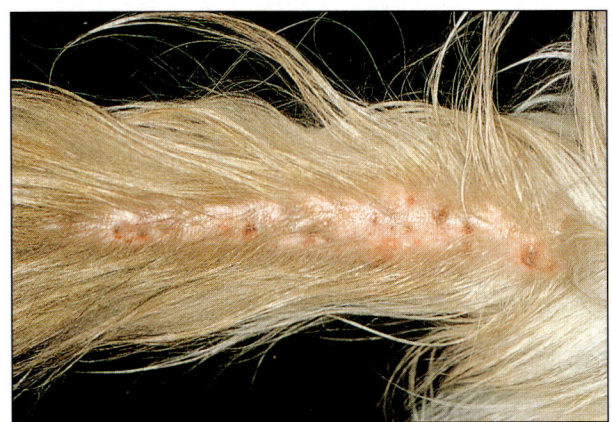

784

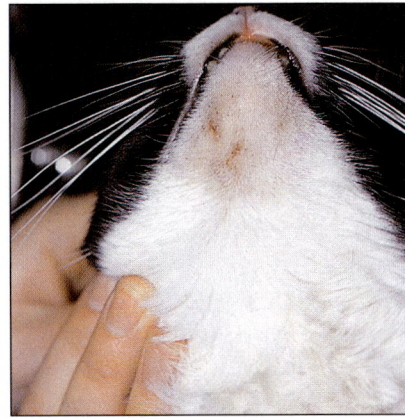

783   Stud tail showing hair loss, greasy skin and comedones. (Illustration from: Herrtage, M.E. (1983). Some feline skin diseases. *Bulletin of the Feline Advisory Bureau*, **21**: 10–11.)

784–786   Feline acne. In most animals the typical lesions (comedones) are difficult to see and clipping may be necessary (**784**) however in more severe cases lesions are obvious (**785** and **786**).

785

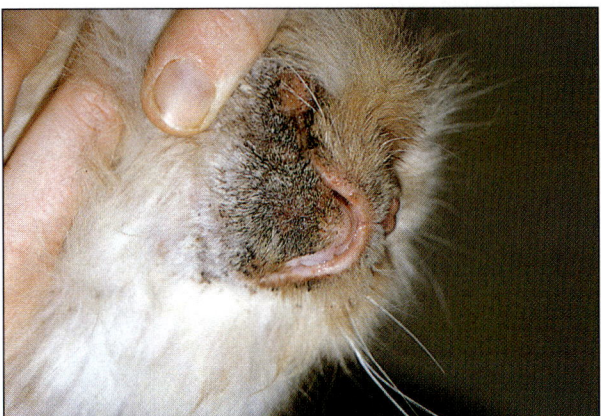

786

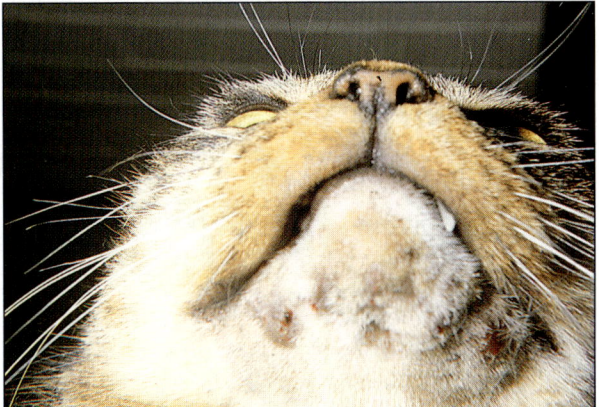

Stud tail

Stud tail is a condition akin to a localised seborrhoea, which occurs in the entire male cat due to the influence of androgens. In the cat an accumulation of sebaceous and apocrine glands is situated along the whole length of the dorsum of the tail, the so-called supracaudal organ. The sebaceous glands continually secrete sebum and this can become excessive in the breeding season due to androgen stimulation. The surface of the skin of the tail becomes greasy, dirt collects, blockage of the follicles with sebum, keratin and debris occurs and secondary bacterial infection often ensues. There is loss of hair over the dorsum of the tail, the skin is inflamed, greasy and crusty and there may be comedone and pustule formation (**783**).

Feline acne

This is a relatively common condition in the cat which usually persists for life, in contrast to the condition in the dog (see Chapter 6). The clinical signs consist of comedones and a 'dirty' appearance to the chin (**784**). In most cases the lesions are confined to the rostral portion of the lower jaw although occasionally more extensive areas will be affected (**785** and **786**).

787

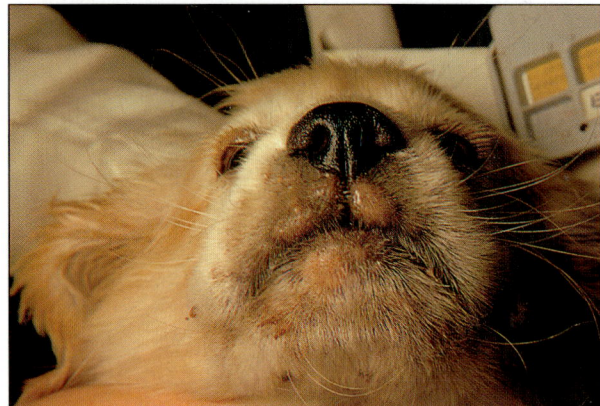

787   Juvenile sterile granulomatous dermatitis and lymphadenitis. Labrador retriever pup illustrating oedematous swelling of the muzzle, eyelids and peripheral pinna.

788

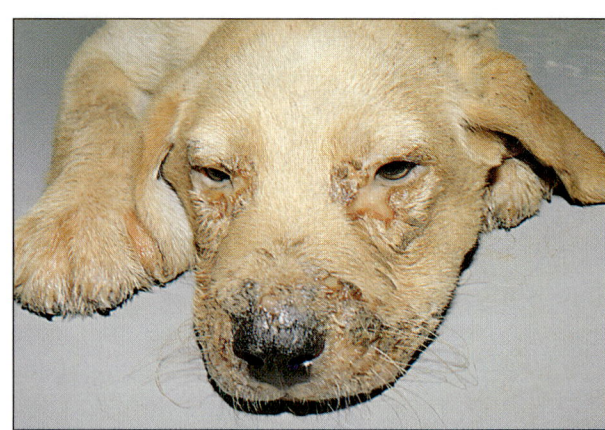

788   Juvenile sterile granulomatous dermatitis and lymphadenitis. Labrador retriever puppy showing purulent discharges and crusting in the muzzle area and around the eyes. Note the oedema of the right front foot due to lymphatic obstruction by the enlarged prescapular lymph node.

789

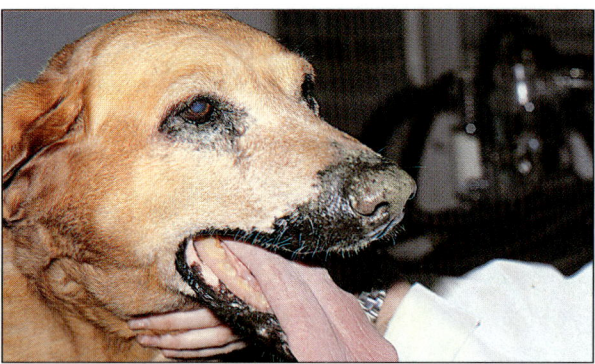

789   Juvenile sterile granulomatous dermatitis and lymphadenitis. Adult Labrador dog showing the disfiguring, hairless, hyperpigmented scarring which is a common sequel to the disease.

Canine

Juvenile sterile granulomatous dermatitis and lymphadenitis

This condition (formerly known as moist juvenile pyoderma, juvenile cellulitis or puppy strangles), is now thought to be immune-mediated. Puppies between three weeks and four months of age are affected. A number of breeds are predisposed including Dachshunds, Labrador retrievers, Golden retrievers and Gordon setters. There is acute onset of oedematous swelling of the lips and around the muzzle, the eyelids and the ears (**787** and **788**). There is often a bilateral purulent otic discharge. Accompanying these changes there is gross enlargement of the regional, and occasionally all the peripheral lymph nodes.[13] In the limbs this may lead to oedema of the extremities. The affected areas of skin become erythematous, thickened and a crust accumulates. Cracks and fissures form on the muzzle and the lips and discharging sinuses

Juvenile sterile granulomatous dermatitis and lymphadenitis is characterised by:
- Age of onset and clinical signs.
- Good response to glucocorticoid treatment.

Differential diagnoses include:
- Nasal pyoderma.
- Angioedema of the head and face.
- Sialadenitis.

Diagnosis can be made by:
- Consideration of the history and clinical signs.
- Regional lymphadenopathy.
- Good response to glucocorticoids/antibiotics.

may develop in these areas. Affected puppies may show systemic signs of pyrexia, anorexia and general malaise. The severe inflammatory process often destroys the hair follicles with resultant hairless, hyperpigmented scarring (**788**).

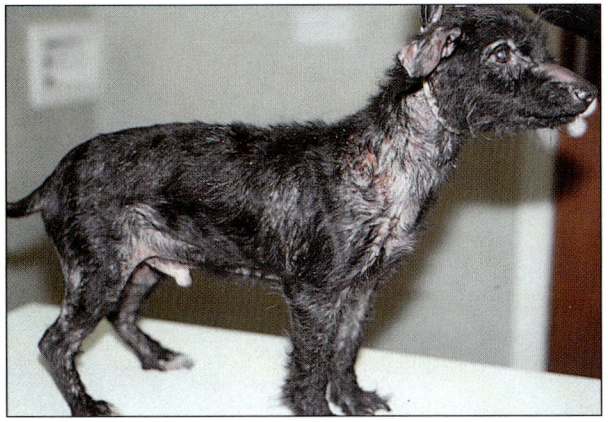
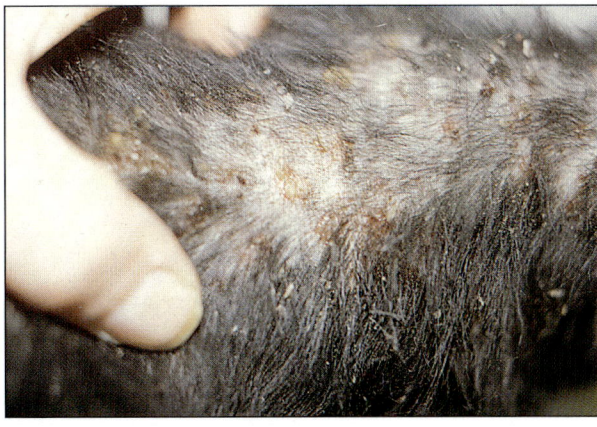

790 and 791   Subcorneal pustular dermatosis. Patchy alopecia on the trunk and face in a cross-bred dog and close up (**791**) illustrating many pustules and focal crusting.

Subcorneal pustular dermatosis

Subcorneal pustular dermatosis is a very rare, chronic skin disorder of dogs of unknown aetiology.[3] The disease is characterised by the formation of superficial, sterile, papulo-pustules associated with pruritus. Miniature Schnauzers may be more susceptible to the disease. It has been suggested that the cause may be immune complex deposition within the superficial subcorneal layers of the epidermis which chemotactically attract neutrophils to form the sterile pustules. However, immunofluorescence testing is negative.

Lesions occur mainly on the trunk but in severe cases the head, especially the bridge of the nose, the feet and the legs may also be involved (**790**). They commence as erythematous macules which then proceed to vesicopapules and then to yellowish pustules, which may be quite large (**791**). The pustules are often transient in nature, usually rupturing within the space of a few hours to leave crusts and epidermal collarettes. These tend to heal slowly from the centre peripherally over the next few weeks often leaving a temporary hyperpigmentation. The disease characteristically pursues a course of remissions and exacerbations. Pruritus varies from non-existent to very severe. Affected dogs are otherwise in good health.

Subcorneal pustular dermatosis is characterised by:
- Recurring crops of transient superficial sterile pustules.
- Varying degrees of pruritus.

Differential diagnoses include:
- Superficial pyoderma.
- Pemphigus foliaceus.

Diagnosis can be made by:
- Consideration of the history and clinical signs.
- Poor response to antibiotics and glucocorticoids.
- Cultures of pustular contents are consistently negative.
- Histopathological examination of biopsy samples of intact pustules.

792

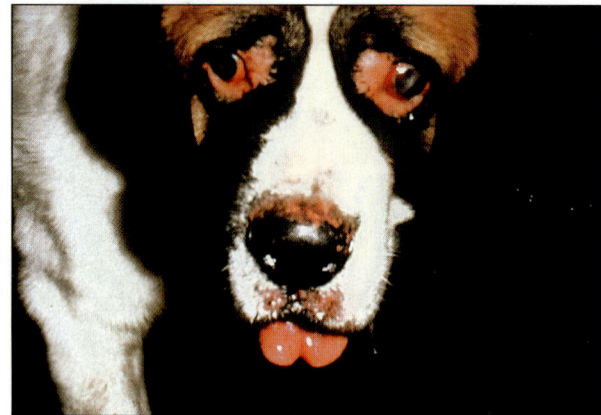

792   Canine Vogt–Koyanagi–Harada-like syndrome in a St. Bernard dog showing depigmentation around muzzle and eyes and uveitis, especially in the left eye.

793

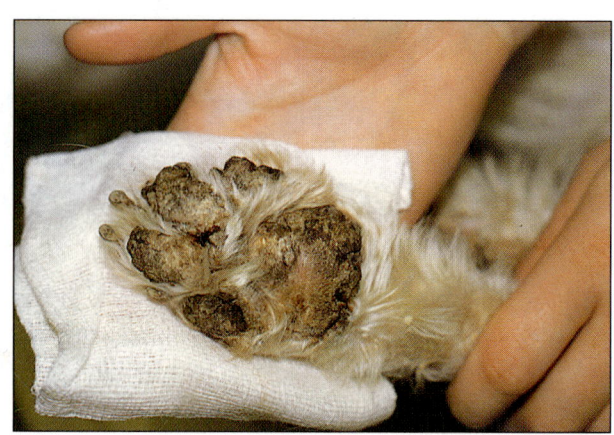

793 and 794   Hepatocutaneous syndrome. Cocker spaniel demonstrating the two classic features of the syndrome; peripheral hyperkeratosis of the footpads and vesiculo-ulcerative lesions in the perineum and groin.

794

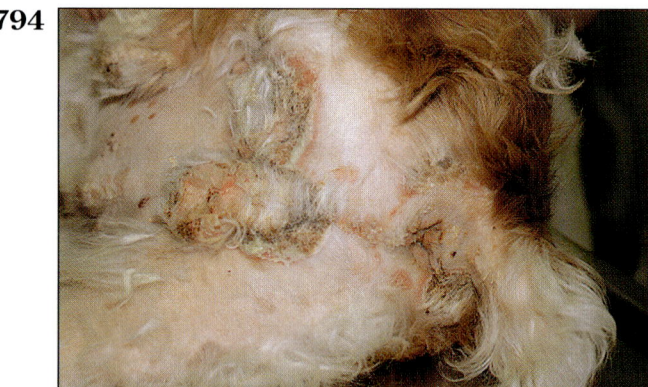

795

795   Hepatocutaneous syndrome. Bearded collie with ulcerated scrotum.

Canine Vogt–Koyanagi–Harada-like syndrome

(CVKH) syndrome is a rare, idiopathic condition in which a granulomatous uveitis is followed by leukoderma.[6] The condition was first reported in young mature Japanese Akitas of either sex but has since occurred in other breeds. It is thought to be due to an autoimmune response to uveal pigment.[7] Clinical signs are acute in onset and consist of a panuveitis together with depigmentation of the eyelids, nose, lips and, more rarely, of the anus and the pads of the feet (**792**).

Hepatocutaneous syndrome

This is a rare dermatosis of uncertain aetiology[4]. The cutaneous lesions are a reflection of internal disease. Although most cases have biochemical and histopathological evidence of hepatic disease this is often associated with, and may be secondary to, pancreatic abnormalities.[5] The cutaneous lesions may result from epidermal protein depletion as a consequence of reduced serum amino acid concentrations, presumably due to hepatic or pancreatic disease. The cutaneous lesions are of an erythematous, ulcerative and crusting dermatosis which have a predilection for the perineum and groin, the foot pads and the lips and face (**793–795**).

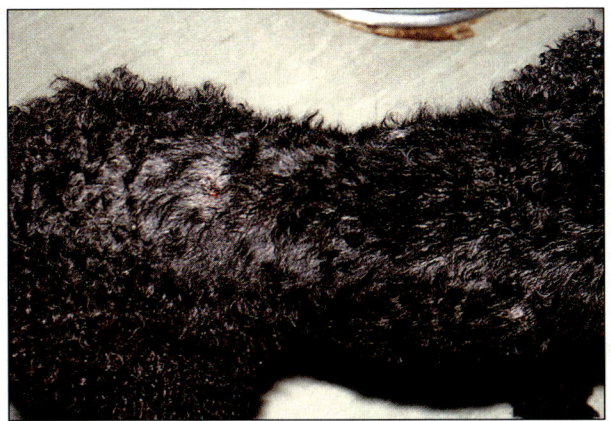
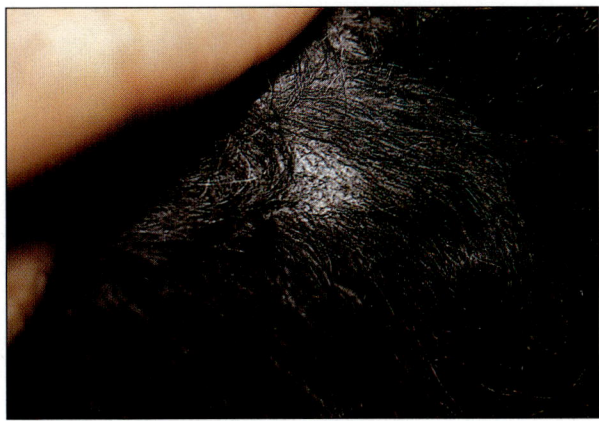

796 and 797   Sebaceous adenitis. An adult Standard Poodle with multifocal patches of alopecia on the dorsal trunk. **797** illustrates one of these lesions. Note the very fine scale. The hairs on the periphery of these lesions are abnormal, being thinner and having lost the crimp of normal hairs.

Sebaceous adenitis

This is a rare disorder that has only been recognised in recent years.[12] The aetiology is unknown. There appears to be a breed predisposition for Standard Poodles, although other breeds have been affected, for example, Hungarian Vizslas, Japanese Akitas and Samoyeds.[11] The disease is non-pruritic and the described cases fall into two syndromes, both characterised by progressive alopecia.[12] In dogs such as the Hungarian Vizsla, the initial lesions are annular areas of alopecia which expand and coalesce until generalised. In breeds with longer hair such as the Standard Poodle the initial lesions are discrete foci of alopecia (**796** and **797**). This is sometimes associated with a fine scale although in some individuals there is severe scaling. The differential diagnosis is extensive and definitive diagnosis is based on histopathological examination of biopsy specimens.

798

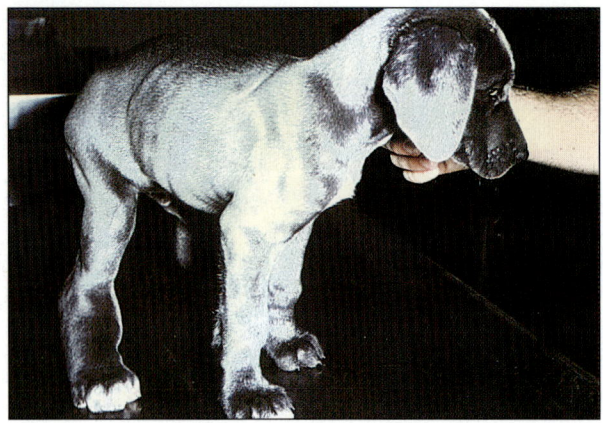

798   Primary lymphoedema in a ten-week-old Weimaraner puppy showing oedematous swelling of the hindlegs below the hocks. The popliteal nodes were not palpable.

Lymphoedema and subcutaneous oedema

Lymphoedema results from a disorder of the lymphatic system leading to oedematous swelling of some part of the body. The condition may be primary, when it is caused by some malformation or developmental defect in the lymph nodes or lymphatics, or secondary when it results from obstruction to the lymph flow by various factors, for example tumour formation, inflammation or trauma. In the primary form, which usually appears within the first three months of life, two structural abnormalities have been incriminated: hypoplasia of lymphatics with or without absence or hypoplasia of regional lymph nodes, and hyperplasia and dilatation of lymphatics. The hindlegs are most frequently affected although other dependent parts, such as the forelegs, the ventrum, the pinnae and the tail may be involved (**798**). There is nonpainful, pitting swelling of the affected part with thickening of the skin, which otherwise appears normal to surface examination. Often the regional lymph nodes cannot be palpated. After a time the affected area may become fibrosed.

Lymphoedema is characterised by:
- Non-painful, pitting swelling of some part of the body.

Differential diagnoses include:
- Other causes of oedema.

Diagnosis can be made by
- Consideration of the history and clinical signs.
- Lymphangiography.
- Biopsy shows hypoplastic or dilated hyperplastic lymphatics.

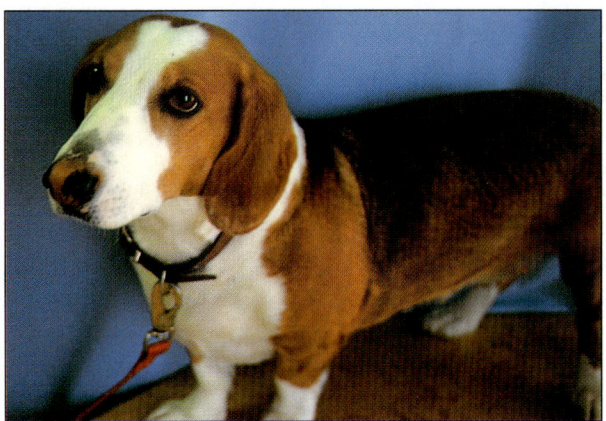
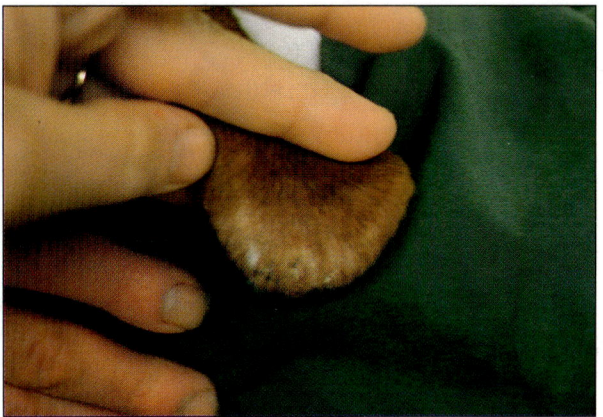

799 and 800   **Ear margin seborrhoea** on the pinna of a Basset hound. (Illustrations courtesy of L. Bellstrom.)

Ear margin seborrhoea

A condition in which greasy plugs form on the hair and skin of the margin of the pinna (**799** and **800**). The condition is reported most frequently in Dachshunds but also occurs in other pendulous-eared breeds and probably represents a defect in keratinisation. Other causes include trauma to or contamination of the ear tips by contact with the ground or food and thrombosis of blood vessels of the pinna.

References

1. Guaguere, E., Hubert, B. and Delabre, C. (1992). Feline pododermatoses. *Veterinary Dermatology*, **3**: 1–11.

2. MacEwan, E. G. and Hess, P. W. (1987). Evaluation of effect of immunomodulation on the feline eosinophilic granuloma complex. *Journal of the American Animal Hospital Association*, **23**: 519–526.

3. McKeever, P. J. and Dahl, M. V. (1977). A disease in dogs resembling human subcorneal pustular dermatosis. *Journal of the American Veterinary Medical Association*, **170**: 704–708.

4. Miller, W. H., Jr., Anderson, W. I. and McCann, J. P. (1991). Necrolytic migratory erythema in a dog with a glucagon-secreting endocrine tumor. *Veterinary Dermatology*, **2**: 179–182.

5. Miller, W. H. Jr, Scott, D. W., Buerger, R. G., Shanley, K. J., Paradis. M., McMurdy, M. A. and Angarano, D. W. (1990). Necrolytic migratory erythema in dogs: a hepatocutaneous syndrome. *Journal of the American Animal Hospital Association*, **26**: 575–581.

6. Morgan, R. V. (1989). Vogt–Koyanagi–Harada syndrome in humans and dogs. *Compendium on Continuing Education*, **11**: 1211–1218.

7. Murphy, C. J. and Bellhorn, R. W. (1991). Anti-retinal antibodies associated with Vogt–Koyanagi–Harada-like syndrome in a dog. *Journal of the American Animal Hospital Association*, **27**: 399–402.

8. Power, H. T. (1990). Eosinophilic granuloma in a family of specific pathogen free cats. *Proceedings of the 6th Annual Congress of the American Academy of Veterinary Dermatology/American College of Veterinary Dermatology*, p. 45.

9. Reedy, L. M. (1982). Results of allergy testing and hyposensitisation in selected feline skin diseases. *Journal of the American Animal Hospital Association*, **18**: 618–623.

10. Rosenkrantz, W. (1987). Eosinophilic granuloma confusion. *Derm Dialogue*, Editorial, Summer, 1987.

11. Rosser, E. J. (1992). Sebaceous adenitis. In: Kirk, R. W. and Bonagura, J. D. (Eds.), *Current Veterinary Therapy*, XI pp. 534–536. W. B. Saunders, Philadelphia.

12. Stewart, L. J. (1990). Newly reported skin disease in the dog. In: DeBoer, D. J. (Ed.), *Veterinary Clinics of North America*, **20**: 1603–1613.

13. White, S. D., Rosychuck, R. A. W., Stewart, L. J., Cape, L. and Hughes, B. J. (1989). Juvenile cellulitis in dogs: 15 cases (1979–1988). *Journal of the American Veterinary Medical Association*, **195**: 1609–16.

Chapter 19:

Zoonotic lesions

Introduction

A number of canine and feline dermatoses are contagious and lesions on human members of the household may occur. The presence of such zoonotic lesions may be of great value in arriving at a diagnosis. In some instances, notably in the case of dermatophytosis due to *Microsporum canis*, the zoonotic lesions are the first indication of disease and it may be a medical practitioner who prompts the owner to present the pet. Not all such cases prove positive and it behoves the veterinary clinician to make a thorough and exhaustive investigation before agreeing with the diagnosis.

Zoonotic disease may result from a number of animal dermatoses but the commonest are due to flea bites. Zoonotic lesions due to *Sarcoptes scabiei* and *Cheyletiella* spp. occur in 30 to 50% of households where animal infection is present.[4] Other parasites that may cause zoonotic disease include *Otodectes cynotis*, *Chirodiscoides caviae* and *Trixacarus caviae*. Micro-organisms inoculated by bites or scratches may result in human disease,

particularly after cat scratch.[5] Recently a dysgonic fermenter type 2 septicaemia has been reported in man as a consequence of a bite wound. The organism is a member of the canine and feline oral flora.[5]

Dermatophytes are regularly a cause of zoonoses but the subcutaneous and systemic fungal infections such as sporotrichosis[1] and blastomycosis are also potentially zoonotic, as is leishmaniasis. Cow pox (an Orthopoxvirus) may be zoonotic.

Patently, human beings get cutaneous diseases that have no connection with the animal's dermatosis and it is necessary to distinguish a zoonotic lesion from psoriasis or atopic dermatitis, for example. A history of onset of skin lesions coincidental with, or at least not before, the onset of animal lesions is suggestive. Zoonotic lesions are usually found in areas of contact. Some of the mites, for example *Sarcoptes scabiei*, may survive on the human host for a short period but, as with cheyletiellosis and bites due to fleas, the lesions resolve once the animal burden is removed.

801

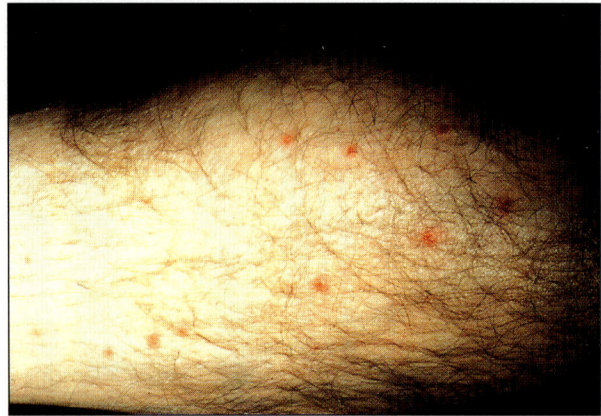

801   Flea bite. Multiple erythematous papules confined to the lower leg.

802

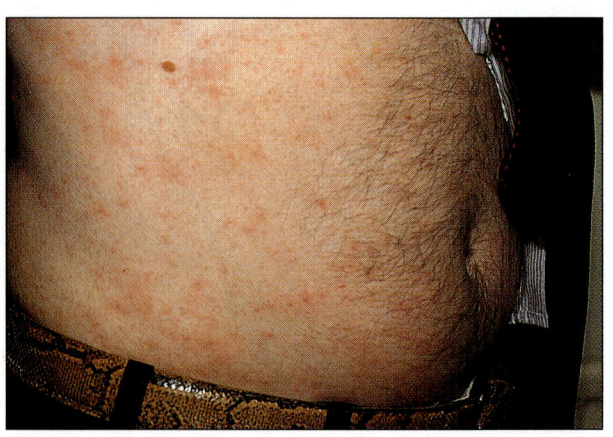

802   Sarcoptic mange lesions on the abdomen. Note that some of the papules are arranged in a linear fashion, a useful sign of sarcoptic mange.

803

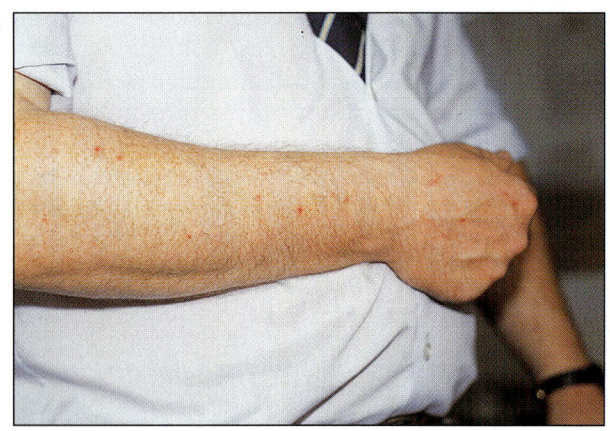

803   Cheyletiellosis. Note that erythematous papules are grouped into twos and threes rather than the random arrangement of flea bite.

Zoonoses due to ectoparasites

Bites due to fleas (usually *Ctenocephalides felis*) are typically confined to the lower legs, as fleas rely on jumping to their host from the floor rather than clambering on the animals and up clothing. Exceptions to this rule may be seen when, for example, the animal sleeps with the owner. The typical lesions are pruritic erythematous papules (**801**). In some cases vesiculation may be seen and a central haemorrhagic punctum may be observed.

Bites due to *Sarcoptes scabiei* and *Cheyletiella* spp. are more generalised in their distribution because mites can climb onto and through clothing. Nonetheless the majority of lesions are in pet contact areas and are usually seen on the lower arms, the waist-line and lower leg. Sarcoptic lesions are pruritic erythematous papules usually arranged in a random pattern although they may be arranged in a linear fashion (**802**). Bites due to *Cheyletiella* spp. whilst similarly distributed are often grouped into twos and threes (**803**). The papular lesions of cheyletiellosis may vesiculate and frequently display a dark necrotic central area.

804

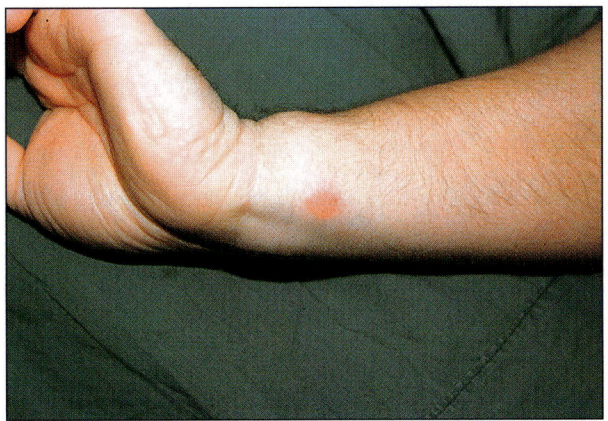

805

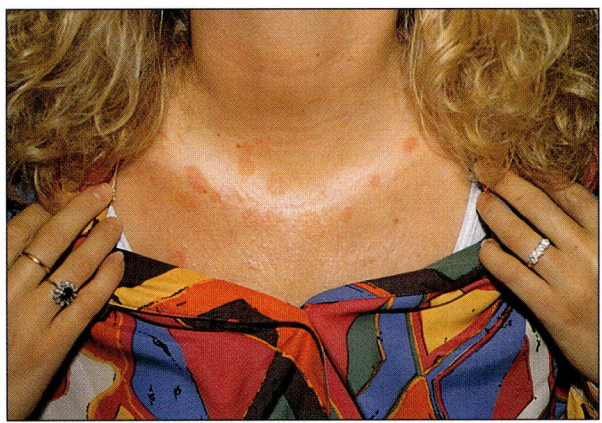

804   Dermatophytosis due to *Microsporum canis*. Note the focal, erythematous nature of the lesion.

805   Dermatophytosis due to *Microsporum canis*. Multiple lesions in the neck region as a consequence of cuddling an infected kitten.

806

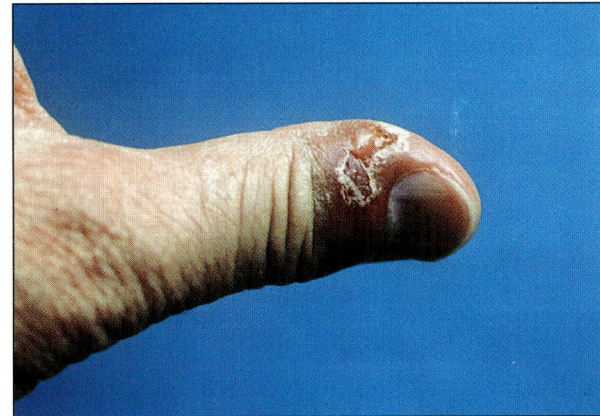

806   Sporotrichosis. Erythematous nodule on the thumb as a result of handling an infected cat without wearing gloves. (Illustration courtesy G. H. Muller.)

Zoonoses due to fungal infections

Dermatophytosis due to *Microsporum canis* is the most common fungal zoonosis. Most infection results from contact with an infected cat, particularly kittens. Transmission usually appears to be by direct contact and thus lesions often are seen on the fore-arm and neck, a result of cuddling the kitten (**804** and **805**). Infection from infected material, such as hair shafts and skin scale, may occur from the environment and appropriate steps to decontaminate the household should be considered. The lesions of human *M. canis* infection are typically a mildly pruritic, erythematous, slightly raised and focal.

Human lesions due to *Sporothrix schenkii* may result from handling material emanating from infected lesions. The initial lesion is an inflammatory papule but ulceration and local lymphadenopathy may follow (**806**).

References

1. Dunston, R. W., Reimann, K. A., Langham, R. F. (1986). Feline sporotrichosis. *Journal of the American Veterinary Medical Association,* **189**: 180–883.

2. Greene, C. E., Lockwood, R. and Goldstein, E. J. C. (1990). Bite and scratch infections. In: Greene, C. E. (Ed.). *Infectious Diseases of the Dog and Cat*, pp. 614–635. W. B. Saunders, Philadelphia.

3. Herbst, J. S., Raffanti, S., Pathy, A. and Zaiac, M. N. (1989). Dysgonic fermenter type 2 septicaemia with purpura fulminans. *Archives of Dermatology*, **125**: 1380–1382.

4. Scott, D. W. and Horne, R. T. (1987). Zoonotic dermatoses of dogs and cats. *Veterinary Clinics of North America*, **17**: 117–144. W. B. Saunders, Philadelphia.

5. Wear, D. J., English, C. K. and Margileth, A. M. (1990). Cat scratch disease. In: Greene, C. E. (Ed.). *Infectious Diseases of the Dog and Cat*, pp. 632–635. W. B. Saunders, Philadelphia.

Index

Page numbers in italic type indicate that a relevant illustration occurs on this page, and those followed by a(t) indicate a table.

melanoma in, 240
prototheocosis in, *128, 129*
pyoderma, fold, in, 92
sebaceous gland hyperplasia in, 222
vitamin A-responsive dermatosis in, 196
Collagenolytic granuloma, 281
Collagenous naevi *see* Naevi, collagenous
Collarettes *see* Epidermal collarettes
Collie,
    actinic dermatitis in, *208*
    dermatomyositis in, *275*
    see also Bearded collie, Border collie *and* Collie cross
Collie cross,
    flea bite hypersensitivity in, *134*
    pemphigus foliaceus in, *158*
    urticaria in, *138*
Collie nose, 208
Colour dilute alopecia *see* Alopecia, colour dilute
Colourpoint cat, acromelanism in, 271
Contact dermatitis,
    allergic *see* Dermatitis, allergic contact
    primary irritant *see* Dermatitis, primary irritant
        contact
Corgi, injection reaction in, *217*
    see also Cardigan corgi *and* Pembroke corgi
Corticoid/creatinine ratio, urinary, 51
Cow pox, zoonotic disease, 291
Creatinine/corticoid ratio, urinary, 51
Crust, 28, *28*
Cryptococcosis, *25, 42*, 130, *130–1*
Cryptococcus neoformans infection *see* Cryptococcosis
Ctenocephalides canis infestation, 54, *55*
Ctenocephalides felis infestation, 54, *55*
    zoonotic disease, 292
CTVT *see* Canine transmissible venereal tumours
Curvularia geniculata, in mycetoma, 126
Cutaneous horn, 250, *250*
Cuterebra spp., in myiasis, 84
Cyst,
    dermoid, 266, *266*
    epidermal origin, 250, *250*
    epitrichial gland, *250*
    ovarian, hyperpigmentation in, *30*
    recognition and significance, 25
    sebaceous, *25*, 250

Dachshund,
    acanthosis nigricans in, 271, *271*
    adrenal neoplasia, 177
    ear margin seborrhoea in, 289
    granulomatous dermatitis and lymphadenitis in, 284, *284*
    pattern baldness in, *264*
    pemphigus foliaceus in, *160*
    pinnal alopecia in, 265
    see also Miniature Dachshund *and* Standard
        Dachshund
Dalmatian,
    atopy in, 145
    dermatitis in,
        acral lick, *255, 256*
        actinic, 208
        exfoliative, *153*

pyoderma, superficial, in, *96*
saliva staining in, *201*
squamous cell carcinoma in, 227, *227*
Demodectic mange *see* Demodicosis
Demodex see Demodicosis
Demodicosis, 73–9
    canine, 9(t), 73
        deep pyoderma in, *100*
        generalised, 74, *75, 76*
        localised, 74, *74*
        otodemodicosis, 76
        pododemodicosis, 76, *76*
    cellulitis in, 102, *102*
    feline, 77, *77, 78*
    gerbil, 79
    hamster, 79, *79*
    pustules in, 20
    skin scrapping in, 39
Dermanyssus gallinae infestation, 79
Dermatitis,
    actinic,
        canine, 208, *208–9*
        feline, 205, *205–7*
    allergic contact, 140, *140–3*
        diagnostic techniques, 48
        hyperpigmentation in, *30*
        papules in, *18*
    atopic *see* Atopy
    canine acral lick, 255, *255–6*
    exfoliative *see* Exfoliative dermatitis
    fly bite, 81, *81*
    heartworm, 86, *86*
    hookworm larval, 85, *85*
    insect bite, 82, *82*
    juvenile sterile, and lymphadenitis, 284, *284*
    miliary *see* Dermatitis, papulocrustous
    neutropic, 251, *251*
    papulocrustous, 136, *136*, 137(t)
    pelodera, 85, 86
    primary irritant contact, 202, *203–4*
    pyotraumatic, 90, *91*, 213
    solar, *201*
    traumatic, 213, *213–6*
        injection reactions, 217, *216–7*
    vesiculobullous, 153, *154*
    see also Pododermatitis
Dermatofibrosis, nodular, 247, *247*
Dermatomyositis,
    familial, 275, *275*
    pustules in, 20
Dermatophagoides spp., in atopy, 144
Dermatosparaxis, 274
Dermoid cyst *see* Cyst, dermoid
Dermoid sinus in Rhodesian Ridgeback dogs, 266, *266*
Devon rex cat, congenital hypotrichosis in, 261, *261*
Dexamethasone test, 51
Diascopy, 34
Dietary intolerance, 149, *149–51*
Dipylidium caninum, in flea bite hypersensitivity, 133
Dirofilaria immitis, in dermatitis, 86, *86*
Discoid lupus erythematosus *see* Lupus erythematosus, discoid
Distemper virus infection *see* Canine distemper virus